New Perspectives in Oral Health for Patients with Special Needs and Compromised Older Adults

New Perspectives in Oral Health for Patients with Special Needs and Compromised Older Adults

Editors

Takahiro Ono
Leonardo Marchini
Anastassia E. Kossioni

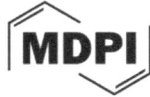

Basel • Beijing • Wuhan • Barcelona • Belgrade • Novi Sad • Cluj • Manchester

Editors

Takahiro Ono
Osaka Dental University
Faculty of Dentistry
Osaka
Japan

Leonardo Marchini
The University of Iowa
College of Dentistry and
Dental Clinics
Iowa City, IA
USA

Anastassia E. Kossioni
National and Kapodistrian
University of Athens
Dental School
Athens
Greece

Editorial Office
MDPI AG
Grosspeteranlage 5
4052 Basel, Switzerland

This is a reprint of articles from the Special Issue published online in the open access journal *Journal of Clinical Medicine* (ISSN 2077-0383) (available at: https://www.mdpi.com/journal/jcm/special_issues/DFEZ7555UH).

For citation purposes, cite each article independently as indicated on the article page online and as indicated below:

Lastname, A.A.; Lastname, B.B. Article Title. *Journal Name* **Year**, *Volume Number*, Page Range.

ISBN 978-3-7258-1963-8 (Hbk)
ISBN 978-3-7258-1964-5 (PDF)
doi.org/10.3390/books978-3-7258-1964-5

© 2024 by the authors. Articles in this book are Open Access and distributed under the Creative Commons Attribution (CC BY) license. The book as a whole is distributed by MDPI under the terms and conditions of the Creative Commons Attribution-NonCommercial-NoDerivs (CC BY-NC-ND) license.

Contents

About the Editors vii

Preface ix

Chikako Hatayama, Kazuhiro Hori, Hiromi Izuno, Masayo Fukuda, Misao Sawada, Takako Ujihashi, et al.
Features of Masticatory Behaviors in Older Adults with Oral Hypofunction: A Cross-Sectional Study
Reprinted from: *J. Clin. Med.* **2022**, *11*, 5902, doi:10.3390/jcm11195902 1

Kentaro Okuno, Ryuichiro Kobuchi, Suguru Morita, Ayako Masago, Masaaki Imaoka and Kazuya Takahashi
Relationships between the Nutrition Status and Oral Measurements for Sarcopenia in Older Japanese Adults
Reprinted from: *J. Clin. Med.* **2022**, *11*, 7382, doi:10.3390/jcm11247382 13

Kazuhiro Murakami, Tasuku Yoshimoto, Kazuhiro Hori, Rikako Sato, Ma. Therese Sta. Maria, Pinta Marito, et al.
Masticatory Performance Test Using a Gummy Jelly for Older People with Low Masticatory Ability
Reprinted from: *J. Clin. Med.* **2023**, *12*, 593, doi:10.3390/jcm12020593 22

Kohei Yamaguchi, Yohei Hama, Hitomi Soeda, Keita Hatano, Mitsuzumi Okada, Ryota Futatsuya and Shunsuke Minakuchi
Factors Associated with Selection of Denture Adhesive Type: A Cross-Sectional Survey
Reprinted from: *J. Clin. Med.* **2023**, *12*, 873, doi:10.3390/jcm12030873 30

Rena Hidaka, Koichiro Matsuo, Tomoka Maruyama, Kyoka Kawasaki, Itsuki Tasaka, Masami Arai, et al.
Impact of COVID-19 on the Surrounding Environment of Nursing Home Residents and Attitudes towards Infection Control and Oral Health Care among Nursing Home Staff in Japan
Reprinted from: *J. Clin. Med.* **2023**, *12*, 1944, doi:10.3390/jcm12051944 39

Linda Slack-Smith, Gina Arena and Lydia See
Rapid Oral Health Deterioration in Older People—A Narrative Review from a Socio-Economic Perspective
Reprinted from: *J. Clin. Med.* **2023**, *12*, 2396, doi:10.3390/jcm12062396 48

Leonardo Marchini and Ronald L. Ettinger
The Prevention, Diagnosis, and Treatment of Rapid Oral Health Deterioration (ROHD) among Older Adults
Reprinted from: *J. Clin. Med.* **2023**, *12*, 2559, doi:10.3390/jcm12072559 57

Hongli Yu, Haruka Fujita, Masako Akiyama, Yuka I. Sumita and Noriyuki Wakabayashi
Prevalence of Possible Dementia in Patients with Maxillofacial Defects and Difficulty of Inserting Obturator in Maxillectomy Patients: Toward Better Provision of Supportive Care
Reprinted from: *J. Clin. Med.* **2023**, *12*, 2722, doi:10.3390/jcm12072722 71

Elisabeth Morén, Pia Skott, Kristina Edman, Nivetha Gavriilidou, Inger Wårdh and Helena Domeij
The Effect of Domiciliary Professional Oral Care on Root Caries Progression in Care-Dependent Older Adults: A Systematic Review
Reprinted from: *J. Clin. Med.* **2023**, *12*, 2748, doi:10.3390/jcm12072748 84

Kalliopi Konstantopoulou and Anastassia E. Kossioni
Association between Oral Hygiene Information Sources and Daily Dental and Denture Care Practices in Urban Community-Dwelling Older Adults
Reprinted from: *J. Clin. Med.* **2023**, *12*, 2881, doi:10.3390/jcm12082881 . . . . **97**

Jhanvi P. Desai and Rohit U. Nair
Oral Health Factors Related to Rapid Oral Health Deterioration among Older Adults: A Narrative Review
Reprinted from: *J. Clin. Med.* **2023**, *12*, 3202, doi:10.3390/jcm12093202 . . . . **110**

Martin Schimmel, Noemi Anliker, Gabriela Panca Sabatini, Marcella Silva De Paula, Adrian Roman Weber and Pedro Molinero-Mourelle
Assessment and Improvement of Masticatory Performance in Frail Older People: A Narrative Review
Reprinted from: *J. Clin. Med.* **2023**, *12*, 3760, doi:10.3390/jcm12113760 . . . . **124**

Gert-Jan van der Putten and Cees de Baat
An Overview of Systemic Health Factors Related to Rapid Oral Health Deterioration among Older People
Reprinted from: *J. Clin. Med.* **2023**, *12*, 4306, doi:10.3390/jcm12134306 . . . . **138**

Frauke Müller, Najla Chebib, Sabrina Maniewicz and Laurence Genton
The Impact of Xerostomia on Food Choices—A Review with Clinical Recommendations
Reprinted from: *J. Clin. Med.* **2023**, *12*, 4592, doi:10.3390/jcm12144592 . . . . **149**

About the Editors

Takahiro Ono

Takahiro Ono graduated from Hiroshima University (Faculty of Dentistry) in 1983 (D.D.S.) and from Osaka University Graduate School of Dentistry in 1987 (Ph.D.). He worked in the Department of Removable Prosthodontics, Gerodontology and Oral Rehabilitation (1988–2014) and then served as a chief professor of the Division of Comprehensive Prosthodontics in Niigata University Graduate School of Medical and Dental Sciences, between 2014 and 2022. Currently, he is a professor at Osaka Dental University (Geriatric Dentistry) and a Professor Emeritus of Niigata University. Between 2014 and 2022, he was invited to be a visiting lecturer at Hokkaido University, Tohoku University, Tokyo Medical and Dental University, Okayama University, Tokushima University, Kyushu University, etc. He also gave invited lectures at universities in Switzerland, Uruguay, Chile, Brazil, China, Indonesia, Thailand, the Philippines, and Taiwan. Dr. Ono has conducted a lot of research work on the development of devices for assessing oro-pharyngeal function and has applied them to clinical and epidemiological studies in collaboration with medicine and food science. He has published more than 120 articles in SCI journals and many textbooks about prosthodontics and dysphagia rehabilitation. He currently serves as a standing director of the Japanese Society of Gerodontology, a past council member of the European College of Gerodontology, a full member of the Store Kro Club (The Society of Oral Physiology), an associate editor of *Gerodontology*, and an Editorial Board Member of the *Journal of Oral Rehabilitation* and the *Journal of Prosthodontic Research*. He received the European College of Gerodontology GABA Research Award in 2006 and the International Association for Dental Research Distinguished Scientist Award (Geriatric Oral Research) in 2018.

Leonardo Marchini

Dr. Marchini (DDS, MSD, PhD) is a Professor and the Chair of the Department of Preventive and Community Dentistry at the University of Iowa College of Dentistry and Dental Clinics. Dr. Marchini's current research focus includes geriatric dentistry and patient satisfaction with dental treatments. He is also interested in researching the best ways to teach dentistry, with a particular interest in geriatric dentistry. He has published seven textbooks, nineteen book chapters, and 197 peer-reviewed articles. One hundred and twenty-five of those articles were included in the Scopus database and have received 1,588 citations (h-index=22). Dr. Marchini also works as a referee for several journals, including the *Special Care in Dentistry Journal*, *Journal of Prosthodontics*, and *Journal of Dental Education*. He has refereed grants for several research agencies worldwide, is a former Editorial Board Member of the *Journal of Dental Education* (2020–2023), and is currently an Editorial Board Member for the *Special Care in Dentistry Journal*, *Journal of Prosthodontics*, and the *Brazilian Dental Science Journal*. He is currently the Immediate Past-President of the Special Care Dentistry Association, a Councilor of the American Dental Education Association's Gerontology and Geriatric Section, a member of the Task and Finish Group for Gerodontology of the European Geriatric Medicine Society, and a former Councilor of the European College of Gerodontology.

Anastassia E. Kossioni

Anastassia Kossioni is Professor of Gerodontology at the Dental School of the National and Kapodistrian University of Athens (NKUA), Greece. She received her DDS and PhD from the NKUA, her MSc in Gerodontics from the Barts and the London School of Medicine and Dentistry (University of London, UK), and her Postgraduate Certificate in Open and Distance Learning from the Hellenic Open University. She is currently Honorary Secretary and Chair of the Education Committee at the European College of Gerodontology (ECG), co-Chair of the Special Interest Group in Gerodontology at the European Geriatric Medicine Society (EuGMS), and Gerodontology coordinator in the European COST action CA21122, PROmoting GeRiAtric Medicine IN countries where it is still eMerGing (PROGRAMMING). She edited the textbook "Gerodontology Essentials for Health Care Professionals" and co-authored several expert opinion papers on oral health promotion in older age. Her research activity is mainly related to the association of oral health with general health in older age, oral health promotion in frail older people, and gerodontology education for dentists and other healthcare professionals.

Preface

Populations are aging worldwide, and this demographic change has major repercussions for healthcare systems. Oral healthcare is no exception. The current cohort of older adults has been able to retain their dentition into old age, which is a positive outcome of modern dentistry. However, as they age, older adults become more susceptible to rapid oral health deterioration (ROHD) due to general medical conditions and care dependency- and socio-economic-related factors. Dentists worldwide need to recognize these factors and be prepared to prevent, diagnose, and treat the consequences of ROHD among the increasing older adult population. At the same time, further research on the relationship between ROHD, general health, and quality of life of older adults is needed. Interdisciplinary research is expected to lead to more efficient and effective health promotion measures.

The following topics were selected for this Special Issue:

- The interrelationship between systemic health factors and ROHD among older adults;
- Oral health factors related to ROHD among older adults;
- Socio-economic factors related to ROHD among older adults;
- Preventing, diagnosing, and treating ROHD among older adults;
- Novel and interdisciplinary approaches to ROHD among older adults;
- The impact of ROHD on the general health and quality of life (QOL).

In response to this call, papers were submitted from all over the world, providing valuable insights into the current state of the art in geriatric dentistry and a glimpse into its future. Looking at the 14 papers that were published, we have deep respect for the work of all authors and are pleased to have been able to create a forum to share these scientific findings and insights.

With population aging accelerating in many countries, more efforts are needed in clinical practice, education, and research in geriatric dentistry. There is little time to stand still, and we hope that this Special Issue will be a source of information that contributes to the advancement of geriatric dentistry.

Takahiro Ono, Leonardo Marchini, and Anastassia E. Kossioni
Editors

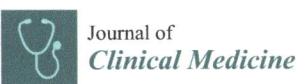

Article

Features of Masticatory Behaviors in Older Adults with Oral Hypofunction: A Cross-Sectional Study

Chikako Hatayama [1,2], Kazuhiro Hori [1,*], Hiromi Izuno [2], Masayo Fukuda [3], Misao Sawada [3], Takako Ujihashi [1,3], Shogo Yoshimura [1], Shoko Hori [1], Hitomi Togawa [1], Fumiko Uehara [1] and Takahiro Ono [1]

[1] Division of Comprehensive Prosthodontics, Faculty of Dentistry & Graduate School of Medical and Dental Sciences, Niigata University, Niigata 951-8514, Japan
[2] Department of Oral Health Sciences, Faculty of Nursing and Health Care, BAIKA Women's University, Osaka 567-8578, Japan
[3] Department of Oral Health Science, Faculty of Health Science, Kobe Tokiwa University, Kobe 653-0838, Japan
* Correspondence: hori@dent.niigata-u.ac.jp; Tel.: +81-25-227-2891; Fax: +81-25-229-3454

Abstract: Although many studies have shown the relationships between oral function and nutrition and health, few reports have investigated the masticatory behaviors of older people. This study aimed to clarify the relationships between oral function and the masticatory behaviors and features of masticatory behaviors with oral hypofunction. A total of 98 community-dwelling independent older adults participated. Seven oral conditions related to oral hypofunction were examined, and the masticatory behaviors when consuming a rice ball were measured. The participants were divided into two groups according to the criteria for oral hypofunction, and the masticatory behaviors were compared. Furthermore, the relationship between masticatory performance and the number of chews was investigated. The chewing rate of the oral hypofunction group was slower than that of the no oral hypofunction group, but there was no difference in the number of chews and chewing time. The decreased tongue–lip motor function group showed a slower chewing rate, and the decreased tongue pressure group showed a smaller number of chews and shorter chewing time. No significant correlation was observed between masticatory performance and behavior. In conclusion, older adults with oral hypofunction chewed slowly due to decreased dexterity, while, even if oral and masticatory function decreased, no compensatory increase in the number of chews was observed.

Keywords: masticatory behaviors; number of chews; oral hypofunction; masticatory performance; oral function

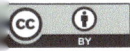

1. Introduction

Various studies to date have shown relationships between healthy life expectancy and oral function [1,2], and between oral function and low nutrition, sarcopenia [3,4], and frailty [5]. In response to this, the Japanese Society of Gerodontology proposed the disease concept of "oral hypofunction" [6], with the aim of preventing severe disease through early diagnosis and the appropriate management of decreased oral function. Seven sub-symptoms and diagnostic criteria were indicated for oral hypofunction: poor oral hygiene, oral dryness, reduced occlusal force, decreased tongue–lip motor function, decreased tongue pressure, decreased masticatory function, and deterioration of swallowing function.

Mastication is the process of grinding food and mixing it with saliva to produce a bolus that can be readily swallowed, and it takes place through the coordination of the various components of oral function [7]. Masticatory function has mainly been evaluated from the perspective of how strongly people can bite (occlusal force) and how efficiently they can crush or mix food (masticatory performance) [8]. At the same time, it was recently pointed out that masticatory behaviors, such as how many times food is chewed and how much time is spent chewing, is important in the prevention of lifestyle-related diseases, such as obesity [9], and aspiration/choking [10]. Such diversification of viewpoints in the evaluation of mastication is essential when addressing the issue of masticatory function in elderly people.

For example, even when a person's masticatory performance or oral function has declined, it would surely be possible to reduce the risk of poor nutrition or choking if there were a greater number of chews at regular mealtimes so that a diverse range of foods could be ingested. In addition, it may perhaps be the case that elderly people with reduced masticatory performance and oral function compensate by increasing the number of chews. However, there have been almost no reports of studies investigating how masticatory behaviors, such as the number of chews, relates to oral function and masticatory function in elderly persons, and the reality of masticatory behaviors in elderly persons with reduced oral function is unknown.

The purpose of the present study was to observe the masticatory behaviors of community-dwelling elderly people when they ingested a prescribed amount of food, in order to explore the relationships of masticatory behaviors with decreased oral function and masticatory performance. We hypothesized that masticatory performance is negatively correlated with the number of chews, and that elderly people with decreased oral function have a greater number of chews, and we attempted to validate this hypothesis.

2. Materials and Methods

2.1. Participants

The present study was designed as an exploratory cross-sectional survey. The participants were 98 elderly people (33 men, 65 women; mean age 74.8 ± 6.3 years) living independently in the community in M City. Recruitment was conducted in senior health classes, and the survey was conducted at the venue of the health classes between September 2018 and October 2021. The inclusion criteria were age 60 years or over, living independently, and a participant in the senior health classes sponsored by the municipal government of M City. The exclusion criteria were history of cerebrovascular disorder, dementia, neuromuscular disease, or head and neck tumor, medication related to oral hypofunction, toothache, significant movement teeth due to severe periodontitis, and missing data. We calculated sample size based on the correlation between number of chews on rice ball and mastication performance. Eight-two participants were required for 80% power, with effect size of 0.5, with a two-sided alfa level of 0.05, for correlation (G*Power 3.1.9.7, Heinrich-Heine-Universität, Düsseldorf, Germany). The objectives and methods of the study were fully explained to the participants, who provided their written, informed consent. The present study was carried out with the approval of the Ethics Committee of Niigata University (approval no. 2017-0230).

2.2. Survey Items

At first, a dentist performed an intraoral examination to investigate the number of remaining teeth, occlusal support, and the presence or absence of dentures. The number of people living together was asked as a social factor. The survey items were the seven items related to oral hypofunction [6], including (1) poor oral hygiene, (2) oral dryness, (3) reduced occlusal force, (4) decreased tongue-lip motor function, (5) decreased tongue pressure, (6) decreased masticatory function, and (7) deterioration of swallowing function, to which was added an eighth item, (8) measurement of masticatory behaviors. For all items, denture wearers were evaluated with their dentures in place.

2.2.1. Poor Oral Hygiene

This was evaluated using a bacterial counter (PHC Corporation, Osaka, Japan) [11] A sterile cotton swab was dipped in distilled water and then rubbed on the tongue at a distance of 1 cm from the center of the dorsum of the tongue using a low-pressure specimen collection device, with the rubbing pressure set at 20 gf. The cotton swab was placed in a measuring cup, and the total number of microorganisms was counted by the bacterial counter. A total microbial count of 6.5 Log10 (CFU/mL) or higher (level 4 or higher) was considered to indicate poor oral hygiene.

2.2.2. Oral Dryness

This was evaluated using an oral moisture checking device (Mucus, Life Co., Ltd., Koshigaya, Japan) [12]. The level of mucosal wetness was measured at the center of the dorsum of the tongue, approximately 10 mm from the apex. For measurement, a dedicated sensor cover was fitted to the sensor, and the sensor was held against the test surface for around 2 s with pressure of about 200 g applied to ensure uniform contact. Measurements were taken three times, and a median value of less than 27.0 was considered to indicate oral dryness.

2.2.3. Occlusal Force

Occlusal force was analyzed using a pressure-sensitive sheet (Dental Prescale II, GC Corporation, Tokyo, Japan) [13] and an analysis device (Bite Force Analyzer, GC Corporation, Tokyo, Japan). The pressure-sensitive sheet was placed in the mouth, and the participant was instructed to clench the teeth for 3 s in the maximum intercuspal position. An occlusal force of less than 500 N was considered to indicate reduced occlusal force.

2.2.4. Tongue–Lip Motor Function

The speed and dexterity of tongue and lip movements were comprehensively evaluated using oral diadochokinesis. Participants were required to pronounce each of the syllables /pa/, /ta/, and /ka/ for 5 s, and the number of pronunciations per second of each syllable was measured using an automatic measuring device (Kenko-kun Handy, Takei Scientific Instruments Co., Ltd., Niigata, Japan) [14]. A count of fewer than 6 repetitions of any of the syllables /pa/, /ta/, or /ka/ per second was considered to represent decreased tongue–lip motor function.

2.2.5. Maximum Tongue Pressure

Maximum tongue pressure was measured using a digital probe for tongue pressure measurement (JMS tongue pressure measuring device TPM-01, JMS Co., Ltd., Hiroshima, Japan) [15]. A balloon fitted to the tongue pressure probe was placed against the anterior part of the palate, and the participant was instructed to voluntarily squash the balloon against the palate using the tongue with maximum force for 7 s. After the participant first practiced and then rested to avoid fatigue, measurements were carried out three times, and the mean value was calculated. Maximum tongue pressure of less than 30 kPa was considered to indicate decreased tongue pressure.

2.2.6. Masticatory Performance

Masticatory performance was measured using a test gummy jelly (UHA Mikakuto Co., Ltd., Osaka, Japan) [16]. The participant was instructed to chew a test gummy jelly (5.50 ± 0.05 g) 30 times and then spit it out onto a gauze, and the condition of the comminuted gummy jelly was compared to a 10-stage visual scale and scored from 0 to 9. A score of 0–2 was considered to indicate decreased masticatory performance.

In addition, the fragments of comminuted gummy jelly were placed in a prescribed box (inner dimensions 140 mm × 95 mm × 36 mm) with black markers (7 mm × 7 mm, distance between a markers-width of 88 mm, length 133 mm), and the increase in surface area of the comminuted gummy jelly was calculated using an imaging method [17].

2.2.7. Swallowing Function

Swallowing function was measured using a swallowing screening questionnaire, the 10-item eating assessment tool (EAT-10) [18]. The participant was required to fill in the questionnaire, and a score of 3 or more was considered to indicate deterioration of the swallowing function.

2.2.8. Masticatory Behaviors

Masticatory behaviors were measured using a device for counting the number of chews (bitescan®, Sharp Corporation, Sakai, Japan; Figure 1) with dedicated software [19]. This device is designed to be worn on the right auricle with an ear hook, which is available in three sizes (S, M, L). The size that best fits the auricle of the participant was selected to enable the built-in sensor to sense the measurement site behind the auricle. For measurement, a Bluetooth connection with a smartphone (SHM05, Sharp Corporation, Sakai, Japan) was confirmed, the bitescan® with the selected ear-hook of appropriate size was placed on the right ear, and calibration was carried out. For the assessment of masticatory behaviors, the participant was asked to eat a 100-g rice ball (seaweed-rolled rice ball, Marusan Co., Ltd., Higashi-Osaka, Japan); no special eating instructions were given. The participants were simply asked to eat a single rice ball as they normally would, and the measurement was carried out until the rice ball was completely swallowed. Measurements were taken at least 2 h after meals.

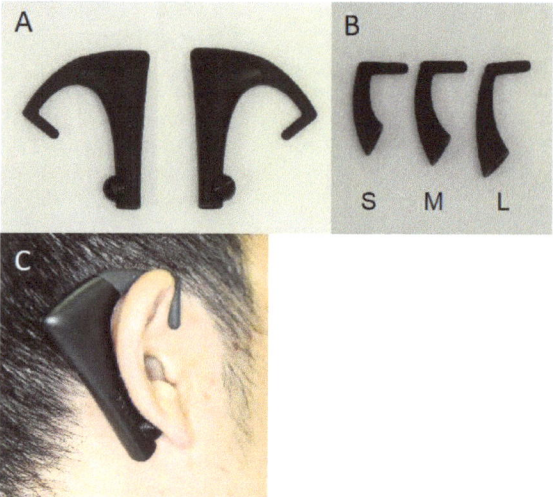

Figure 1. A wearable device for counting the number of chews (bitescan®). (**A**) Main unit; (**B**) ear-hooks for size adjustment; (**C**) bitescan® when worn.

As parameters of masticatory behaviors, the number of chews, the number of chews per bite, the chewing rate, and the total chewing time were evaluated. The masticatory behavior items were defined as follows:

- Number of chews (no.): The total number of chewing cycles during the time to eat 1 rice ball.
- Number of chews per bite (no.): Mean number of chews per bite which is an uptake action.
- Chewing rate (no./min): The number of chews per minutes calculated by dividing by total chewing time.
- Total chewing time (s): The time taken to eat 1 rice ball.

2.3. Analysis

Each participant was examined in accordance with the criteria for the seven sub-symptoms of oral hypofunction, and they were considered to have oral hypofunction if they had three of the seven items [6]. The participants were divided into two groups based on the oral hypofunction diagnostic criteria and the criteria for each of the seven sub-symptoms of oral hypofunction, and the masticatory behaviors of each group were compared using the Mann–Whitney U test. The relationship between masticatory performance and the number of chews was examined using Spearman's correlation coefficient. SPSS Statistics 23.0 (IBM) was used for statistical analysis, and the significance level was set at $p < 0.05$.

3. Results

3.1. Participants' Oral Condition and Oral Hypofunction

A total of 113 individuals applied for this study, and 101 met the inclusion and exclusion criteria. Three participants were excluded from the analysis due to withdrawal of consent, and finally 98 participants were included in the analysis.

The number of remain teeth, occlusal status, and usage of removable denture of the participants are shown in Table 1. In addition, the age, height, body weight number of people living together are also presented in Table 1.

Table 1. Information of the participants.

			All		Male		Female	
		n (%)	98	(100)	33	(33.7)	65	(66.3)
Age (y)		mean (SD)	74.8	(6.3)	74.6	(6.1)	75.0	(6.5)
Oral hypofunction		n (%)	71	(72.4)	23	(69.7)	48	(73.8)
Height (cm)		mean (SD)	156.7	(3.3)	165.1	(2.0)	148.4	(4.7)
Body weight (kg)		mean (SD)	59.4	(1.5)	63.8	(3.3)	55.0	(1.8)
Number of remain teeth		mean (SD)	21.6	(7.8)	22.1	(6.9)	21.4	(8.3)
Occlusal status	Eichner A	n (%)	53	(54.2)	15	(45.5)	38	(58.5)
	Eichner B	n (%)	22	(22.9)	9	(27.2)	13	(20.0)
	Eichner C	n (%)	23	(22.9)	9	(27.2)	14	(21.5)
N of participants using removal denture		n (%)	38	(38.8)	14	(42.4)	24	(36.9)
N of people living together		n (SD)	2.2	(1.2)	2.3	(1.3)	2.1	(1.1)

Of the 98 participants, 71 (23 men, 48 women, 75.8 ± 6.2 years) had oral hypofunction, and 27 (10 men, 17 women, 72.5 ± 6.0 years) did not (Table 1). Those with oral hypofunction were significantly older than those without, with oral hypofunction present in 32 (65.3%) early-stage elderly people (aged 65–74, 49 persons) and 39 (80.0%) late-stage elderly people (aged 75 and older, 49 persons). The group of participants with poor oral hygiene (91 persons, 92.9%) was largest, and those with deterioration of swallowing function (10 persons, 10.2%) were smallest in number (Table 2).

Table 2. The masticatory behaviors in consuming a rice ball between the participants with and without oral hypofunction and subcategory.

		n	Number of Chews (Cycles)			Number of Chews Per Bite (Cycles)			Chewing Rate (Cycles/min)			Total Chewing Time (s)		
			Median	IQR	P*	Median	IQR	P*	Median	IQR	P*	Median	IQR	P*
Oral hypofunction	Yes	71	240	(171–280)	0.975	26.5	(17.2–38.8)	0.259	77.0	(66.8–85.0)	0.035	173	(131–216)	0.477
	No	27	228	(160–341)		29.3	(19.0–51.0)		81.0	(75.0–92.0)		156	(121–226)	
Poor oral hygiene	Yes	91	232	(168–280)	0.327	27.0	(18.0–44.0)	0.644	78.7	(70.7–88.0)	0.200	165	(127–207)	0.161
	No	7	262	(169–313)		24.0	(22.0–28.2)		72.1	(66.0–81.0)		210	(156–258)	
Oral dryness	Yes	56	230	(161–274)	0.208	27.2	(18.7–38.5)	0.892	79.5	(73.3–87.8)	0.277	163	(128–195)	0.088
	No	42	251	(171–308)		26.2	(18.8–45.5)		75.9	(65.0–84.5)		186	(125–252)	
Reduced occlusal force	Yes	43	234	(159–281)	0.747	27.0	(17.2–40.8)	0.652	77.0	(65.0–85.9)	0.235	170	(129–216)	0.836
	No	55	232	(171–281)		26.2	(19.0–45.0)		80.0	(72.0–88.0)		169	(126–223)	
Decreased tongue pressure	Yes	43	262	(180–297)	0.046	27.0	(21.0–44.0)	0.506	77.9	(70.7–83.0)	0.266	193	(151–242)	0.010
	No	55	225	(139–268)		23.2	(18.6–40.8)		80.0	(68.0–90.5)		155	(121–192)	
Decreased tongue-lip motor function	Yes	55	230	(139–277)	0.229	17.1	(16.8–43.6)	0.594	75.0	(66.0–83.0)	0.003	169	(127–210)	0.783
	No	43	234	(180–316)		19.0	(18.7–40.8)		82.5	(75.0–90.7)		164	(129–223)	
Decreased masticatory function	Yes	15	241	(180–313)	0.653	25.7	(19.6–32.4)	0.531	74.3	(66.0–84.0)	0.354	169	(131–250)	0.421
	No	83	232	(160–281)		27.0	(18.6–44.7)		79.0	(70.7–88.0)		169	(125–202)	
Deterioration of swallowing function	Yes	10	251	(218–267)	0.651	29.7	(22.3–47.4)	0.439	80.5	(63.7–91.8)	0.972	186	(154–212)	0.372
	No	88	232	(162–287)		26.4	(18.2–39.4)		78.0	(71.0–86.2)		164	(126–221)	

*: Mann–Whitney's U test, IQR: interquartile range.

3.2. Comparison of Masticatory Behaviors in Participants with and without Oral Hypofunction

The number of chews (mean ± standard deviation {median}) was 236 ± 103 {233} for participants overall, with no significant difference between the oral hypofunction group (230 ± 89 {240}) and the non-oral hypofunction group (254 ± 133 {228}) ($p = 0.975$) (Table 2).

The number of chews per bite was 32.7 ± 22.1 {26.6} for participants overall, with no significant difference between the oral hypofunction group (30.7 ± 20.3 {26.5}) and the non-oral hypofunction group (37.9 ± 26.0 {29.3}) ($p = 0.259$).

The chewing rate was 77.5 ± 15.0 {78.0} cycles/min for participants overall, with the oral hypofunction group (75.4 ± 13.9 {77.0} cycles/min) significantly slower than the non-oral hypofunction group (83.1 ± 16.4 {81.0} cycles/min) ($p = 0.035$).

The total chewing time was 177 ± 69 {169} s for participants overall, with no significant difference between the oral hypofunction group (176 ± 62 {173} s) and the non-oral hypofunction group (180 ± 87 {156} s) ($p = 0.477$).

3.3. Comparison of Masticatory Behaviors by Oral Hypofunction Sub-Symptoms

The analysis of masticatory behaviors by each sub-symptom of oral hypofunction is shown in Table 2.

In the decreased tongue pressure group ($n = 43$), the number of chews (255 ± 97 {262}) was significantly greater than in the non-decreased tongue pressure group ($n = 55$) (221 ± 106 {225}), and total chewing time (194 ± 68 {193} s) was significantly longer than in the non-decreased tongue pressure group (164 ± 68 {155} s).

In the decreased tongue–lip motor function group ($n = 55$), the chewing rate (73.7 ± 14.2 {75.0} cycles/min) was significantly slower than in the non-decreased tongue–lip motor function group ($n = 43$) (82.4 ± 14.6 {82.5} chews/min).

For all other sub-symptoms, there were no significant differences in masticatory behaviors between the groups with and without the sub-symptom.

3.4. Relationship between Masticatory Performance and Number of Chews

No significant correlation was found between masticatory performance (amount of increase in surface area of comminuted gummy jelly) and the number of chews when consuming a rice ball (Figure 2; $r = 0.055$, $p = 0.600$).

No significant correlation was found between masticatory performance (amount of increase in surface area of comminuted gummy jelly) and the number of chews when consuming a rice ball (Spearman's correlation coefficient: $r = 0.055$, $p = 0.600$).

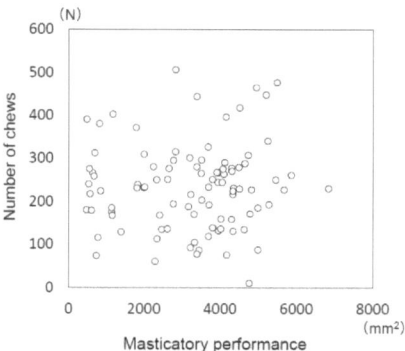

Figure 2. Relationship between masticatory performance and the number of chews when consuming a rice ball.

4. Discussion

The present study is the first attempt to objectively measure masticatory behaviors and masticatory performance in independent, community-dwelling, older adults to explore the relationship between the two and also to examine how they are affected by oral hypofunction. The results showed that older adults with oral hypofunction, and in particular elderly people with decreased tongue–lip motor function, have a slower chewing rate, and that older adults with decreased tongue pressure have a greater number of chews and longer total chewing time. In addition, no significant correlation was seen between masticatory performance and the number of chews. These findings show the relationship between oral function and masticatory behaviors in older adults, providing basic data for approaches to dealing with those with declining oral function.

4.1. Measurement of Masticatory Behaviors

To extend healthy life expectancy, it is essential to prevent elderly people from falling into the cycle of frailty through low nutrition [20]. It has been reported that people with an inadequate ability to form a food bolus tend to avoid fibrous foods or meat, thus losing variety from their diet [21]. Formation of the food bolus within the mouth requires not only conservation of the remaining teeth, but also maintenance of oral functions, such as tongue function and occlusal force. Various methods of assessment of oral function have, therefore, been devised to enable the management of oral function in older adults.

The prevention of frailty in older adults needs to be approached not just from the perspective of oral function, but also through the assessment of regular dietary behavior and provision of appropriate guidance. For example, it has been reported in edentulous individuals that prosthodontic treatment alone does not result in sufficient improvement in diet and nutritional intake, and the treatment needs to be accompanied by guidance on food selection and nutritional intake [22]. At the same time, masticatory behaviors, such as number and rate of chews at mealtimes, are important for the selection of a wide range of foods and safe swallowing through appropriate bolus formation. While there have been various educational campaigns encouraging people to eat slowly and chew their food thoroughly [23], little has been known to date about the extent to which older adults masticate their food when ingesting.

One reason for the scarcity of reports on the number of chews is the difficulty of accurate and convenient measurement. Studies to date have used a device to measure jaw movement [24] or a muscle activity meter [25,26] to measure the number of chews, but such devices are cumbersome and require measurement to be carried out in a laboratory, so they are unsuitable for surveying large numbers of people. Studies have also been carried out by measuring the number of chews through direct observation of participants at mealtimes or by video recording mealtimes and then measuring masticatory behaviors [27]. However, such measurement environments may differ from regular mealtimes.

We studied the masticatory behaviors using bitescan®, a wearable device that measures the number of chews [19]. This device is simply placed on the right ear, and it monitors the changes in the skin surface behind the auricle that accompany masticatory movements. It is connected to a smartphone via Bluetooth to measure parameters relating to masticatory behaviors, so there is no need to restrain the participant in any way. We previously confirmed that the device has sufficient measurement accuracy [19], and we used it to study masticatory behaviors in healthy adults [28,29].

In the present study, masticatory behaviors were measured using rice balls. Rice balls are among the most popular and frequently consumed foods in Japan, and as well as being made at home, they are readily available from supermarkets and convenience stores. It has been reported that the ingestion method, such as the eating utensils used, affects the number of chews [30], but rice balls are generally eaten out of the hands. Furthermore, it is difficult to evaluate the number of chews per bite with a small amount of food that can be ingested in one bite. In the present study, rice balls were used because there is little influence from participants' preferences or the method of ingestion, rice balls need to be masticated, there is a reasonable amount to be ingested, and measurements can be made under uniform conditions. Based on measurements of 99 healthy adults, it was reported that the number of chews, the number of bites, the number of chews per bite, and the chewing rate with a single rice ball used in the present study all show significant positive correlations with the same parameters during usual meals for an entire day [29].

4.2. Oral Hypofunction

Of the 98 participants in the present study, 72.4% had oral hypofunction. Looking at prior studies of oral hypofunction [4,5,31–34], the reported prevalence shows a wide range, from 43% [31] to 63% [32,34]. The participants of these studies included not just different age groups, but also community-dwelling elderly persons [4,5,31,33,34] and older adults who were visiting a dental clinic [32], with the incidence in community-dwelling older adults often reported in the range of 50–60%. The results of the present study seem to show a somewhat high proportion of participants with oral hypofunction. However, all prior reports indicate that the incidence of oral hypofunction increases with age [31,32,34], and the same trend was seen in the present study. In addition, looking at the sub-symptoms, it may be seen that the incidences of poor oral hygiene [33,34] and decreased tongue–lip motor function [4,31,32,34] are often high. In the present study as well, there were many older adults with poor oral hygiene, which may have resulted in a higher incidence of oral hypofunction. In the case of participants who were visiting a dental clinic, it could be assumed that they had some kind of oral complaint [32]. However, in the case of older adults who visited a dental clinic for a regular check-up, they may be less likely to have oral hypofunction as a result of dental treatment or poor oral hygiene thanks to their oral hygiene management. In the present study, the participants were independent older adults aged 60 years or older who participated in the senior health classes sponsored by the municipal government of M City, and not patients who were visiting a dental clinic. However, though there were a few participants who complained of problems with dentures or poor oral status, there were also participants receiving regular oral hygiene care at their regular dental clinic. The present study did not investigate dental visit history or oral symptoms, but there is a need for studies that survey these items in order to adjust the participants for analysis in the future.

4.3. The Characteristics of Masticatory Behaviors in Older Adults with Oral Hypofunction (and Its Sub-Symptoms)

The results of the present study showed the number of chews (median value) to be 240 in the oral hypofunction group and 228 in the non-oral hypofunction group, with no significant difference between the two. This result suggests that there is no increase in the number of chews to compensate for the decline in oral function. At the same time, the number of chews per bite in the oral hypofunction group was 26.5, which was slightly less than the number in the non-oral hypofunction group (29.3), although the difference was not significant. In addition, though the chewing rate was significantly slower in the oral hypofunction group than in the non-oral hypofunction group, there was no significant difference between the oral hypofunction group and the non-oral hypofunction group in the total chewing time to eat 1 rice ball. It therefore appears that, even though older adults with oral hypofunction masticated a rice ball more slowly, they had fewer chews per bite, with the result that there was no difference between the oral hypofunction group and the non-oral hypofunction group in the overall number of chews or total chewing time. This suggests that bolus formation may be inadequate in older adults with oral hypofunction, which would indicate a risk of choking or incomplete absorption of nutrients. It appears that older adults with oral hypofunction not only need dental treatment and improvement or management of oral function, but also guidance in taking their time over meals and chewing their food well.

Older adults with decreased tongue–lip motor function showed a significantly slower chewing rate than those without this sub-symptom. Decreased tongue–lip motor function is a condition in which the speed and dexterity of tongue and lip movements are reduced due to neuromuscular system dysfunction. This results in incomplete bolus formation and spills during mastication, which impact negatively on mastication and swallowing consequently limiting the types and amount of food that can be ingested. In addition, decreased tongue–lip motor function can cause problems with articulation and speech. Speech disorders in older adults can lead to social deterioration, not just because they cause difficulties in communication, but also because they can lead to the affected person being reluctant to meet others or avoiding going out. Since participants in the decreased tongue–lip motor function group had a slower chewing rate, total chewing time would be expected to be longer. However, there was no difference in total chewing time between the decreased tongue–lip motor function group and the non-decreased group. It may therefore be conjectured that, even though these participants were chewing slowly, they either swallowed the food soon without adequate mastication, or else there was a large amount of food per bite.

In addition, in the decreased tongue pressure group, the number of chews (262) and the total chewing time (193 s) were significantly greater than in the non-decreased tongue pressure group (number of chews: 225, total chewing time: 155 s). The tongue plays an important role in mastication, swallowing, and pronunciation, and the measured values for these items decrease when the muscle strength of the suprahyoid muscle group declines [35]. In particular, dexterity of tongue movement and muscle strength are essential at each stage of the masticatory and swallowing process, starting with transport of food taken into the anterior part of the mouth to the molars (stage I transport), followed by the mixing of food fragments crushed by the molars with saliva, formation of the bolus (processing), transport of the bolus to the oropharynx (stage II transport), and then the subsequent ejection of the bolus and maintenance of swallowing pressure when the swallowing reflex occurs [36]. There have been prior reports of the relationships of decreased tongue pressure to activities of daily living (ADL) [37] and dysphagia [38]. It has also been reported that decreased tongue pressure is associated with longer mealtimes [39] and the intake of formula diet [40], suggesting that decreased tongue pressure also affects the form of food that can be ingested. In the present study as well, elderly people with decreased tongue pressure showed an increased number of chews and longer total chewing time in order to form a bolus adequately, suggesting that decreased tongue pressure affects bolus formation.

4.4. Relationship between Masticatory Behaviors and Masticatory Performance

Since masticatory performance was thought to be closely related to masticatory behaviors, in the present study, masticatory performance was evaluated not only by the score method, but also by an imaging method to evaluate the increase in surface area of comminuted gummy jelly in order to give a detailed evaluation. With the evaluation of masticatory performance using a test gummy jelly, the significant relationship between the score method and imaging was previously demonstrated [17,41]. In the present study, no significant correlation was found between increased surface area of the comminuted gummy jelly and number of chews of a rice ball.

To date, there have only been a few studies investigating the relationship between masticatory performance and number of chews. Some of these have reported no association [42–44], which is the same result as the present study, but one study reported a negative association, with a greater number of chews in participants with low masticatory performance [45].

Many of these reports had participants with a wide age range, from young to old [44,45]. In addition, a variety of foods was used for evaluation, such as peanuts [42,43], carrots [45], and gummy jelly [44], and it therefore appears that the results are greatly influenced by the food.

Although the measurement conditions in the survey may have influenced the results, attention should be given to the finding that there are elderly people with both low masticatory performance and low number of chews. Such elders are at risk of choking, as well as defective digestion or absorption of nutrients, suggesting the need to not only restore occlusal support and improve the oral environment through dental treatment, but also to pay attention to their daily masticatory behaviors and, where necessary, provide guidance on chewing habits.

4.5. Limitations and Future Study

In this study, we did not investigate the degree of periodontal disease or the history of dental caries though the applicant who had toothache or significant movement teeth were excluded. Even if there is no pain, caries and periodontal disease might affect chewing behavior. Although it is thought that the participants' oral condition lacks homogeneity, in this study we analyzed oral function as an explanatory variable.

In addition, the bitescan® should have been used for a full day or several days to assess daily masticatory behaviors. However, since some older adults have difficulty using a smartphone or wearable device, masticatory behaviors were evaluated with a single rice ball at the research site. If improvements could be made to the bitescan® to allow simple self-monitoring by older adults, we would like to conduct surveys of masticatory behaviors at everyday meals.

In the future, a large survey of mastication behaviors would further clarify the details of mastication behaviors according to oral conditions and age in the elderly persons. We also want to investigate the relationship between mastication behaviors and nutritional status. Furthermore, we plan to examine the effects of mastication behaviors modification on the health of the elderly people.

Although these are possible limitations, the present study is the first to investigate masticatory behaviors in older adults in detail through the number of chews, chewing time, and chewing rate. In addition, it was possible to clarify characteristics, such as the slower chewing rate in older adults with decreased oral function. We believe that these results show some of the detailed aspects of mastication in older adults with decreased oral function. Elderly people with decreased oral and masticatory functions should be given masticatory instruction in addition to rehabilitation and dental treatment. The results of this study are considered to be useful as indices for mastication instruction.

5. Conclusions

In older adults living independently in the community, the chewing rate of the oral hypofunction group was significantly slower than that of the non-oral hypofunction group, but no difference was observed between the groups in the number of chews or total chewing time. In particular, the decreased tongue–lip motor function group showed a significantly slower chewing rate, and the decreased tongue pressure group showed a significantly higher number of chews and significantly longer total chewing time. These results indicate that decline in oral function affects masticatory behaviors. At the same time, older adults with decreased oral or masticatory function showed no compensatory increase in the number of chews, suggesting that functional decline may increase the risk of choking or affect digestion and the absorption of nutrients. These results suggest the need for guidance on mastication that covers individual oral functions.

Author Contributions: Conceptualization, K.H.; methodology, C.H., K.H. and H.I.; formal analysis, C.H. and K.H.; investigation, C.H., K.H., H.I., M.F., M.S., T.U., S.Y., S.H., H.T. and F.U.; resources, K.H., H.I. and M.F.; data curation, K.H.; writing—original draft preparation, C.H.; writing—review and editing, K.H.; supervision, T.O.; project administration, K.H., H.I. and M.F.; funding acquisition, T.O. All authors have read and agreed to the published version of the manuscript.

Funding: This work was funded by Research Program for Health Behavior Modification by Utilizing IoT, Japan Agency for Medical Research and Development.

Institutional Review Board Statement: The study was conducted in accordance with the Declaration of Helsinki, and approved by the Ethics Committee of Niigata University (approval no. 2017-0230).

Informed Consent Statement: Informed consent was obtained from all participants involved in the study.

Data Availability Statement: The data presented in this study are available on request from the corresponding author. The data are not publicly available due to ethical restrictions.

Acknowledgments: We would like to express our deep gratitude to Yasuyuki Nishikawa and Naoto Shigenobu and all the staff of the Osaka YMCA for their cooperation.

Conflicts of Interest: The authors declare no conflict of interest associated with this manuscript.

References

1. Matsuyama, Y.; Aida, J.; Watt, R.G.; Tsuboya, T.; Koyama, S.; Sato, Y.; Kondo, K.; Osaka, K. Dental Status and Compression of Life Expectancy with Disability. *J. Dent. Res.* **2017**, *96*, 1006–1013. [CrossRef] [PubMed]
2. Watanabe, Y.; Okada, K.; Kondo, M.; Matsushita, T.; Nakazawa, S.; Yamazaki, Y. Oral health for achieving longevity. *Geriatr. Gerontol. Int.* **2020**, *20*, 526–538. [CrossRef] [PubMed]
3. Hatta, K.; Ikebe, K. Association between oral health and sarcopenia: A literature review. *J. Prosthodont. Res.* **2021**, *65*, 131–136. [CrossRef]
4. Kugimiya, Y.; Iwasaki, M.; Ohara, Y.; Motokawa, K.; Edahiro, A.; Shirobe, M.; Watanabe, Y.; Obuchi, S.; Kawai, H.; Fujiwara, Y.; et al. Relationship between Oral Hypofunction and Sarcopenia in Community-Dwelling Older Adults: The Otassha Study. *Int. J. Environ. Res. Public Health* **2021**, *18*, 6666. [CrossRef] [PubMed]
5. Yoshida, M.; Hiraoka, A.; Takeda, C.; Mori, T.; Maruyama, M.; Yoshikawa, M.; Tsuga, K. Oral hypofunction and its relation to frailty and sarcopenia in community-dwelling older people. *Gerodontology* **2022**, *39*, 26–32. [CrossRef]
6. Minakuchi, S.; Tsuga, K.; Ikebe, K.; Ueda, T.; Tamura, F.; Nagao, K.; Furuya, J.; Matsuo, K.; Yamamoto, K.; Kanazawa, M.; et al. Oral hypofunction in the older population: Position paper of the Japanese Society of Gerodontology in 2016. *Gerodontology* **2018**, *35*, 317–324. [CrossRef] [PubMed]
7. Palmer, J.B.; Rudin, N.J.; Lara, G.; Crompton, A.W. Coordination of mastication and swallowing. *Dysphagia* **1992**, *7*, 187–200. [CrossRef] [PubMed]
8. Goncalves, T.; Schimmel, M.; van der Bilt, A.; Chen, J.; van der Glas, H.W.; Kohyama, K.; Hennequin, M.; Peyron, M.A.; Woda, A.; Leles, C.R.; et al. Consensus on the terminologies and methodologies for masticatory assessment. *J. Oral Rehabil.* **2021**, *48*, 745–761. [CrossRef]
9. Otsuka, R.; Tamakoshi, K.; Yatsuya, H.; Murata, C.; Sekiya, A.; Wada, K.; Zhang, H.M.; Matsushita, K.; Sugiura, K.; Takefuji, S.; et al. Eating fast leads to obesity: Findings based on self-administered questionnaires among middle-aged Japanese men and women. *J. Epidemiol.* **2006**, *16*, 117–124. [CrossRef]
10. Berzlanovich, A.M.; Fazeny-Dorner, B.; Waldhoer, T.; Fasching, P.; Keil, W. Foreign body asphyxia: A preventable cause of death in the elderly. *Am. J. Prev. Med.* **2005**, *28*, 65–69. [CrossRef]
11. Kikutani, T.; Tamura, F.; Takahashi, Y.; Konishi, K.; Hamada, R. A novel rapid oral bacteria detection apparatus for effective oral care to prevent pneumonia. *Gerodontology* **2012**, *29*, e560–e565. [CrossRef] [PubMed]
12. Yamada, H.; Nakagawa, Y.; Nomura, Y.; Yamamoto, K.; Suzuki, M.; Watanabe, N.Y.; Saito, I.; Seto, K. Preliminary results of moisture checker for Mucus in diagnosing dry mouth. *Oral Dis.* **2005**, *11*, 405–407. [CrossRef] [PubMed]
13. Suzuki, T.; Kumagai, H.; Watanabe, T.; Uchida, T.; Nagao, M. Evaluation of complete denture occlusal contacts using pressure-sensitive sheets. *Int. J. Prosthodont.* **1997**, *10*, 386–391.
14. Yamada, A.; Kanazawa, M.; Komagamine, Y.; Minakuchi, S. Association between tongue and lip functions and masticatory performance in young dentate adults. *J. Oral Rehabil.* **2015**, *42*, 833–839. [CrossRef] [PubMed]
15. Hayashi, R.; Tsuga, K.; Hosokawa, R.; Yoshida, M.; Sato, Y.; Akagawa, Y. A novel handy probe for tongue pressure measurement. *Int. J. Prosthodont.* **2002**, *15*, 385–388.
16. Nokubi, T.; Yoshimuta, Y.; Nokubi, F.; Yasui, S.; Kusunoki, C.; Ono, T.; Maeda, Y.; Yokota, K. Validity and reliability of a visual scoring method for masticatory ability using test gummy jelly. *Gerodontology* **2013**, *30*, 76–82. [CrossRef]
17. Salazar, S.; Hori, K.; Uehara, F.; Okawa, J.; Shibata, A.; Higashimori, M.; Nokubi, T.; Ono, T. Masticatory performance analysis using photographic image of gummy jelly. *J. Prosthodont. Res.* **2020**, *64*, 48–54. [CrossRef]
18. Belafsky, P.C.; Mouadeb, D.A.; Rees, C.J.; Pryor, J.C.; Postma, G.N.; Allen, J.; Leonard, R.J. Validity and reliability of the Eating Assessment Tool (EAT-10). *Ann. Otol. Rhinol. Laryngol.* **2008**, *117*, 919–924. [CrossRef]
19. Hori, K.; Uehara, F.; Yamaga, Y.; Yoshimura, S.; Okawa, J.; Tanimura, M.; Ono, T. Reliability of a novel wearable device to measure chewing frequency. *J. Prosthodont. Res.* **2021**, *65*, 340–345. [CrossRef]
20. Fried, L.P.; Tangen, C.M.; Walston, J.; Newman, A.B.; Hirsch, C.; Gottdiener, J.; Seeman, T.; Tracy, R.; Kop, W.J.; Burke, G.; et al. Frailty in older adults: Evidence for a phenotype. *J. Gerontol. Ser. A Biol. Sci. Med. Sci.* **2001**, *56*, M146–M156. [CrossRef]
21. Zhu, Y.; Hollis, J.H. Tooth loss and its association with dietary intake and diet quality in American adults. *J. Dent.* **2014**, *42*, 1428–1435. [CrossRef] [PubMed]
22. Amagai, N.; Komagamine, Y.; Kanazawa, M.; Iwaki, M.; Jo, A.; Suzuki, H.; Minakuchi, S. The effect of prosthetic rehabilitation and simple dietary counseling on food intake and oral health related quality of life among the edentulous individuals: A randomized controlled trial. *J. Dent.* **2017**, *65*, 89–94. [CrossRef] [PubMed]

23. Doi, T.; Hinode, D.; Nakae, H.; Yoshioka, M.; Matsuyama, M.; Iga, H.; Fukushima, Y. Relationship between Chewing Behavior and Oral Conditions in Elementary School Children Based on the "Chewing 30" Program: An Intervention Study. *J. Dent. Health* **2016**, *66*, 438–444. [CrossRef]
24. Le Reverend, B.; Saucy, F.; Moser, M.; Loret, C. Adaptation of mastication mechanics and eating behaviour to small differences in food texture. *Physiol. Behav.* **2016**, *165*, 136–145. [CrossRef]
25. Mioche, L.; Bourdiol, P.; Martin, J.F.; Noel, Y. Variations in human masseter and temporalis muscle activity related to food texture during free and side-imposed mastication. *Arch. Oral Biol.* **1999**, *44*, 1005–1012. [CrossRef]
26. van der Bilt, A.; Abbink, J.H. The influence of food consistency on chewing rate and muscular work. *Arch. Oral Biol.* **2017**, *83*, 105–110. [CrossRef]
27. Goto, T.; Nakamich, A.; Watanabe, M.; Nagao, K.; Matsuyama, M.; Ichikawa, T. Influence of food volume per mouthful on chewing and bolus properties. *Physiol. Behav.* **2015**, *141*, 58–62. [CrossRef]
28. Yoshimura, S.; Hori, K.; Uehara, F.; Hori, S.; Yamaga, Y.; Hasegawa, Y.; Akazawa, K.; Ono, T. Relationship between body mass index and masticatory factors evaluated with a wearable device. *Sci. Rep.* **2022**, *12*, 4117. [CrossRef]
29. Uehara, F.; Hori, K.; Hasegawa, Y.; Yoshimura, S.; Hori, S.; Kitamura, M.; Akazawa, K.; Ono, T. Impact of masticatory behaviors measured with wearable device on metabolic syndrome: Cross-sectional study. *JMIR Mhealth Uhealth* **2022**, *10*, e30789. [CrossRef]
30. Sun, L.; Ranawana, D.V.; Tan, W.J.; Quek, Y.C.; Henry, C.J. The impact of eating methods on eating rate and glycemic response in healthy adults. *Physiol. Behav.* **2015**, *139*, 505–510. [CrossRef]
31. Iwasaki, M.; Motokawa, K.; Watanabe, Y.; Shirobe, M.; Ohara, Y.; Edahiro, A.; Kawai, H.; Fujiwara, Y.; Kim, H.; Ihara, K.; et al. Oral hypofunction and malnutrition among community-dwelling older adults: Evidence from the Otassha study. *Gerodontology* **2022**, *39*, 17–25. [CrossRef] [PubMed]
32. Hatanaka, Y.; Furuya, J.; Sato, Y.; Uchida, Y.; Shichita, T.; Kitagawa, N.; Osawa, T. Associations between Oral Hypofunction Tests, Age, and Sex. *Int. J. Environ. Res. Public Health* **2021**, *18*, 256. [CrossRef] [PubMed]
33. Nakamura, M.; Hamada, T.; Tanaka, A.; Nishi, K.; Kume, K.; Goto, Y.; Beppu, M.; Hijioka, H.; Higashi, Y.; Tabata, H.; et al. Association of Oral Hypofunction with Frailty, Sarcopenia, and Mild Cognitive Impairment: A Cross-Sectional Study of Community-Dwelling Japanese Older Adults. *J. Clin. Med.* **2021**, *10*, 1626. [CrossRef] [PubMed]
34. Shimazaki, Y.; Nonoyama, T.; Tsushita, K.; Arai, H.; Matsushita, K.; Uchibori, N. Oral hypofunction and its association with frailty in community-dwelling older people. *Geriatr. Gerontol. Int.* **2020**, *20*, 917–926. [CrossRef]
35. Yamaguchi, K.; Hara, K.; Nakagawa, K.; Yoshimi, K.; Ariya, C.; Nakane, A.; Furuya, J.; Tohara, H. Ultrasonography Shows Age-related Changes and Related Factors in the Tongue and Suprahyoid Muscles. *J. Am. Med. Dir. Assoc.* **2021**, *22*, 766–772. [CrossRef]
36. Hiiemae, K.M.; Palmer, J.B. Food transport and bolus formation during complete feeding sequences on foods of different initial consistency. *Dysphagia* **1999**, *14*, 31–42. [CrossRef]
37. Tsuga, K.; Yoshikawa, M.; Oue, H.; Okazaki, Y.; Tsuchioka, H.; Maruyama, M.; Yoshida, M.; Akagawa, Y. Maximal voluntary tongue pressure is decreased in Japanese frail elderly persons. *Gerodontology* **2012**, *29*, e1078–e1085. [CrossRef]
38. Yoshida, M.; Kikutani, T.; Tsuga, K.; Utanohara, Y.; Hayashi, R.; Akagawa, Y. Decreased tongue pressure reflects symptom of dysphagia. *Dysphagia* **2006**, *21*, 61–65. [CrossRef]
39. Namasivayam, A.M.; Steele, C.M.; Keller, H. The effect of tongue strength on meal consumption in long term care. *Clin. Nutr.* **2016**, *35*, 1078–1083. [CrossRef]
40. Liu, H.Y.; Chen, J.H.; Hsu, K.J.; Yao, C.T.; Chen, P.H.; Hsiao, S.Y.; Lin, C.L. Decreased Tongue Pressure Associated with Aging, Chewing and Swallowing Difficulties of Community-Dwelling Older Adults in Taiwan. *J. Pers. Med.* **2021**, *11*, 653. [CrossRef]
41. Murakami, K.; Hori, K.; Yoneda, H.; Sato, N.; Suwanarpa, K.; Sta Maria, M.T.; Marito, P.; Nokubi, T.; Ono, T. Compatibility of two types of gummy jelly tests for detecting decreased masticatory function. *Gerodontology* **2021**, *39*, 10–16. [CrossRef] [PubMed]
42. Yurkstas, A. Compensation for inadequate mastication. *Br. Dent. J.* **1951**, *91*, 261–262. [PubMed]
43. Dahlberg, B. The masticatory habits; an analysis of the number of chews when consuming food. *J. Dent. Res.* **1946**, *25*, 67–72. [CrossRef] [PubMed]
44. Ohno, K.; Fujita, Y.; Ohno, Y.; Takeshima, T.; Maki, K. The factors related to decreases in masticatory performance and masticatory function until swallowing using gummy jelly in subjects aged 20–79 years. *J. Oral Rehabil.* **2020**, *47*, 851–861. [CrossRef] [PubMed]
45. Zhu, Y.; Hollis, J.H. Differences in chewing behaviors between healthy fully dentate young and older adults assessed by electromyographic recordings. *Int. J. Food Sci. Nutr.* **2015**, *66*, 452–457. [CrossRef] [PubMed]

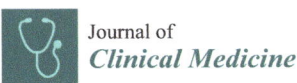

Article

Relationships between the Nutrition Status and Oral Measurements for Sarcopenia in Older Japanese Adults

Kentaro Okuno [1,*], Ryuichiro Kobuchi [1], Suguru Morita [1,2], Ayako Masago [1], Masaaki Imaoka [1] and Kazuya Takahashi [1]

[1] Department of Geriatric Dentistry, Osaka Dental University, 1-8, Kuzuhahanazono-cho, Hirakata-shi 573-1121, Japan
[2] Department of Dentistry and Oral-Maxillofacial Surgery, Chikaishi Hospital, Medical Corporation Touhoukai, 2-46, Hikari-machi, Gifu-shi 502-0901, Japan
* Correspondence: okuno-kentaro-ig@alumni.osaka-u.ac.jp; Tel./Fax: +81-66910-1050

Abstract: Introduction: The purpose of the present study was to clarify the relationships between the risk of malnutrition as a preliminary stage of malnutrition and overall and oral measurements for sarcopenia in older Japanese adults. Methods: Forty-five participants (79.7 ± 6.1 years) were included in the analysis. The nutrition status of the participants was assessed using the Mini Nutritional Assessment-Short Form (MNA-SF) and classified into two groups: normal and at risk of malnutrition. Overall measurements for sarcopenia in the present study were the skeletal muscle mass index, grip strength, and walking speed, while oral measurements were the cross-sectional area of the geniohyoid muscle, tongue pressure (TP), and oral diadochokinesis. Results: MNA-SF correlated with TP ($r = 0.347$, $p = 0.019$). We observed decreases of 5.7 kPa in TP and 3.9 kg/cm^2 in BMI in the at risk of malnutrition group. A multiple regression analysis of parameters contributing to the risk of malnutrition identified TP as an independent variable ($β = 0.913$, $p = 0.042$). Conclusions: The present results demonstrate that the risk of malnutrition is associated with TP as an oral measurement for sarcopenia, but not overall measurements for sarcopenia. Therefore, low TP may be related with the risk of malnutrition.

Keywords: nutrition; sarcopenia; tongue pressure

1. Introduction

Older adults are at risk of malnutrition due to a decline in physiological function with aging and socioeconomic and psycho-behavioral factors [1]. Malnutrition is a risk factor for sarcopenia, which is characterized by the loss of skeletal muscle mass and strength, thereby reducing the basal metabolic rate in a negative chain reaction that lowers energy consumption and nutrient intake [2]. Sarcopenia may occur secondary to a systemic disease, particularly one that induces inflammatory processes (e.g., malignancy, inflammatory bowel diseases, malabsorption and malnutrition, physical inactivity, or organ failure). The emerging concept of the "gut–muscle axis" needs to be adequately described in the pathogenesis of sarcopenic dysphagia, taking into account the key role of inflammation and the gut microbiota in the development of muscle wasting [3]. The mechanisms underlying a low nutritional status involve a decline in oral function, which plays an important role in food intake; therefore, the deterioration of oral function in older adults worsens their nutritional status [4–6].

Among the tissues involved in oral function, the tongue plays an important role in swallowing and speech. Our research group examined the muscle mass, muscle strength, and motor function of the tongue in assessments of oral sarcopenia. Oral measurements for sarcopenia were identified as the cross-sectional area of the geniohyoid muscle (CSG), tongue pressure (TP), and oral diadochokinesis (ODK), and all endpoints of oral sarcopenia were influenced by overall measurements for sarcopenia [7].

Based on these findings, we hypothesized that oral measurements for sarcopenia may precede overall measurements for sarcopenia and contribute to the risk of malnutrition, the preliminary stage of malnutrition. The purpose of the present study was to clarify the relationships between the risk of malnutrition as a preliminary stage of malnutrition and overall and oral measurements for sarcopenia in older Japanese adults.

2. Materials and Methods

2.1. Participants

The present study was designed as a cross-sectional survey. Participants were selected from the database of our previous study [7]. Inclusion criteria were the nutrition status assessed by the Mini Nutritional Assessment-Short Form (MNA-SF) showing a normal status and risk of malnutrition. Exclusion criteria were age < 70 years, pacemaker wearers, non-ambulatory patients, an inability to communicate, and a malnutrition status assessed by MNA-SF. We calculated sample size based on the correlation between MNA-SF and tongue power in a previous study [7]. Twenty-six participants were required for 80% power, with an effect size of 0.5, with a two-sided alfa level of 0.05, for correlation (G*Power 3.1, Heinrich-Heine- Universität, Düsseldorf, Germany). Fifty-four participants from the database of our previous study were candidates for the present study. Three participants were excluded due to malnutrition and six for being younger than 70 years old. Therefore, 45 participants were ultimately analyzed in the present study (Figure 1). The Ethics Committee of Osaka Dental University approved the present study (Approval No. 110970).

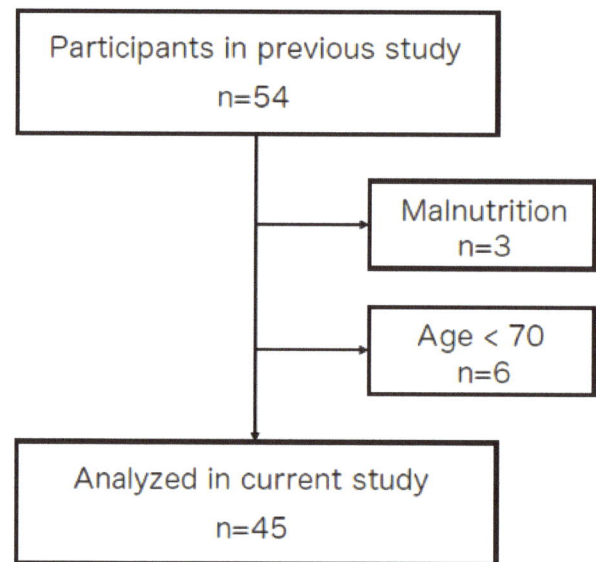

Figure 1. A diagram of study participants. Participants were selected from the database of our previous study [7]. Among 54 participants, 9 were excluded due to malnutrition and being younger than 70 years old; therefore, 45 participants were ultimately analyzed in the present study.

2.2. Basic Information

Interviews with participants and clinical records provided information on age, sex, basic diseases, medical history, and medications. Body mass index (BMI) was calculated as weight divided by height squared. The Barthel Index was used to assess basic daily activities and, thus, functional independence in daily life [8]. Interviews with participants using the questionnaire on Eating Assessment Tool-10 (EAT-10) [9] were used to evaluate eating and swallowing functions.

2.3. Nutritional Risk Assessment

Interviews with participants using MNA-SF [10] were conducted to evaluate their nutritional status. MNA-SF includes the following six domains: appetite loss (0–2 points), weight loss (0–3 points), mobility (0–2 points), stress/acute disease (0 or 2 points), neuropsychological impairment (0–2 points), and BMI (0–3 points). If it was not possible to weigh a patient, calf circumference was used as a substitute for BMI (0 or 3 points). According to the total score of MNA-SF, patients were classified into three categories: malnourished (0–7 points), at risk of malnutrition (8–11 points), or a normal nutritional status (12–14 points).

2.4. Overall Measurements for Sarcopenia

A bioelectrical impedance analysis of skeletal muscle masses in the extremities was performed and used to calculate the skeletal muscle mass index (SMI). In Body S10 (In Body Japan, Tokyo, Japan) was used for these measurements, which were conducted in a standing position with electrodes attached to the thumbs and middle fingers of both hands and ankles of both legs. Patients were asked to remain quiet and still during measurements. Standard values for SMI reductions in males and females were previously reported to be ≤ 7.0 and <5.4 kg/m^2, respectively [11].

A digital grip strength tester (Takei Scientific Instruments Co., Ltd., Yashiroda Akiha-Ku Niigata City, Japan) was employed to assess grip strength (GS). The second joint of the index finger was adjusted at a right angle to the grip of the strength tester, and participants held the tester without shaking their arm. Measurements were conducted in duplicate alternating between the left and right hands, and the maximum value was used as GS. Standard values for GS reductions in males and females were previously reported to be <26 and <18 kgf, respectively [11].

Walking speed (WS) was assessed over a distance of 9 m, which comprised 2 m at the start and end points as a preparatory route and 5 m for the measurement of WS [12]. Participants were asked to walk as usual without knowledge of the measurement being performed. The start and 2-, 7-, and 9 m (goal) points were marked. The measurement started when one foot touched the 2 m point and ended when one foot touched the 7 m point. The calculation of WS involved dividing 5 m by the measured time. Measurements were conducted in duplicate, with the faster WS being used as the measured value. The standard value for a WS reduction in both males and females was previously reported to be <0.8 m/s [11].

2.5. Oral Measurements for Sarcopenia

CSG, a muscle that plays a role in swallowing function [13], was evaluated as an indicator of muscle mass in oral measurements for sarcopenia. An ultrasonic diagnostic system was employed to examine the geniohyoid muscle [14]. Each participant was seated in a comfortable posture on a reclining chair at an angle of 30° from the floor. A 3.5 MHz convex probe ultrasonic diagnostic system (Miruco®; Nippon Sigmax Co., Ltd., Tokyo, Japan) was attached perpendicularly to the lower surface of the geniohyoid muscle in the center of the mouth floor such that it did not touch thyroid cartilage and its surface was in close contact with the bottom of the jaw. Ultrasonic gel was used at an amount that did not compress soft tissue under the probe. The hyoid bone and mandible with acoustic shadows and the geniohyoid muscle attached to both were shown in the B-mode sagittal cross-sectional plane (frequency: 3.5 MHz) on a single screen, and the resting state was saved as a still image. Ultrasound images stored in the ultrasound diagnostic device were loaded onto a personal computer. The geniohyoid muscle depicted between the mandible and hyoid bone on ultrasound images was plotted using Image J software, followed by evaluations of the surrounding area. Ultrasonography and CSG measurements were conducted by the same examiner (RK).

A JMS tongue-measuring instrument was used to assess TP as an indicator of muscle strength in oral measurements for sarcopenia [15]. Following a calibration, the upper and lower front teeth held the concave part of the TP probe in place, while the examiner held the probe. Measurements were conducted as previously reported. After sufficient training, each participant pressed and crushed the vinyl bulge at the tip of the probe against the palate with maximum tongue force. Measurements were conducted in triplicate with a sufficient rest period between measurements. The average of three measurements was used as TP.

ODK is an indicator of motor function in oral measurements for sarcopenia [16]. The task performed by participants involved pronouncing /ta/ accompanied by the movement of the tongue tip. Each participant repeated the task as rapidly as possible in five seconds and took breaths where needed. Measurements were conducted in triplicate using the calculator method with a sufficient rest period between measurements. The ODK value of /ta/ was calculated as the mean number of pronunciations per second in three measurements.

2.6. Statistical Analysis

MNA-SF, SMI, GS, WS, CSG, TP, and ODK were assessed by Pearson's correlation coefficient because of normal distributions using the Shapiro–Wilk test. According to the MNA-SF classification, participants were classified into the at risk of malnutrition group and normal nutritional status group. The *t*-test was used to investigate the significance of differences in age, BMI, SMI, GS, WS, CSG, TP, and ODK between the normal status group and the at risk of malnutrition group (significance level: <0.05). A multivariable logistic regression analysis was conducted with the risk of malnutrition as the dependent variable and SMI, GS, WS, CSG, TP, and ODK as independent variables (significance level: <0.05). A stepwise forward selection procedure was also used to assess the effects of different variables and identify important explanatory variables. Statistical analyses were conducted using SPSS Statistics 22 (IBM, Armonk, NY, USA).

3. Results

The data of 45 participants (14 males and 31 females, mean age of 79.7 ± 6.1 years) were analyzed in the present study. Table 1 shows basic information on each participant. Mean BMI was 21.9 ± 3.2 kg/cm^2, which was within the normal range. The mean Barthel Index (99.1 ± 2.9) was high, indicating that participants were living independently. Mean values for overall and oral measurements for sarcopenia were within standard values. Muscle mass and strength as well as motor function were assessed in relation to overall and oral measurements for sarcopenia.

Table 1. Characteristics of the study population.

Variable	All (n = 45)
Age (years)	79.7 ± 6.1
Sex (%)	Male (31.1) Female (68.9)
BMI (kg/m^2)	21.9 ± 3.2
BI	99.1 ± 2.9
MNA-sf	11.6 ± 1.8
EAT-10	2.2 ± 3.1
SMI (kg/m^2)	6.1 ± 1.1
GS (kgf)	22.6 ± 6.9
WS (m/s)	1.03 ± 0.28
CSG (mm^2)	235.2 ± 60.5
TP (Kpa)	28.3 ± 7.6
ODK (/s)	5.9 ± 0.8

Data are shown as the mean $\pm$ SD. BMI: body mass index; BI: Barthel index; MNA-sf: Mini Nutritional Assessment-Short Form; EAT-10: eating assessment tool-10; SMI: skeletal muscle mass index; GS: grip strength; WS: walking speed; CSG: cross-sectional area of the geniohyoid muscle; TP: tongue pressure; ODK: oral diadochokinesis of /ta/.

Table 2 shows the relationships among MNA-SF, SMI, GS, WS, CSG, TP, and ODK. TP strength was 0.347 higher with each unit of increase in the value for MNA-SF (r = 0.347, $p = 0.019$). In terms of the relationship between overall and oral measurements for sarcopenia, a correlation was noted between SMI and CSG (r = 0.529, $p = 0.000$), GS and TP (r = 0.422, $p = 0.004$), and WS and ODK (r = 0.531, $p = 0.000$). A moderate correlation was found between overall and oral measurements for sarcopenia.

Table 2. Bivariate simple correlation analysis of MNA-sf and overall and oral measurements for sarcopenia.

n = 45	ODK	TP	CSG	WS	GF	SMI	MNA-sf
MNA-sf	0.278	0.347 *	0.091	0.264	0.126	0.224	1
SMI	0.384 **	0.411 **	0.529 **	0.278	0.793 **	1	
GS	0.337 *	0.422 **	0.335 *	0.293	1		
WS	0.531 **	0.475 **	0.116	1			
CSG	0.344 *	0.498 **	1				
TP	0.420 **	1					
ODK	1						

Coefficients of correlation were calculated with Pearson's product moment correlation coefficient for parametric values. ** $p < 0.01$ * $p < 0.05$. MNA-sf: Mini Nutritional Assessment-Short Form; SMI: skeletal muscle mass index; GS: grip strength; WS: walking speed; CSG: cross-sectional area of the geniohyoid muscle; TP: tongue pressure; ODK: oral diadochokinesis of /ta/.

Table 3 shows comparisons of age, BMI, and the parameters of overall and oral measurements for sarcopenia between the normal nutrition and at risk of malnutrition groups. We observed decreases of 5.7 kPa in TP and 3.9 kg/cm^2 in BMI in the at risk of malnutrition group (BMI: 23.8 ± 2.1 kg/cm^2 vs. 19.9 ± 3.0 kg/cm^2, $p = 0.000$; TP: 30.6 ± 7.6 kPa vs. 25.9 ± 7.0 kPa, $p = 0.035$). Participants in the at risk of malnutrition group were slightly thin and had low tongue strength. There were no correlations among the parameters of overall measurements for sarcopenia (SMI, GS, and WS) between the groups.

Table 3. Comparisons of overall and oral measurements for sarcopenia between the normal and at risk of malnutrition groups.

	Normal	At Risk of Malnutrition	p
n	23	22	
Age	80.0 ± 6.4	79.5 ± 6.0	0.786
Sex %Male	26.0%	36.0%	0.468
BMI	23.8 ± 2.1	19.9 ± 3.0	0.000
SMI	6.3 ± 1.0	5.8 ± 1.0	0.112
GS	23.4 ± 6.8	21.7 ± 7.0	0.414
WS	1.1 ± 0.2	0.9 ± 0.3	0.054
CSG	246.5 ± 66.2	223.3 ± 52.9	0.202
TP	30.6 ± 7.6	25.9 ± 7.0	0.035
ODK	6.0 ± 0.9	586 ± 0.8	0.278

The *t*-test. BMI: body mass index; SMI: skeletal muscle mass index; GS: grip strength; WS: walking speed; CSG: cross-sectional area of the geniohyoid muscle; TP: tongue pressure; ODK: oral diadochokinesis of /ta/.

Parameters contributing to the risk of malnutrition were examined using a multiple regression analysis, which was conducted with the risk of malnutrition as the dependent variable and overall (SMI, GS, and WS) and oral (CSG, TP, and ODK) measurements for sarcopenia as independent variables. The results obtained identified TP as an independent variable ($\beta = 0.913$, $p = 0.042$) (Table 4). Among the parameters of overall and oral measurements for sarcopenia examined, only TP was associated with the risk of malnutrition.

Table 4. Multiple regression analysis of the risk of malnutrition.

Independent Variable	β	Wald	p
Tongue pressure	0.913	4.117	0.042

4. Discussion

Basic information and the endpoints of overall and oral measurements for sarcopenia were investigated in the present study to elucidate their relationships with the nutrition status in older community-dwelling individuals. The results obtained revealed a correlation between MNA-SF as a diagnostic index of the nutrition status and TP as an oral measurement for sarcopenia. TP was 5.7 kPa lower in the at risk of malnutrition group than in the normal nutrition group. There were no correlations among the parameters of overall measurements for sarcopenia between the normal nutrition and at risk of malnutrition groups.

Malnutrition is a risk factor for sarcopenia because a decrease in muscle mass reduces the basal metabolic rate in a negative chain reaction that results in lower energy consumption and lower nutrient intake [2]. Demographic and socioeconomic factors, psycho-behavioral factors, and the nutritional status accelerate this negative chain, which a previous study termed the cycle of frailty [17]. Sarcopenia is considered 'primary' (or age-related) when no other specific cause is evident, and 'secondary' when causal factors other than aging are present. Sarcopenia may occur secondary to a systemic disease, particularly one that induces inflammatory processes (e.g., malignancy, inflammatory bowel diseases, malabsorption and malnutrition, physical inactivity, or organ failure). The emerging concept of the "gut–muscle axis" needs to be adequately described in the pathogenesis of sarcopenic dysphagia, taking into account the key role of inflammation and the gut microbiota in the development of muscle wasting [3]. In the present study, we focused on the status of the risk of malnutrition.

Parameters between overall and oral measurements for sarcopenia moderately correlated. SMI, an indicator of muscle mass in overall measurements for sarcopenia, correlated with CSG, an indicator of muscle mass in oral measurements for sarcopenia, TP, an indicator of muscle strength in oral measurements for sarcopenia, correlated with ODK, an indicator of muscle dexterity measurements implying neurological integrity in oral measurements for sarcopenia. This result showed the relevance between overall and oral measurements for sarcopenia, which is consistent with our previous findings [7].

A relationship has been reported between oral function and the nutrition status. An analysis of more than 5000 Japanese older adults revealed that TP decreased with advancing age in both males and females [18]. Mean (years) TP measurements in male participants were 34.0 (65–69), 32.2 (70–74), 30.8 (75–79), 28.4 (80–84), and 24.4 ($\geq$85) kPa, while the corresponding values in female participants were 31.5 (65–69), 30.5 (70–74), 29.6 (75–79), 28.4 (80–84), and 26.4 ($\geq$85) kPa. In the present study, the mean age was 79 years and mean TP was 28.3 kPa in both sexes, which were consistent with previously reported values [17].

In terms of TP in patients with dysphagia, mean TP with a dysphagia diet in patients with acute stroke was 21.7 kPa [19]. However, Maeda et al. [20] reported that the cut-off value of TP for decreased swallowing function was lower than 20 kPa because mean TP was 25.3 kPa in patients without dysphagia and 14.7 kPa in those with dysphagia. These findings suggest that the nutrition status is worse in patients with dysphagia; therefore, these patients may have a malnutrition status. In the present study, participants in the at risk of malnutrition group had an EAT-10 score of 1.9, which was below the cut-off value and, thus, they were a population without dysphagia. TP in the risk of malnutrition group in the present study—which was 25.9 kPa and, thus, was slightly higher than that in groups with dysphagia in previous studies—was appropriate for a population at risk of malnutrition.

A relationship was previously reported between the risk of malnutrition and TP in community-dwelling older individuals in Taiwan [21]. TP positively correlated with

MNA scores and did not significantly differ between the normal nutrition and at risk of malnutrition groups. However, when participants were divided into four subgroups based on the quartiles of TP and age and sex were adjusted for, the subgroup in the third quartile had a significantly higher risk (OR = 4.85) of malnutrition. The present study also demonstrated that TP correlated with MNA-SF (r = 0.347), which was smaller in the at risk of malnutrition group (TP: 30.6 ± 7.6 kPa vs. 25.9 ± 7.0 kPa), and this was consistent with previous findings. Expect for TP, the correlations between other parameters (CSG, ODK, SMI, GF, and WS) and the MNA-SF score were weak. The nutrition status of participants in the present study was either normal or at risk of malnutrition, and participants with malnutrition were excluded because the focus of the present study was the risk of malnutrition as a preliminary stage of malnutrition. This may be the reason for the weak correlation with the MNA-SF score and is a limitation of the present study.

Previous studies reported a relationship between oral function and CSG. Shimizu et al. [22] measured the mass of the geniohyoid muscle in perioperative patients using ultrasonography. The findings obtained revealed significant reductions in the area of the geniohyoid muscle after surgery (preoperative = 203 mm^2, postoperative day 7 = 176 mm^2, and postoperative day 14 = 174 mm^2). Moreover, the postoperative percent decrease in the area of the geniohyoid muscle was greater on average in the poor oral intake group than in the good oral intake group, and a significant difference was observed on postoperative day 14. Patient characteristics, namely, a mean age of 70.6 years and BMI of 21.2 kg/cm^2, were similar to those of the participants in the present study. However, the MNA-sf score in the previous study was 7 points, which is borderline between malnutrition, and lower than that (11.6 points) in the present study. Patients had esophageal, gastric, small bowel, or colon cancer. The populations in the previous and present studies appeared to be similar before surgery and, thus, the area of the geniohyoid muscle was also similar (203 mm^2 preoperatively in the Shimizu study [21] vs. 223.3 mm^2 in the at risk of malnutrition group in the present study). Another study [23] reported the areas of the geniohyoid muscle as 136.3 mm^2 in patients with sarcopenic dysphagia and 154.4 mm^2 in those without. The cut-off value to detect sarcopenic dysphagia was previously reported to be 116.6 mm^2. The population of the previous study was older and slightly thinner, with a mean age of 82.1 years and BMI of 20.0 kg/cm^2, than the participants in the present study, and included patients with dysphagia. Therefore, participants in the present study were healthier older adults than those in previous studies. The area of the geniohyoid muscle was 223.3 mm^2 in the at risk of malnutrition group in the present study, which was an appropriate value for a population at risk of malnutrition.

In the present study, TP, the indicator of muscle strength in oral measurements for sarcopenia, was significantly smaller in the at risk of malnutrition group, whereas the parameters of overall measurements for sarcopenia (SMI, GS, and WS) did not significantly differ between the groups. Participants in the at risk of malnutrition group were slightly thinner and had low tongue strength. There were no correlations among the parameters of overall measurements for sarcopenia between the groups. A multiple regression analysis of the parameters contributing to the risk of malnutrition was conducted and identified TP as a significant factor (β = 0.913, p = 0.042), but not other parameters, including SMI, GS, WS, CSG, and ODK. These results suggest a relationship between the risk of malnutrition and TP in older adults as oral measurements for sarcopenia, but not overall measurements for sarcopenia. Weak tongue strength may be associated with the hypoactivity of masticatory muscles and affect the food intake balance, thereby increasing the risk of malnutrition, the preliminary stage of malnutrition.

There are a number of limitations in this study that need to be addressed. Since this was a cross-sectional analysis, a prospective cohort study on the causal relationship between TP and malnutrition that ideally includes a malnutrition group is needed. In the present study, the majority of participants lived independently; therefore, they were in the state of normal nutrition or at risk of malnutrition, while few had malnutrition. Furthermore, we did not perform a sex-specific analysis because the sample size was small. The feature of the nutrition status and the standard values for muscle mass and strength differed between males and females. As previously mentioned, the sample size of the present study was small. Regarding the correlation, twenty-six participants were required based on calculation software and a requisite number of participants was obtained for this study. However, in regard to the t-test between two groups, the sample size of the present study was small, because 128 patients were required according to the software. This suggests the possibility that in larger studies other parameters may display significant differences, especially walking speed ($p = 0.054$). In the future, a large number of participants, including the same number of males and females, and multilevel states of nutrition (normal, at risk of malnutrition, and malnutrition) need to be examined in a prospective cohort study.

5. Conclusions

The present study demonstrated that the risk of malnutrition was associated with TP in older adults as oral measurements for sarcopenia, but not overall measurements for sarcopenia. Therefore, low TP may be related with the risk of malnutrition, the preliminary stage of malnutrition.

Author Contributions: K.O. contributed to data collection, analysis, and interpretation, and assisted in the preparation of the manuscript. All other authors contributed to the analysis and interpretation of data, and critically reviewed the manuscript. All authors approved the final version of the manuscript and agree to be accountable for all aspects of the work in ensuring that questions related to the accuracy or integrity of any part of the work are appropriately investigated and resolved. All authors have read and agreed to the published version of the manuscript.

Funding: This study was funded by the Japan Society of Gerodontology (Grant Number: 2019-001).

Institutional Review Board Statement: This study was conducted according to the Declaration of Helsinki. All procedures involving human individuals have been approved by the Ethics Committee of Osaka Dental University (Approval No.110970).

Informed Consent Statement: Informed consent was obtained from all participants involved in the study.

Data Availability Statement: The data presented in this study are available on request from the corresponding author. The data are not publicly available due to ethical restrictions.

Acknowledgments: We appreciate the participants of this study and medical staff members at the Department of Geriatric Dentistry, Osaka Dental University Dental Hospital, for their cooperation.

Conflicts of Interest: The authors declare that they have no competing interests.

References

1. Yamada, M.; Arai, H. Predictive Value of Frailty Scores for Healthy Life Expectancy in Community-Dwelling Older Japanese Adults. *J. Am. Med. Dir. Assoc.* **2015**, *16*, 1002-e7. [CrossRef]
2. Xue, Q.L.; Bandeen-Roche, K.; Varadhan, R.; Zhou, J.; Fried, L.P. Initial manifestations of frailty criteria and the development of frailty phenotype in the Women's Health and Aging Study II. *J. Gerontol. A Biol. Sci. Med. Sci.* **2008**, *63*, 984–990. [CrossRef]
3. Chen, K.C.; Jeng, Y.; Wu, W.T.; Wang, T.G.; Han, D.S.; Özçakar, L.; Chang, K.V. Sarcopenic Dysphagia: A Narrative Review from Diagnosis to Intervention. *Nutrients* **2021**, *13*, 4043. [CrossRef]
4. Hironaka, S.; Kugimiya, Y.; Watanabe, Y.; Motokawa, K.; Hirano, H.; Kawai, H.; Kera, T.; Kojima, M.; Fujiwara, Y.; Ihara, K.; et al. Association between oral, social, and physical frailty in community-dwelling older adults. *Arch. Gerontol. Geriatr.* **2020**, *89*, 104105. [CrossRef]
5. Ikebe, K.; Gondo, Y.; Kamide, K.; Masui, Y.; Ishizaki, T.; Arai, Y.; Inagaki, H.; Nakagawa, T.; Kabayama, M.; Ryuno, H.; et al. Occlusal force is correlated with cognitive function directly as well as indirectly via food intake in community-dwelling older Japanese: From the SONIC study. *PLoS ONE* **2018**, *13*, e0190741. [CrossRef]
6. Ohta, M.; Imamura, Y.; Chebib, N.; Schulte-Eickhoff, R.M.; Allain, S.; Genton, L.; Mojon, P.; Graf, C.; Ueda, T.; Müller, F. Oral function and nutritional status in non-acute hospitalised elders. *Gerodontology* **2022**, *39*, 74–82. [CrossRef] [PubMed]
7. Kobuchi, R.; Okuno, K.; Kusunoki, T.; Inoue, T.; Takahashi, K. The relationship between sarcopenia and oral sarcopenia in elderly people. *J. Oral. Rehabil.* **2020**, *47*, 636–642. [CrossRef]
8. Mahoney, F.I.; Barthel, D.W. Functional evaluation. The Barthel index. *Md. State Med. J.* **1965**, *14*, 61–65. [PubMed]

9. Belafsky, P.C.; Mouadeb, D.A.; Rees, C.J.; Pryor, J.C.; Postma, G.N.; Allen, J.; Leonard, R.J. Validity and reliability of the Eating Assessment Tool (EAT-10). *Ann. Otol. Rhinol. Laryngol.* **2008**, *117*, 919–924. [CrossRef] [PubMed]
10. Van Nes, M.C.; Herrmann, F.R.; Gold, G.; Michel, J.P.; Rizzoli, R. Does the mini nutritional assessment predict hospitalization outcomes in older people? *Age Ageing* **2001**, *30*, 221–226. [CrossRef]
11. Chen, L.K.; Liu, L.K.; Woo, J.; Assantachai, P.; Auyeung, T.W.; Bahyah, K.S.; Chou, M.Y.; Chen, L.Y.; Hsu, P.S.; Krairit, O.; et al. Sarcopenia in Asia: Consensus report of the Asian Working Group for Sarcopenia. *J. Am. Med. Dir. Assoc.* **2014**, *15*, 95–101. [CrossRef] [PubMed]
12. Cesari, M.; Kritchevsky, S.B.; Penninx, B.W.; Nicklas, B.J.; Simonsick, E.M.; Newman, A.B.; Tylavsky, F.A.; Brach, J.S.; Satterfield, S.; Bauer, D.C.; et al. Prognostic value of usual gait speed in well-functioning older people—Results from the Health, Aging and Body Composition Study. *J. Am. Geriatr. Soc.* **2005**, *53*, 1675–1680. [CrossRef] [PubMed]
13. Fukumoto, Y.; Ikezoe, T.; Yamada, Y.; Tsukagoshi, R.; Nakamura, M.; Mori, N.; Kimura, M.; Ichihashi, N. Skeletal muscle quality assessed from echo intensity is associated with muscle strength of middle-aged and elderly persons. *Eur. J. Appl. Physiol.* **2012**, *112*, 1519–1525. [CrossRef] [PubMed]
14. Shimizu, S.; Hanayama, K.; Metani, H.; Sugiyama, T.; Abe, H.; Seki, S.; Hiraoka, T.; Tsubahara, A. Retest reliability of ultrasonic geniohyoid muscle measurement. *Jpn. J. Compr. Rehabil. Sci.* **2016**, *7*, 55–60. [CrossRef]
15. Tsuga, K.; Yoshikawa, M.; Oue, H.; Okazaki, Y.; Tsuchioka, H.; Maruyama, M.; Yoshida, M.; Akagawa, Y. Maximal voluntary tongue pressure is decreased in Japanese frail elderly persons. *Gerodontology* **2012**, *29*, e1078–e1085. [CrossRef]
16. Takeuchi, N.; Sawada, N.; Ekuni, D.; Morita, M. Oral diadochokinesis is related to decline in swallowing function among community-dwelling Japanese elderly: A cross-sectional study. *Aging. Clin. Exp. Res.* **2021**, *33*, 399–405. [CrossRef]
17. Fried, L.P.; Tangen, C.M.; Walston, J.; Newman, A.B.; Hirsch, C.; Gottdiener, J.; Seeman, T.; Tracy, R.; Kop, W.J.; Burke, G.; et al. Frailty in older adults: Evidence for a phenotype. *J. Gerontol. A Biol. Sci. Med. Sci.* **2001**, *56*, M146–M156. [CrossRef]
18. Iwasaki, M.; Ohara, Y.; Motokawa, K.; Hayakawa, M.; Shirobe, M.; Edahiro, A.; Watanabe, Y.; Awata, S.; Okamura, T.; Inagaki, H.; et al. Population-based reference values for tongue pressure in Japanese older adults: A pooled analysis of over 5000 participants. *J. Prosthodont. Res.* **2022**, *Epub ahead of print*. [CrossRef]
19. Nakamori, M.; Ishikawa, K.; Imamura, E.; Yamamoto, H.; Kimura, K.; Ayukawa, T.; Mizoue, T.; Wakabayashi, S. Relationship between tongue pressure and dysphagia diet in patients with acute stroke. *PLoS ONE* **2021**, *16*, e0252837. [CrossRef]
20. Maeda, K.; Akagi, J. Decreased tongue pressure is associated with sarcopenia and sarcopenic dysphagia in the elderly. *Dysphagia* **2015**, *30*, 80–87. [CrossRef]
21. Chang, K.V.; Wu, W.T.; Chen, L.R.; Wang, H.I.; Wang, T.G.; Han, D.S. Suboptimal Tongue Pressure Is Associated with Risk of Malnutrition in Community-Dwelling Older Individuals. *Nutrients* **2021**, *13*, 1821. [CrossRef] [PubMed]
22. Shimizu, S.; Hanayama, K.; Nakato, R.; Sugiyama, T.; Tsubahara, A. Ultrasonographic evaluation of geniohyoid muscle mass in perioperative patients. *Kawasaki Med. J.* **2016**, *42*, 47–56.
23. Ogawa, N.; Mori, T.; Fujishima, I.; Wakabayashi, H.; Itoda, M.; Kunieda, K.; Shigematsu, T.; Nishioka, S.; Tohara, H.; Yamada, M.; et al. Ultrasonography to Measure Swallowing Muscle Mass and Quality in Older Patients with Sarcopenic Dysphagia. *J. Am. Med. Dir. Assoc.* **2018**, *19*, 516–522. [CrossRef] [PubMed]

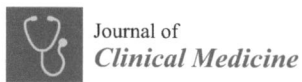 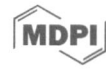

Article

Masticatory Performance Test Using a Gummy Jelly for Older People with Low Masticatory Ability

Kazuhiro Murakami [1], Tasuku Yoshimoto [1], Kazuhiro Hori [1,*], Rikako Sato [1], Ma. Therese Sta. Maria [1,2], Pinta Marito [1,3], Hinako Takano [1], Aye Mya Mya Khaing [1], Takashi Nokubi [4] and Takahiro Ono [1,5]

1. Division of Comprehensive Prosthodontics, Faculty of Dentistry and Graduate School of Medical and Dental Sciences, Niigata University, Niigata 951-8514, Japan
2. Department of Prosthodontics, College of Dentistry, Manila Central University, Caloocan 1400, Philippines
3. Department of Prosthodontics, Faculty of Dentistry, Universitas Indonesia, Jakarta 10430, Indonesia
4. Osaka University, Suita 565-0871, Japan
5. Department of Geriatric Dentistry, Osaka Dental University, Osaka 540-0008, Japan
* Correspondence: hori@dent.niigata-u.ac.jp; Tel.: +81-25-227-2891; Fax: +81-25-229-3454

Abstract: Evaluation of masticatory ability has become more important in an aging society because decreased masticatory ability has the potential to affect the general health of older people. A new masticatory performance test, intended for older people with low masticatory ability, has been developed using gummy jelly half the size of that used in the conventional masticatory performance test. This study aimed to investigate the compatibility between the new and conventional tests and the adaptation of the new test. The new test using the 8-grade visual score with half-size gummy jelly was performed among 137 removable denture wearers (mean age 75.8 ± 9.0 years) with low masticatory performance (a score of ≤4 on a conventional test). The correlation between the scores of half-size gummy jelly (VS-H) in the new test and those of full-size gummy jelly (VS) in the conventional test was evaluated. VS-H among the groups divided by VS were also compared. A strong positive correlation was detected between VS-H and VS (r_s = 0.70). In groups with VS of 0 and 1, VS-H values were widely distributed from 0 to 7. There were significant differences in VS-H between the groups with VS of 0–2 but no significant differences in VS-H between the groups with VS of 2–4. Therefore, the masticatory performance test using half-size gummy jelly is suitable for a detailed evaluation of masticatory ability in older people with low masticatory ability when their visual score of full-size gummy jelly in the conventional test is 2 or less.

Keywords: gummy jelly; masticatory performance; oral function; mastication

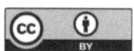

1. Introduction

Mastication is a very complex process in which various oral organs such as teeth, tongue, cheeks, temporomandibular joint, and masticatory muscles work together [1,2], and it is an indispensable part of nutrient intake. Aging-associated environmental changes in the oral cavity such as tooth loss [3], loss of tongue muscle strength [4], and reduced masticatory muscle mass [5] decrease masticatory ability. Decreased masticatory ability leads to the deterioration of eating habits [6] and has the potential to be one of the causes of metabolic syndrome [7], malnutrition [8], and the occurrence of aspiration pneumonia [9]. Thus, it is increasingly becoming important to quantify, objectively evaluate, and detect deterioration of masticatory ability in the super-aged society.

The comminution test is a popular method for evaluating masticatory ability, and is a method for evaluating masticatory performance based on the degree to which food crushes after biting [10]. The comminution tests have been developed in the past using various test foods such as nuts and carrots [11]. However, the type and shape of test food are very important factors when developing a comminution test that corresponds to the characteristics of older people, such as the large individual differences in oral conditions and the high percentage of people wearing dentures.

So far, we have focused on the following properties of gummy jelly: (1) gummy samples are homogeneous, (2) there is no pain even if a bit fragment becomes stuck between the denture and the mucous membrane, (3) its adhesiveness is low and it does not adhere to the denture or teeth, and (4) its mechanical properties as foodstuffs can be freely adjusted. We previously developed a method for evaluating masticatory performance by measuring the increased surface area of the chewed pieces of a gummy sample after a participant had chewed it 30 times and spat it out (Figure 1) [12]. This evaluation method has been used in various situations, such as the evaluation of prosthetic treatment outcomes [13] and epidemiological studies of oral function in older people [14]. However, especially in older patients wearing complete dentures, there are many cases in which gummy samples cannot be sheared off due to a significant decrease in occlusal force [15] and masticatory muscle mass [5]. It is difficult to correctly evaluate the differences in masticatory ability among these older people, minute changes in the masticatory ability within individuals, and the effects of prosthetic treatment and oral function training. Therefore, we developed a masticatory performance test for older people with low masticatory ability [16].

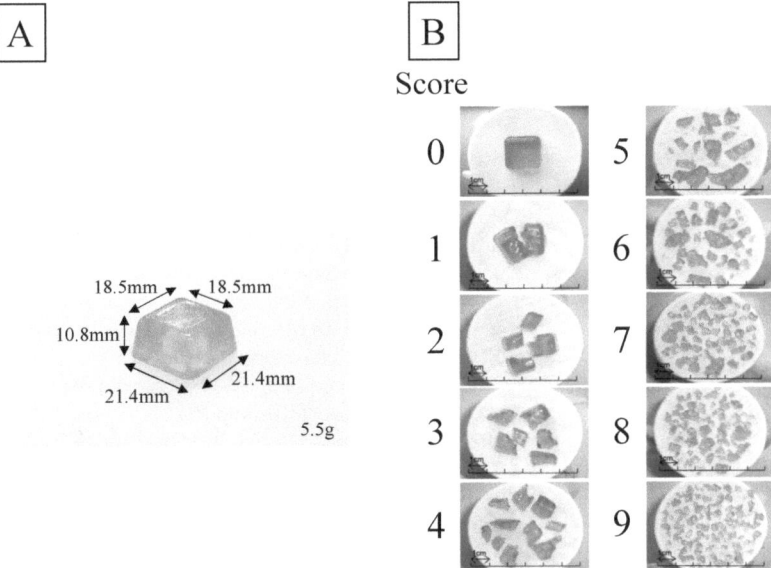

Figure 1. Evaluation of masticatory performance with full-size test gummy jelly. (**A**) A sample of the full-size test gummy jelly. (**B**) The visual scoring table of full-size test gummy jelly. Only patients with the visual score of 4 or less were included in this study.

This new method is based on the property that for the same food sample, smaller sizes are easier to bite. The test sample in the new method is a "half-size gummy jelly," which contains the same material as a full-size gummy jelly that has been used in the conventional test but has only half the volume. For this method, similar to the conventional method [12], the crushing of the gummy jelly after chewing 30 times is visually evaluated as a chewing performance score from 0 to 7 using a score table. In the previous report, the validity of a score chart for the half-size gummy jelly method has been verified [16]. However, the relationship between the masticatory performance scores evaluated via this method and the conventional method is unclear. Further, the suitable cutoff score of the conventional method has not been investigated in relation to the use of the newly developed method.

Therefore, in this study, we aimed to evaluate the relationship between the masticatory performance scores obtained using the half-size gummy jelly and the full-size gummy jelly, targeting older people with low masticatory ability. In addition, we aimed to examine the adaptations to the new masticatory performance test. Here, we hypothesized that a positive correlation exists between masticatory performance scores obtained using half-size gummy jelly and full-size gummy jelly.

2. Materials and Methods

2.1. Participants

The study participants were denture wearers aged 65 years or older with a conventional masticatory performance test score of 4 or less (Figure 1) and who visited the Department of Removable Prosthodontics and General Dentistry at the Niigata University Medicine and Dental Hospital from 2015 to 2021 for dental maintenance. The exclusion criteria were oral/facial pain at the examination, severe periodontitis, severe symptom of temporomandibular disorders, jaw defect or dysphagia, neuromuscular disease, and an inability to follow the instructions of the operator due to conditions such as dementia. All study participants received an explanation of the purpose of this study in advance and only participated after providing informed consent.

Assuming that the correlation between the results of two types of masticatory performance tests was to be analyzed, the optimum sample size was determined to be 134 using G*Power (Universität Düsseldorf, Düsseldorf, Germany) with a statistical power of 0.95 and an effect size of 0.3. This study was conducted in accordance with the guidelines of the Declaration of Helsinki. The study protocol was approved by the Ethics Committee of the Faculty of Dentistry, Niigata University (approval no. 2015-3038).

2.2. Data Collection

The participants were seated in a reclining chair such that their Frankfurt plane was parallel to the ground, and the conventional gummy test was administered once [12]. The participants were asked to freely chew 5.5 g of full-size test gummy jelly (UHA Mikakuto, Osaka, Japan) 30 times without swallowing, and then spit it out on a piece of gauze spread out in a paper cup. Next, the piece of gauze and the saliva adhering to the chewed sample were removed with running water. Then, the degree of crushing of the sample was evaluated by the pre-trained examiner using a 10-level score table (Figure 1); this score was defined as the visual score (VS) of masticatory performance. VS of 4 was considered to correspond to the average of the bottom 25% group of older people in terms of masticatory performance [17].

After measuring VS, for participants with VS of 4 or less, a half-size gummy test [15] was administered once. Participants were asked to chew 2.75 g of gummy jelly (a half-size gummy jelly, UHA Mikakuto, Osaka, Japan) 30 times in the same steps as in the conventional method. Then, the degree of crushing of the sample was evaluated using an eight-level score table (Figure 2); this score was defined as the visual score by half-size gummy jelly (VS-H). A resting period of 1 min was provided between measurements, and the participants were asked to gargle several times.

The following basic information was also investigated: the participant's age, sex, number of remaining teeth, and the Eichner index [18], a classification system for occlusal support.

2.3. Statistical Analysis

Spearman's rank correlation coefficient was used to examine the relationship between VS-H and VS. In addition, participants were classified into five groups (0, 1, 2, 3, 4) according to the VS value, and the Kruskal–Wallis test was used to compare VS-H values among groups. The Mann–Whitney U test with Bonferroni correction was performed for multiple comparisons. The statistical analyses were performed using SPSS Statistics version 25 (IBM Japan, Tokyo, Japan) at a significance level of 5%.

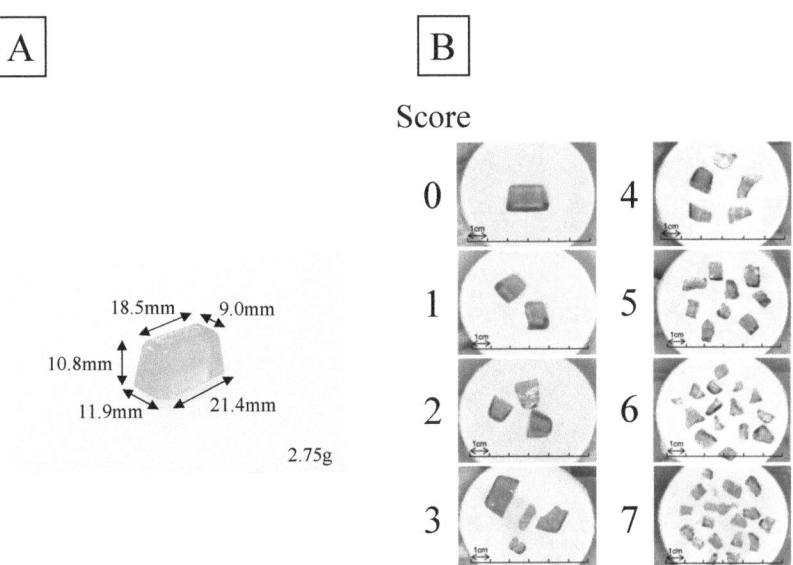

Figure 2. Evaluation of masticatory performance with half-size test gummy jelly. (**A**) A sample of the half-size test gummy jelly. (**B**) The visual scoring table of half-size test gummy jelly. The gummy jelly used in this new test is half the size of that used in the conventional test (Figure 1A), and the score table is different from that of the conventional test (Figure 1B).

3. Results

3.1. Participant Characteristics

A total of 137 participants (52 males, 85 females; average age 75.8 ± 9.0 years) were included in this study. The average number of remaining teeth among the participants was 8.3 ± 7.8. Regarding the Eichner index [18], there were 2 participants in group A (all occlusal contacts in the posterior region were preserved), 48 participants in group B (missing one or more occlusal contacts in the posterior region), and 87 participants in group C (loss of maxillary occlusal contact). Seventy-five participants (54.7%) wore complete dentures. Table 1 details the baseline characteristics of the participants.

3.2. Relationship between the Two Types of Gummy Jelly Regarding Masticatory Performance

A strong positive correlation was observed between VS-H and VS (r_s = 0.70) (Figure 3). However, among participants with VS of 0 and 1, VS-H values were widely distributed from 0 to 5 and 1 to 7, respectively.

3.3. Comparison of Masticatory Performances between the Half-Size Gummy Test and The Conventional Gummy Test

Figure 4 shows the results obtained in the comparison of VS-H between groups classified by VS value. The group with a VS of 0 showed a lower VS-H value than the other groups (VS of 1 to 4) and a significant difference was observed. The group with a VS of 1 showed a lower VS-H value than the groups with VS values of 2, 3, and 4, and significant differences were observed. However, no significant differences were observed among groups with VS values of 2, 3, and 4.

Table 1. Baseline characteristics of the participants.

Characteristics		Total (n = 137)
Age		
	65–74	55
	75–84	61
	≥85	21
Sex		
	Male	52
	Female	85
Number of remaining teeth		
	0	38
	1–9	44
	10–19	39
	≥20	16
Eichner index		
	Group A	2
	Group B	48
	Group C	87
Denture use		
	PD alone	62
	CD alone	43
	CD and PD	32

PD, partial denture; CD, complete denture.

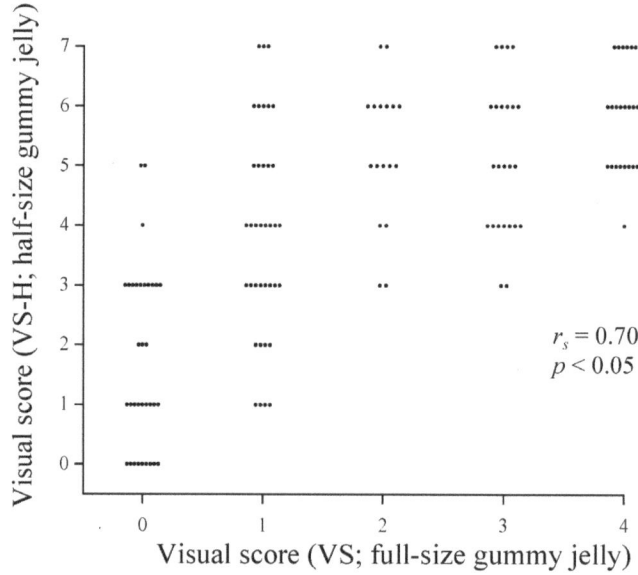

Figure 3. Relationship between masticatory performances determined using the two types of gummy jelly. The cluster of dots indicates the number of participants. The visual score showed a positive correlation between the test with half-size gummy jelly and that with full-size gummy jelly. Spearman's ranked correlation coefficient ($p < 0.05$).

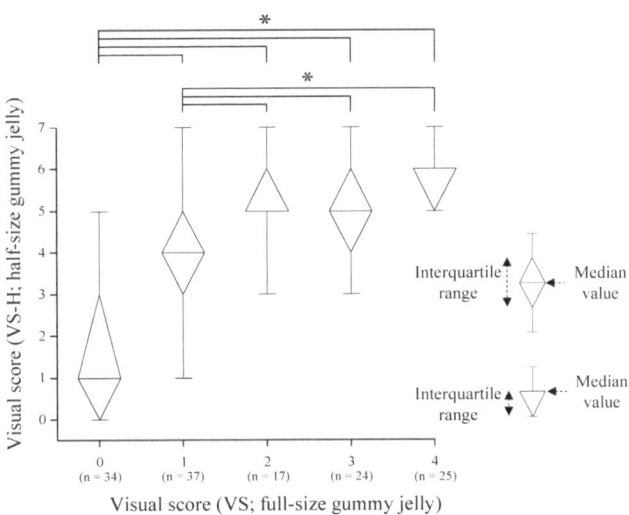

Figure 4. Differences in visual score (VS-H; half-size gummy jelly) among the different visual score groups (VS; full-size gummy jelly). VS-H significantly increased as VS increased from 0 to 2. There were no significant differences in VS-H and VS values of 2 to 4. Kruskal–Wallis test and post hoc test with Bonferroni's correction (*: $p < 0.05$).

4. Discussion

The purpose of this study was to evaluate the relationship between the masticatory performance scores obtained using half-size gummy jelly and those obtained using full-size gummy jelly. Further, we clarified the applicable range of participants for the new method of evaluating masticatory performance. Although many methods have been developed to evaluate masticatory ability [10], to the best of our knowledge, this is the first study to evaluate a method of masticatory ability assessment that focuses on participants with low masticatory ability.

The present study revealed a strong positive correlation between VS-H and VS. This was because the test samples for both tests comprised gummy foods with the same ingredients and composition. In addition, the evaluation methods of both tests were based on the same measurement principle of the degree to which the test sample was crushed. The previous study which evaluated the compatibility of two tests of masticatory ability using gummy jellies of different sizes and hardness reported that the test results showed a positive correlation, which supports the findings of the present study [19].

VS-H was widely distributed from 0 to 7 even in participants with a VS of 0 or 1, that is, participants whose test specimens could not be cut at all or could only be divided into two. Previous studies have shown that tooth loss reduces occlusal force [15] and masseter muscle mass [5] in older people. Salazar et al. also reported that the median masticatory performance among patients with new complete dentures corresponded to a VS of 1 [13]. Kosaka et al. reported that the average masticatory performance of patients in the Eichner index group C corresponded to a VS of 2 [14]. Since approximately half of the participants in this study wore complete dentures, many participants could not break the conventional gummy jelly at all. However, the cross-sectional area of the half-size gummy jelly was approximately half that of the gummy jelly used in the conventional method. Therefore, the force required to break the gummy jelly could be smaller than that of the gummy jelly used in the conventional method, making it easier to crush. This might have led to a widely distributed VS-H even in participants with a VS of 0 or 1. Therefore, VS-H has the potential for evaluating the masticatory performance of participants with a VS of 0 or 1 in detail.

On the other hand, the half-size gummy jelly was easier to crush than the full-size gummy jelly used in the conventional method; thus, it was confirmed that the score reached a plateau as the VS increased. In the present study, we divided the participants according to the VS value and compared the VS-H. Among participants with a VS of 0 to 2, VS-H increased in a stepwise manner; however, there were no significant differences in VS-H between the VS 2 group and the VS 3 and 4 groups. In other words, for participants with a VS of 3 or higher, it is possible that the VS-H will not differ due to the ceiling effect. These discussions on the ease of crushing gummy may be clarified by measuring mastication with electromyography in the future study.

Our study had several limitations. First, this study only included older adults with VS values between 0 and 4, the lower half of the VS of the conventional gummy test. To explore the range of participants suitable for the test with half-size gummy jelly, it may have been necessary not to limit the VS values among participants in this manner. However, the ceiling effect in VS-H was observed when the VS was between 2 and 4, suggesting that there was no problem with this selection criterion. In addition, in this study, we did not confirm the reproducibility and inter-rater reliability of the masticatory performance test using half-size gummy jelly. However, high reproducibility and inter-rater reliability have been confirmed for conventional masticatory performance test with full-size gummy jelly [12]. Thus, it is highly likely that the new method, which employs the same evaluation method except for the size of the test sample, would have yielded similar results.

Despite these limitations, the masticatory performance test using half-size gummy jelly has the potential to become an evaluation tool that can further stratify masticatory ability among participants with a VS of 2 or less. Previous studies have reported that decreased bolus-forming ability affects the occurrence of food aspiration and aspiration pneumonia [9,20]. Therefore, it is possible that the new method can be used as an indicator in the evaluation of aspiration risk and the selection of nursing care foods for people with dysphagia. In recent years, evidence has been accumulated not only for evaluating the deterioration of oral function but also for treatment and training aimed at maintaining and improving oral function [21–23]. In these treatments, the conventional masticatory performance test as well as the new method can be used to evaluate minute changes in the masticatory ability of older people with decreased masticatory function. In the future, we will evaluate changes in VS and VS-H in the treatments, including denture treatment and oral function training among older people with low masticatory ability.

5. Conclusions

There was a positive correlation between the masticatory performance scores obtained using the two gummy jellies. However, among participants with a masticatory performance score exceeding 2 with the conventional gummy jelly, a ceiling effect was observed in the masticatory performance score obtained using the half-size gummy jelly. The masticatory performance test using half-size gummy jelly is suitable for a detailed evaluation of the masticatory ability of participants with low masticatory ability who have a score of 2 or less in the conventional masticatory performance test.

Author Contributions: Conceptualization, K.H. and T.O.; methodology, K.M., K.H. and T.O.; formal analysis, K.M., T.Y. and K.H.; investigation, K.M., T.Y., R.S., M.T.S.M., P.M., H.T. and A.M.M.K.; writing—original draft, K.M.; writing—review & editing, K.H., T.N. and T.O. All authors have read and agreed to the published version of the manuscript.

Funding: This study was supported by JSPS KAKENHI, grant number 20H03877C.

Institutional Review Board Statement: This study was conducted in accordance with the guidelines of the Declaration of Helsinki. The study protocol was approved by the Niigata University School of Dentistry Ethics Committee (approval no. 2015-3038).

Informed Consent Statement: Informed consent was obtained from all participants involved in the study.

Data Availability Statement: The data that support the findings of this study are available from the corresponding author upon reasonable request.

Conflicts of Interest: The authors declare no conflict of interest.

References

1. Hiiemae, K.; Heath, M.R.; Heath, G.; Kazazoglu, E.; Murray, J.; Sapper, D.; Hamblett, K. Natural bites, food consistency and feeding behaviour in man. *Arch. Oral Biol.* **1996**, *41*, 175–189. [CrossRef] [PubMed]
2. Peck, C.C. Biomechanics of occlusion—Implications for oral rehabilitation. *J. Oral Rehabil.* **2016**, *43*, 205–214. [CrossRef] [PubMed]
3. Ikebe, K.; Matsuda, K.; Kagawa, R.; Enoki, K.; Yoshida, M.; Maeda, Y.; Nokubi, T. Association of masticatory performance with age, gender, number of teeth, occlusal force and salivary flow in Japanese older adults: Is ageing a risk factor for masticatory dysfunction? *Arch. Oral Biol.* **2011**, *56*, 991–996. [CrossRef] [PubMed]
4. Morita, K.; Tsuka, H.; Kato, K.; Mori, T.; Nishimura, R.; Yoshida, M.; Tsuga, K. Factors related to masticatory performance in healthy elderly individuals. *J. Prosthodont. Res.* **2018**, *62*, 432–435. [CrossRef] [PubMed]
5. Newton, J.P.; Yemm, R.; Abel, R.W.; Menhinick, S. Changes in human jaw muscles with age and dental state. *Gerodontology* **1993**, *10*, 16–22. [CrossRef]
6. Inomata, C.; Ikebe, K.; Kagawa, R.; Okubo, H.; Sasaki, S.; Okada, T.; Takeshita, H.; Tada, S.; Matsuda, K.; Kurushima, Y.; et al. Significance of occlusal force for dietary fibre and vitamin intakes in independently living 70-year-old Japanese: From SONIC Study. *J. Dent.* **2014**, *42*, 556–564. [CrossRef]
7. Fushida, S.; Kosaka, T.; Nakai, M.; Kida, M.; Nokubi, T.; Kokubo, Y.; Watanabe, M.; Miyamoto, Y.; Ono, T.; Ikebe, K. Lower Masticatory Performance Is a Risk for the Development of the Metabolic Syndrome: The Suita Study. *Front. Cardiovasc. Med.* **2021**, *8*, 752667. [CrossRef]
8. Okada, K.; Enoki, H.; Izawa, S.; Iguchi, A.; Kuzuya, M. Association between masticatory performance and anthropometric measurements and nutritional status in the elderly. *Geriatr. Gerontol. Int.* **2010**, *10*, 56–63. [CrossRef]
9. Hase, T.; Miura, Y.; Nakagami, G.; Okamoto, S.; Sanada, H.; Sugama, J. Food bolus-forming ability predicts incidence of aspiration pneumonia in nursing home older adults: A prospective observational study. *J. Oral Rehabil.* **2020**, *47*, 53–60. [CrossRef]
10. Goncalves, T.; Schimmel, M.; van der Bilt, A.; Chen, J.; van der Glas, H.W.; Kohyama, K.; Hennequin, M.; Peyron, M.A.; Woda, A.; Leles, C.R.; et al. Consensus on the terminologies and methodologies for masticatory assessment. *J. Oral Rehabil.* **2021**, *48*, 745–761. [CrossRef]
11. Bates, J.F.; Stafford, G.D.; Harrison, A. Masticatory function—A review of the literature: III. Masticatory performance and efficiency. *J. Oral Rehabil.* **1976**, *3*, 57–67. [CrossRef]
12. Nokubi, T.; Yoshimuta, Y.; Nokubi, F.; Yasui, S.; Kusunoki, C.; Ono, T.; Maeda, Y.; Yokota, K. Validity and reliability of a visual scoring method for masticatory ability using test gummy jelly. *Gerodontology* **2013**, *30*, 76–82. [CrossRef]
13. Salazar, S.; Hasegawa, Y.; Kikuchi, S.; Kaneda, K.; Yoneda, H.; Nokubi, T.; Hori, K.; Ono, T. The impact of a newly constructed removable denture on the objective and subjective masticatory function. *J. Prosthodont. Res.* **2021**, *65*, 346–352. [CrossRef] [PubMed]
14. Kosaka, T.; Ono, T.; Kida, M.; Kikui, M.; Yamamoto, M.; Yasui, S.; Nokubi, T.; Maeda, Y.; Kokubo, Y.; Watanabe, M.; et al. A multifactorial model of masticatory performance: The Suita study. *J. Oral Rehabil.* **2016**, *43*, 340–347. [CrossRef]
15. Schimmel, M.; Memedi, K.; Parga, T.; Katsoulis, J.; Muller, F. Masticatory Performance and Maximum Bite and Lip Force Depend on the Type of Prosthesis. *Int. J. Prosthodont.* **2017**, *30*, 565–572. [CrossRef]
16. Ono, T.; Yasui, S.; Kaneda, K.; Kikuchi, S.; Kida, M.; Kosaka, T.; Kikui, M.; Maeda, Y.; Nokubi, T. Development of visual scoring method using a half size gummy jelly for evaluating masticatory performance. *J. Masticat. Health Soc.* **2016**, *26*, 9–13. (In Japanese)
17. Kikui, M.; Ono, T.; Kokubo, Y.; Kida, M.; Kosaka, T.; Yamamoto, M.; Nokubi, T.; Watanabe, M.; Maeda, Y.; Miyamoto, Y. Relationship between metabolic syndrome and objective masticatory performance in a Japanese general population: The Suita study. *J. Dent.* **2017**, *56*, 53–57. [CrossRef]
18. Eichner, K. Renewed examination of the group classification of partially edentulous arches by Eichner and application advices for studies on morbidity statistics. *Stomatol. DDR* **1990**, *40*, 321–325. (In German)
19. Murakami, K.; Hori, K.; Yoneda, H.; Sato, N.; Suwanarpa, K.; Sta Maria, M.T.; Marito, P.; Nokubi, T.; Ono, T. Compatibility of two types of gummy jelly tests for detecting decreased masticatory function. *Gerodontology* **2022**, *39*, 10–16. [CrossRef]
20. Feinberg, M.J.; Ekberg, O. Videofluoroscopy in elderly patients with aspiration: Importance of evaluating both oral and pharyngeal stages of deglutition. *AJR Am. J. Roentgenol.* **1991**, *156*, 293–296. [CrossRef]
21. Matsuo, K.; Kito, N.; Ogawa, K.; Izumi, A.; Kishima, M.; Itoda, M.; Masuda, Y. Improvement of oral hypofunction by a comprehensive oral and physical exercise programme including textured lunch gatherings. *J. Oral Rehabil.* **2021**, *48*, 411–421. [CrossRef] [PubMed]
22. Iyota, K.; Mizutani, S.; Kishimoto, H.; Oku, S.; Tani, A.; Yatsugi, H.; Chu, T.; Liu, X.; Kashiwazaki, H. Effect of Isometric Tongue Lifting Exercise on Oral Function, Physical Function, and Body Composition in Community-Dwelling Older Individuals: A Pilot Study. *Gerontology* **2022**, *68*, 644–654. [CrossRef] [PubMed]
23. Takano, S.; Yamaguchi, K.; Nakagawa, K.; Yoshimi, K.; Nakane, A.; Okumura, T.; Tohara, H. Effect of isometric exercises on the masseter muscle in older adults with missing dentition: A randomized controlled trial. *Sci. Rep.* **2021**, *11*, 7285. [CrossRef] [PubMed]

Disclaimer/Publisher's Note: The statements, opinions and data contained in all publications are solely those of the individual author(s) and contributor(s) and not of MDPI and/or the editor(s). MDPI and/or the editor(s) disclaim responsibility for any injury to people or property resulting from any ideas, methods, instructions or products referred to in the content.

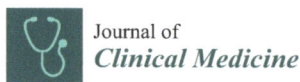 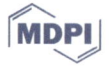

Article

Factors Associated with Selection of Denture Adhesive Type: A Cross-Sectional Survey

Kohei Yamaguchi, Yohei Hama *, Hitomi Soeda, Keita Hatano, Mitsuzumi Okada, Ryota Futatsuya and Shunsuke Minakuchi

Department of Gerodontology and Oral Rehabilitation, Graduate School of Medical and Dental Sciences, Tokyo Medical and Dental University, Tokyo 113-8549, Japan
* Correspondence: y.hama.gerd@tmd.ac.jp; Tel.: +81-3-5803-5856

Abstract: The type of denture adhesive, cream or home-liner, chosen by regular denture adhesive users and oral conditions contributing to this selection require elucidation. The factors associated with denture adhesive selection were investigated through a face-to-face survey on oral and denture conditions. Age, sex, oral moisture, masticatory performance, retention and stability of the removable denture, ridge shape, mucosal thickness, and duration of denture use were examined in cream and home-liner-type denture adhesive users who did not regularly visit a dentist. Univariate analysis and multivariate analyses were performed. There were 38 and 40 cream-type and home-liner-type adhesive users, respectively. The type of denture adhesive was significantly associated with the oral moisture value, retention, ridge shape, mucosal thickness, and duration of denture use in univariate analyses. The residual ridge conditions with large factor loadings for ridge shape and mucosal thickness and duration of denture use were significantly related to the denture adhesive selection in multivariate logistic analysis. The residual ridge conditions and duration of denture use were significant factors in the selection of cream- and home-liner-type denture adhesives. These results can provide appropriate guidance based on the adhesives patients without dental supervision are more likely to choose.

Keywords: denture adhesive; home-liner; residual ridge condition; duration of denture use

Citation: Yamaguchi, K.; Hama, Y.; Soeda, H.; Hatano, K.; Okada, M.; Futatsuya, R.; Minakuchi, S. Factors Associated with Selection of Denture Adhesive Type: A Cross-Sectional Survey. *J. Clin. Med.* **2023**, *12*, 873. https://doi.org/10.3390/jcm12030873

Academic Editors: Takahiro Ono, Leonardo Marchini and Anastassia E. Kossioni

Received: 15 December 2022
Revised: 11 January 2023
Accepted: 18 January 2023
Published: 21 January 2023

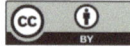

Copyright: © 2023 by the authors. Licensee MDPI, Basel, Switzerland. This article is an open access article distributed under the terms and conditions of the Creative Commons Attribution (CC BY) license (https://creativecommons.org/licenses/by/4.0/).

1. Introduction

Japan has become a super-aged society, and the number of older adults is expected to increase in the future [1]. Although the number of remaining teeth in older adults has been increasing [2], previous surveys in Japan reported that the removable denture usage rate was approximately 30% among 1,875 older adults living in a community with an average age of 66.7 years [3] and approximately 40% among 1272 people with an average age of 69.7 years [4]. These studies indicate that there are still many people who use removable dentures. Furthermore, various types of denture adhesives are known, including cream, home-liner, powder, and sheet types. Cream, powder, and sheet types are categorized as narrowly defined denture adhesives. A web-based survey of 1,470 denture wearers in Japan reported that 21.6% of participants used denture adhesives, of which 66.7% used the cream type, followed by the liner type (23.3%) [5]. Another web-based study has reported that 23.3% of denture wearers use denture adhesives, with 79.7% using the cream type and 16.2% using the liner type [6]. Thus, users of these two types of denture adhesives exist to some extent in Japan.

Denture adhesives are sold at drug shops in Japan, and anyone can buy and use denture adhesives on their own initiative. The cream type is classified as a denture adhesive in the narrow sense of the term and exhibits adhesive properties when mixed with saliva between the mucous surface of the denture base and subfloor mucosa. It has high fluidity and spreads thinly; therefore, it is less likely to cause changes in the occlusal vertical dimension. The thinner the denture adhesive, the greater the adhesion strength [7]. Generally, the cream type must be cleaned at daily intervals and should not be used for more than one day. On the other hand, the home-liner type is a highly viscous material that fills the gap between the denture base mucosa surface and the subfloor mucosa. The home-liner-type adhesive can be used for a few days, but there is no published evidence stating this.

The effects of cream-type denture adhesives include improvement in the stability of well-fitting dentures [8], masticatory performance [9], patient satisfaction, mandibular movement during chewing [10], and denture retention [11]. Risks of using denture adhesives include residual ridge resorption, denture stomatitis, *Candida* infection, and oral flora imbalance [12]. Although there is little longitudinal research, one study has reported that there is no problem with microorganisms for a 2-month period of use [13]. There are currently no long-term progress reports in the literature. It has also been shown that the home-liner-type denture adhesive improves patient satisfaction and masticatory performance by filling the gap between the denture and mucosa due to natural bone resorption and providing a cushioning effect [14–16]. The risk of using it includes occlusal misalignment, which may cause residual ridge resorption [17,18]. Therefore, since each denture adhesive has its particular advantages and disadvantages, dentists must instruct patients to use denture adhesives correctly. Dentists need to understand the denture adhesive more likely to be selected by people and the conditions under which this selection is performed to provide guidance according to the tendency of selection.

A previous study, a web-based survey of 1470 denture wearers, did not identify any significant factors related to the type of denture adhesive selection [5]. In another web-based survey of denture adhesive use, 59.9% of respondents chose "Saw in the pharmacy/drugstore/store" and 19.3% chose "Saw an advertisement" as their reason for choosing a denture adhesive product [6]. This is only a subjective answer by the users, and thus, objective factors, of which the respondents themselves may be unaware, were not investigated. Therefore, the present study was conducted to examine the objective factors related to denture adhesive selection by conducting a face-to-face survey of oral and denture conditions. The null hypothesis of this study was that oral and denture conditions were not related to the selection of denture adhesive type. The purpose of this study was to identify the factors involved in the selection of cream- and home-liner-type denture adhesives among individuals who use denture adhesives on a daily basis.

2. Materials and Methods

2.1. Participant Characteristics

Participants in this study were recruited via e-mail sent to those registered with the research companies. The inclusion criteria were as follows: age 50 years or older, use of a cream or home-liner type of denture adhesives at least once a week, more than 6 months of use, no regular visits to the dentist, not currently undergoing dental treatment, and consent to face-to-face measurement. Participants in Eichner classification groups A and B1 and those using intermediary defect dentures were excluded. Written consent was obtained from all participants at the time of measurement. This study was approved by the Ethics Review Committee of Tokyo Medical and Dental University (D2018-057).

2.2. Measurements

2.2.1. Oral Moisture

Using an oral moisture checker (Mucus; Life Co., Ltd., Saitama, Japan), the mucosal wetness of the tongue was measured thrice at the center of the tongue, and the median score was used as the "mucus value" to evaluate the oral moisture [19].

2.2.2. Masticatory Performance

Color-changeable chewing gum (Mastication Check Gum; Lotte Co., Ltd., Tokyo, Japan) was used to evaluate the masticatory performance without denture adhesives. The gum was chewed 100 times, with one chew per second, without specifying the chewing side or using denture adhesives. The chewed gum was pressed using two glass slabs to a 1.5 mm thickness. The L*, a*, and b* values (CIELAB color system) of the sample were measured using a colorimeter (CR13; Konica Minolta Sensing, Tokyo, Japan) at the center and at 3 mm to the top, bottom, left, and right of the center, and the average value was obtained. The masticatory ability evaluation value (MPIG) was calculated using ΔE [20,21].

$$\Delta E = \sqrt{(L^* - 72.3)^2 + (a^* - (-14.9))^2 + (b^* - 33.0)^2} \quad (1)$$

$$\text{MPIG} = \frac{1}{9.55 \times 10^{-3}} \ln\left(\frac{-2.85 \times 10^7}{\Delta E - 73.2} - 1\right) - 1.35 \times 10^3 \quad (2)$$

(L*, a*, b*: coordinates in CIELAB color space).

A higher MPIG indicates higher masticatory performance.

2.2.3. Retention and Stability

Denture retention and stability were evaluated according to Kapur's classification [22]. Kapur scored the denture retention, stability, and ridge shape. The retention criterion is scored as follows: 0, no retention (when a denture is seated in its place, it displaces itself); 1, minimum retention (when a denture offers slight resistance to vertical pull and little or no resistance to lateral force); 2, moderate retention (when a denture offers moderate resistance to lateral force); 3, good retention (when a denture offers maximum resistance to vertical pull and sufficient resistance to lateral force). Scores of 0 and 1 were defined as "not enough" and 2 and 3 as "good". The stability criterion is scored as follows: 0, no stability (when a denture base demonstrates extreme rocking on its supporting structures under pressure); 1, some stability (when a denture base demonstrates moderate rocking on its supporting structures under pressure); 2, sufficient stability (when a denture base demonstrates slight or no rocking on its supporting structures under pressure). Scores of 0 and 1 were defined as "not enough" and 2 as "good".

2.2.4. Residual Ridge and Mucosal Thickness

The residual ridge was evaluated according to Kapur's classification [22]. The ridge shape was classified as V-shaped, flat, depressed, or U-shaped. Mucosal thickness was classified as thin, normal, or thick by manipulation. These were evaluated by one prosthodontist with at least 10 years of clinical experience.

2.2.5. Duration of Denture Use

The questionnaire asked about the duration of denture use (more or less than three years).

2.3. Statistical Analysis

The Shapiro–Wilk test was performed to evaluate the normality of the data. To check the differences between the two groups of cream- and home-liner-type users, Wilcoxon's rank-sum test was performed for age, and chi-squared tests were performed for sex and denture type.

2.3.1. Univariate Analysis

Logistic regression analysis was performed with the type of denture adhesive as the objective variable and mucus value and MPIG as independent variables.

A chi-squared test was performed with the type of denture adhesive as the objective variable and the ridge shape, mucosal thickness, retention, stability, and duration of denture use were used as independent variables.

2.3.2. Multivariate Analysis

Exploratory factor analysis was performed to consolidate variables. Factor analysis was performed on the correlation matrix, and the maximum likelihood method was used.

Factor loadings were adjusted using varimax rotation to make the analysis easier. To determine the number of factors, the Kaiser–Guttman criterion was used up to a factor with an eigenvalue greater than 1 and selected factors that contained items with an absolute factor loading of at least 0.3. Multivariate logistic regression analysis was performed on three different factors resulting from the exploratory factor analysis, with age and sex as independent variables and the denture adhesive type as the dependent variable.

All statistical significance levels were set at $p = 0.05$, and the statistical software JMP8.0 (SAS Institute, Cary, NC, USA) was used.

3. Results

3.1. Characteristics of Participants

Among the respondents, 88 registrants agreed to participate and be measured face-to-face, and 10 participants were excluded because they had used denture adhesives for less than 6 months. The participants' characteristics are listed in Table 1. No significant differences were found in age, sex, type of denture, or masticatory performance between the types of denture adhesives. Significant differences were found only in oral moisture.

Table 1. Characteristics of participants.

	Cream	Home-Liner	p-Value
N	38	40	
Mean age, years (SD)	70.5 (5.9)	69.5 (8.0)	0.95 [a]
Sex			
Male	29	23	0.08 [b]
Female	9	17	
Type of denture			
Partial	14	15	0.95 [b]
Complete	24	25	
Oral moisture	27.5 [26, 28.9]	26.9 [26, 27.9]	**0.04** [a]
Masticatory performance	104 [83.4, 122]	110 [90.6, 132]	0.29 [a]

[a]: Wilcoxon rank sum test; [b]: Pearson's chi-squared test. SD, standard deviation. If either the upper or lower arch was edentulous, the patient was categorized as having a complete denture. Oral moisture and masticatory performance data are presented as median (25th percentile, 75th percentile). Bold faces denote significance ($p < 0.05$).

3.1.1. Univariate Analysis

Table 2 shows the logistic regression analysis results with the denture adhesive type as the objective variable and mucus value and MPIG as independent variables. Significant associations were found for the mucus value.

Table 2. Logistic regression analysis with the type of denture adhesive as a dependent variable.

Independent Variables	OR [95%CI]	p-Value
Oral moisture	1.31 [1.02–1.76]	**0.03**
Masticatory performance	0.99 [0.98–1.01]	0.35

OR [95%CI]: odds ratio (95% confidence interval). Boldface denotes significance ($p < 0.05$).

The results of the chi-squared test are shown in Table 3. Significant differences were found in denture retention, ridge shape, mucosal thickness, and duration of denture use.

Table 3. Pearson's chi-squared test with denture adhesive as a dependent variable.

Independent Variables	Cream	Home-Liner	Cream Ratio	OR [95%CI]	p-Value
Retention of denture					
Not enough	16	7	69.6%	0.29 [0.10–0.82]	**0.01**
Good	22	33	40.0%		
Stability of denture					
Not enough	24	22	52.2%	0.71 [0.29–1.77]	0.46
Good	14	18	43.8%		
Ridge shape					
V-shaped, flat, depressed	13	26	33.3%	3.57 [1.40–9.08]	**<0.01**
U-shaped	25	14	64.1%		
Mucosal thickness					
Thin	1	17	5.6%	27.3 [3.41–220]	**<0.01**
Normal, thick	37	23	61.7%		
Duration of denture use					
>3 years	36	25	59.0%	0.09 [0.02–0.44]	**<0.01**
<3 years	2	15	11.8%		

OR [95% CI]: odds ratio (95% confidence interval); Boldface denotes significance ($p < 0.05$).

3.1.2. Exploratory Factor Analysis

Table 4 shows the factor loadings resulting from exploratory factor analysis of the 7 univariate independent variables. These were aggregated into 3 factors with eigenvalues greater than 1, with a cumulative contribution of 62.6%. The items with an absolute factor loading of 0.3 or greater were the retention of denture and stability of denture (Factor 1), ridge shape and mucosal thickness (Factor 2), and duration of denture use (Factor 3).

Table 4. Exploratory factor analysis.

Independent Variables.	Factor Loadings after Rotation		
	Factor 1	Factor 2	Factor 3
Oral moisture	0.18	0.25	−0.07
Masticatory performance	0.02	0.01	0.27
Retention of denture	**0.44**	−0.19	0.06
Stability of denture	**1.00**	0.07	0.06
Ridge shape	−0.05	**0.64**	−0.01
Mucosal thickness	−0.03	**0.76**	−0.06
Duration of denture use	0.09	−0.22	**0.97**

Boldface denotes an absolute value > 0.3.

3.1.3. Multivariate Analysis

A multivariate logistic regression analysis was performed on Factors 1, 2, and 3, with age and sex as the independent variables and denture adhesive type as the dependent variable (Table 5). Significant associations were found between Factors 2 and 3.

Table 5. Multivariate adjusted logistic regression analyses with denture adhesive type as the dependent variable.

Independent Variables	OR [95% CI]	p-Value
Factor 1 (retention and stability)	0.72 [0.39–1.29]	0.27
Factor 2 (residual ridge condition)	5.50 [2.40–15.8]	**<0.01**
Factor 3 (duration of denture use)	0.40 [0.18–0.76]	**<0.01**
Age	1.01 [0.92–1.11]	0.86
Sex (male/female)	1.50 [0.42–5.59]	0.51

Boldface denotes significance ($p < 0.05$). OR [95% CI]: odds ratio (95% confidence interval).

4. Discussion

This is the first study to examine the factors associated with the selection of cream- and home-liner denture adhesives by evaluating the oral and denture conditions among those who used denture adhesives on a daily basis. This study found significant factors associated with the selection of the type of denture adhesive, and these results are useful for predicting the adhesive a patient is likely to choose without supervision and in providing appropriate guidance.

Denture adhesives should be used only for the minimally required period of time under the supervision of a dentist [12]. The choice of denture adhesive for patients under supervision is likely to be heavily influenced by the dentist's instructions. Therefore, patients who do not see a dentist regularly and who choose their own denture adhesives should be targeted to examine the factors associated with the selection of the type of denture adhesive.

The results of this study may also be useful in educating patients who visit the dental clinic regarding denture adhesives as it will allow one to predict the denture adhesive they may choose in the future. Moreover, in a previous web survey, 28.5% of denture adhesive users had not visited a dentist for more than 1 year [5]. This group of non-dentist visiting denture adhesive users should not be ignored, and it would be useful to know the tendencies related to their selection of denture adhesive.

In this study, those who had started using denture adhesives for less than 6 months were excluded. It has been reported that the most common reasons for choosing denture adhesives were "Saw the product in the pharmacy/drugstore/store" (59.9%) followed by "Saw an advertisement" (19.3%) [6]. However, it can be assumed that those who are still using a denture adhesive after 6 months are aware of its effectiveness, regardless of the subjective reason for their initial choice of adhesive. Therefore, it is meaningful to examine the relationship between the type of adhesive the individual chooses to use and objective evaluation in this study.

As mentioned above, a previous study using a web-based questionnaire failed to identify factors related to the selection of denture adhesive type [5]. This in-person study focused on oral and denture conditions. Considering the different characteristics of the cream or home-liner type, the following measurement items were selected as possible factors related to the selection of denture adhesives. First, considering that the purpose of denture adhesives is to improve retention the oral moisture value was measured, which is related to denture retention [23]. One of the main purposes of a prosthesis is to improve the masticatory function; thus, the masticatory performance without denture adhesives was evaluated as a criterion of denture quality. As another evaluation for dentures, Kapur's classification [22] was used, which is used in denture adhesive research to evaluate retention and stability [16]. Furthermore, as denture-supporting tissue is associated with the selection of the type of denture adhesives, the residual ridge shape and mucosal thickness were evaluated with reference to Kapur's classification. Finally, dentures may become incompatible over time [24,25] due to residual ridge resorption and incongruity in an occlusal relationship. Therefore, the duration of denture use of the present denture was considered in a comprehensive evaluation of dentures.

Logistic regression analysis showed that participants with higher mucus values are more likely to use the cream-type adhesive (Table 2). The cream-type adhesive would be suitable for those with a high oral moisture content as it mixes with saliva to increase the viscosity. Pearson's chi-squared test showed that the usage rate of cream-type denture adhesive users was significantly higher for those with a U-shaped ridge, normal mucosal thickness, not enough denture retention, and more than 3 years of denture use (Table 3). It is possible that participants with unfavorable ridge shapes or thin mucosa selected viscoelastic home-liner-type adhesives to prevent pain. It is also natural that they would choose cream-type adhesives with viscous properties when the retention is insufficient. The results indicated that cream-type denture adhesives were more likely to be used by long-term denture users.

This study included 38 cream-type and 40 home-liner-type users. The sample size was originally planned to be approximately 70 subjects in each group, assuming 7 items were to be used in the multivariate analysis. However, the COVID-19 pandemic made it difficult to secure the planned sample size. Therefore, exploratory factor analysis was conducted to consolidate the independent variables.

Using exploratory factor analysis, the factors were aggregated into three, and each factor was interpreted based on the number of factor loadings. Factor 1 was referred to as "retention and stability" because of the large factor loadings for the retention and stability of dentures. In other words, Factor 1 is high when the retention and stability of dentures are good. Factor 2 was named the "residual ridge condition" because of the large factor loadings of the mucosal thickness and the ridge shape. Factor 2 is high when the mucosal thickness is thick and the ridge shape is good. Factor 3 was the "duration of denture use" because it has a large factor loading only for the duration of denture use. Factor 3 was high for less than 3 years of denture use.

In the multivariate analysis, the residual ridge condition and duration of denture use were significant. In other words, the better the residual ridge condition and the longer the duration of denture use, the greater the probability of using the cream type. After adjusting for age, sex, and denture condition, the results of the multivariate analysis were similar to those of the univariate analysis for residual ridge condition. Unfortunately, no studies have directly compared cream-type and home-liner-type adhesives and evaluated the differences in their properties and effects. Therefore, we have discussed studies that independently evaluated creams and home-liners. A previous study reported that the use of liner-type denture adhesive greatly improved the retention, masticatory ability, self-confidence in social activities, and satisfaction of participants, especially among those with poor supporting tissues (Kapur index) and those who reported poor retention of their previous dentures [16]. This result is one reason why the use of liner-type denture adhesives was more likely among those with poor ridge conditions in the present study. From a clinical standpoint, the choice of viscoelastic home-liner-type adhesives for sharp ridges and thin mucosa may make sense.

In addition, the probability of usage of a cream-type adhesive was higher when Factor 3 was small. No study has examined the effect of cream-type adhesives on the duration of denture use; however, cream-type adhesives may have an improvement effect, at least from the patient's subjective point of view, on dentures in long-term users. Of course, continued use of denture adhesives in denture wearers without dentist supervision is not recommended, but dentists should be aware that long-term denture wearers tend to choose creams when using denture adhesives and should instruct them to go to a dental clinic first instead of immediately choosing a cream-type denture adhesive.

This study has several limitations. First, sampling bias is possible. The participants were selected from those who self-registered on a website as a sample of the population that uses denture adhesives on a daily basis. Participation was therefore limited to those who could access the internet. As a result, the participants were independent elderly people who had high information literacy skills and did not have severe problems related to activities of daily living. In addition, the participants were those who did not currently make regular dental visits and may differ from those under dental supervision in terms of health literacy and other factors. Second, the study did not assess the subjective reasons for choosing the denture adhesive type. The price of denture adhesives may also be included as a reason for selection. Although this study focused on objective measures to examine factors associated with the selection of the type of denture adhesive, it would have been more meaningful and applicable to a clinical setting if the subjective reasons for denture adhesive selection by each adhesive user had been also included. Finally, this study did not examine differences in effects or side effects. These factors are also important to understand and need to be examined in the future.

From the above, the null hypothesis was rejected, and it was shown that denture conditions such as retention, stability, and duration of denture use were related to the selection of denture adhesive. In other words, denture wearers with a poor residual ridge condition were more likely to select a home liner, and denture wearers with a long duration of denture use were more likely to select a cream type. These results are significant for providing guidance regarding the adhesive a patient is likely to choose when they suspend dental supervision in the future or when they are not currently under dental supervision. Further research will be conducted to determine the reasons why the residual ridge condition and duration of denture use are related to the selection of the type of denture adhesives, including subjective factors.

Author Contributions: Conceptualization, Y.H.; methodology, Y.H.; formal analysis, K.Y.; investigation, K.Y., Y.H., K.H., M.O. and R.F.; resources, H.S.; data curation, M.O. and R.F.; writing—original draft preparation, K.Y.; writing—review and editing, Y.H.; visualization, K.Y.; supervision, S.M.; project administration, S.M.; funding acquisition, Y.H. All authors have read and agreed to the published version of the manuscript.

Funding: This research was funded by Kobayashi Pharmaceutical Co., Ltd.

Institutional Review Board Statement: This study was approved by the Ethics Review Committee of Tokyo Medical and Dental University (D2018-057).

Informed Consent Statement: Informed consent was obtained from all subjects involved in the study.

Data Availability Statement: Not applicable.

Acknowledgments: This study was supported by a grant from Kobayashi Pharmaceutical Co., Ltd. The study sponsor had no role in the study design, collection, analysis, and interpretation of the data, in the writing of the report, or in the decision to submit the paper for publication.

Conflicts of Interest: The authors declare no conflict of interest.

References

1. Cabinet Office Tokyo. Chart 1-1-1—Trends in Ageing Population and Projection for the Future. In *Annual Report on the Ageing Society 2021 [Summary]*; Cabinet Office Tokyo: Tokyo, Japan, 2021; p. 3.
2. Ministry of Health, Labour and Welfare; Health Policy Bureau. *Statistical Tables of the Survey of Dental Diseases 2016*; Ministry of Health, Labour and Welfare: Tokyo, Japan; Health Policy Bureau: Tokyo, Japan, 2016.
3. Kosaka, T.; Ono, T.; Kida, M.; Kikui, M.; Yamamoto, M.; Yasui, S.; Nokubi, T.; Maeda, Y.; Kokubo, Y.; Watanabe, M.; et al. A multifactorial model of masticatory performance: The Suita study. *J. Oral Rehabil.* **2016**, *43*, 340–347. [CrossRef] [PubMed]
4. Hama, Y.; Kubota, C.; Moriya, S.; Onda, R.; Watanabe, Y.; Minakuchi, S. Factors related to removable denture use in independent older people: A cross-sectional study. *J. Oral Rehabil.* **2020**, *47*, 998–1006. [CrossRef] [PubMed]
5. Bo, T.M.; Hama, Y.; Akiba, N.; Minakuchi, S. Utilization of denture adhesives and the factors associated with its use: A cross-sectional survey. *BMC Oral Health* **2020**, *20*, 194. [CrossRef] [PubMed]
6. Okazaki, Y.; Abe, Y.; Dainobu, K.; Iwaguro, S.; Kato, R.; Tsuga, K. A web-based survey of denture adhesive use among denture wearers 40 years of age and older. *J. Oral Sci.* **2020**, *63*, 98–100. [CrossRef] [PubMed]
7. Kano, H.; Kurogi, T.; Shimizu, T.; Nishimura, M.; Murata, H. Viscosity and adhesion strength of cream-type denture adhesives and mouth moisturizers. *Dent. Mater. J.* **2012**, *31*, 960–968. [CrossRef]
8. Munoz, C.A.; Gendreau, L.; Shanga, G.; Magnuszewski, T.; Fernandez, P.; Durocher, J. A clinical study to evaluate denture adhesive use in well-fitting dentures. *J. Prosthodont.* **2012**, *21*, 123–129. [CrossRef]
9. De Oliveira Junior, N.M.; Rodriguez, L.S.; Mendoza Marin, D.O.; Paleari, A.G.; Pero, A.C.; Compagnoni, M.A. Masticatory performance of complete denture wearers after using two adhesives: A crossover randomized clinical trial. *J. Prosthet. Dent.* **2014**, *112*, 1182–1187. [CrossRef]
10. Marin, D.O.; Leite, A.R.; Paleari, A.G.; Rodriguez, L.S.; Oliveira Junior, N.M.; Pero, A.C.; Compagnoni, M.A. Effect of a denture adhesive on the satisfaction and kinesiographic parameters of complete denture wearers: A cross-over randomized clinical trial. *Braz. Dent. J.* **2014**, *25*, 391–398. [CrossRef]
11. Ozcan, M.; Kulak, Y.; de Baat, C.; Arikan, A.; Ucankale, M. The effect of a new denture adhesive on bite force until denture dislodgement. *J. Prosthodont.* **2005**, *14*, 122–126. [CrossRef]
12. Slaughter, A.; Katz, R.V.; Grasso, J.E. Professional attitudes toward denture adhesives: A Delphi technique survey of academic prosthodontists. *J. Prosthet. Dent.* **1999**, *82*, 80–89. [CrossRef]
13. Ozkan, Y.K.; Ucankale, M.; Ozcan, M.; Uner, N. Effect of denture adhesive on the micro-organisms in vivo. *Gerodontology* **2012**, *29*, 9–16. [CrossRef] [PubMed]

14. Udo-Yamakawa, A.; Kawai, Y. Effects of home and office care denture reliners on maxillary complete dentures. *Gerodontology* **2010**, *27*, 141–146. [CrossRef] [PubMed]
15. Uysal, H.; Altay, O.T.; Alparslan, N.; Bilge, A. Comparison of four different denture cushion adhesives—A subjective study. *J. Oral Rehabil.* **1998**, *25*, 209–213. [CrossRef] [PubMed]
16. Koronis, S.; Pizatos, E.; Polyzois, G.; Lagouvardos, P. Clinical evaluation of three denture cushion adhesives by complete denture wearers. *Gerodontology* **2012**, *29*, e161–e169. [CrossRef] [PubMed]
17. Woelfel, J.B.; Berg, T., Jr.; Mann, A.W.; Kreider, J.A. Documented Reports of Bone Loss Caused by Use of a Denture Reliner. *J. Am. Dent. Assoc.* **1965**, *71*, 23–34. [CrossRef]
18. Tautin, F.S. Home reliners—Where we have failed. *J. Prosthet. Dent.* **1971**, *25*, 19–20. [CrossRef] [PubMed]
19. Takahashi, F.; Koji, T.; Morita, O. The usefulness of an oral moisture checking device (Moisture Checker for Mucus). *Nihon Hotetsu Shika Gakkai Zasshi* **2005**, *49*, 283–289. [CrossRef]
20. Hama, Y.; Kanazawa, M.; Minakuchi, S.; Uchida, T.; Sasaki, Y. Properties of a color-changeable chewing gum used to evaluate masticatory performance. *J. Prosthodont. Res.* **2014**, *58*, 102–106. [CrossRef]
21. Hama, Y.; Hosoda, A.; Komagamine, Y.; Gotoh, S.; Kubota, C.; Kanazawa, M.; Minakuchi, S. Masticatory performance-related factors in preschool children: Establishing a method to assess masticatory performance in preschool children using colour-changeable chewing gum. *J. Oral Rehabil.* **2017**, *44*, 948–956. [CrossRef]
22. Kapur, K.K. A clinical evaluation of denture adhesives. *J. Prosthet. Dent.* **1967**, *18*, 550–558. [CrossRef]
23. Niedermeier, W.H.; Krämer, R. Salivary secretion and denture retention. *J. Prosthet. Dent.* **1992**, *67*, 211–216. [CrossRef] [PubMed]
24. Tallgren, A. The continuing reduction of the residual alveolar ridges in complete denture wearers: A mixed-longitudinal study covering 25 years. *J. Prosthet. Dent.* **2003**, *89*, 427–435. [CrossRef] [PubMed]
25. Atwood, D.A. Reduction of residual ridges: A major oral disease entity. *J. Prosthet. Dent.* **1971**, *26*, 266–279. [CrossRef] [PubMed]

Disclaimer/Publisher's Note: The statements, opinions and data contained in all publications are solely those of the individual author(s) and contributor(s) and not of MDPI and/or the editor(s). MDPI and/or the editor(s) disclaim responsibility for any injury to people or property resulting from any ideas, methods, instructions or products referred to in the content.

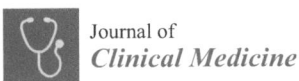 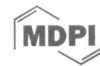

Article

Impact of COVID-19 on the Surrounding Environment of Nursing Home Residents and Attitudes towards Infection Control and Oral Health Care among Nursing Home Staff in Japan

Rena Hidaka [1], Koichiro Matsuo [1,*], Tomoka Maruyama [1], Kyoka Kawasaki [1], Itsuki Tasaka [1], Masami Arai [2], Satoshi Sakoda [3], Kazunori Higuchi [4], Erina Jinno [5], Tsuyoshi Yamada [6] and Shunsuke Minakuchi [7]

1. Department of Oral Health Sciences for Community Welfare, Graduate School of Medical and Dental Sciences, Tokyo Medical and Dental University, 1-5-45 Yushima, Bunkyo, Tokyo 113-8549, Japan
2. M's Dental Clinic, 3F Kitashinagawa 21 Building, 1-1-15 Kitashinagawa, Shinagawa, Tokyo 140-0001, Japan
3. Sakoda Dental Clinic, 6F Li-Ka 1920, 19-40 Chuoumachi, Kagoshima, Kagoshima 890-0053, Japan
4. Minnano Dental Clinic, 1F Cainzmall, 3-152 Nijinooka, Tokoname 479-0849, Japan
5. White Smile Dental Clinic, 2F Mituinoritake Building, 1-4-15 Noritake, Chuo, Nagoya 453-0014, Japan
6. Shinshiraoka Oral Rehabilitation & Dental Clinic, 7-14-14 Shinshiraoka, Shiraoka 349-0212, Japan
7. Department of Gerodontology and Oral Rehabilitation, Graduate School of Medical and Dental Sciences, Tokyo Medical and Dental University, Tokyo 113-8549, Japan
* Correspondence: matsuo.ohcw@tmd.ac.jp; Tel.: +81-3-5803-4548

Abstract: The environments of nursing home staff and residents have dramatically changed since the onset of the COVID-19 pandemic, with greater demand for infection control. This study aimed to clarify the changes and regional differences in the surrounding environment of nursing home residents as well as the working environment of staff, including oral health care, after the spread of SARS-CoV-2. A self-administered questionnaire survey was sent to nursing staff at about 40 nursing homes in different areas of Japan in September and October 2021. The questionnaire consisted of items centered around: (1) the surrounding environment of nursing home residents, (2) awareness and attitudes towards daily work among staff, and (3) attitudes to and procedures for oral health care among staff. A total of 929 respondents included 618 (66.5%) nursing care workers and 134 (14.4%) nurses. Regarding changes in resident daily life, 60% of staff perceived decreases in psychosocial and physical function after the start of the pandemic due to limited family communication and recreational activities, especially in urban areas. Concerning infection control, most respondents adopted routines of disinfecting hands before and after their duties. Oral health care was part of the regular duties of over 80% of respondents. Many participants answered that the frequency and time of oral health care only slightly changed after the onset of COVID-19, but many also reported disinfecting hands both before and after oral health care, particularly in rural areas. Our findings suggested that the COVID-19 pandemic decreased the daily living activities of residents, leading to psychosocial and physical decline, especially in urban areas. The results also indicated that the spread of SARS-CoV-2 triggered improvements in the awareness and attitudes towards infection control in daily work, including oral health care, among nursing care staff, notably in rural areas. Such an effect may contribute to a more positive perception of oral health care infection measures after the pandemic.

Keywords: COVID-19; nursing home; infection control; oral health care

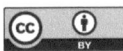

1. Introduction

The spread of the novel coronavirus infection has drastically changed daily life in the medical and nursing care setting since the beginning of 2020 [1–3]. In particular, older adults with systemic disorders have a higher mortality risk from COVID-19 [4–7].

Since COVID-19 was easily transmitted by asymptomatic pathogen carriers, its complete prevention was a struggle in nursing care facilities, which led to mass infection of frail older adults. To reduce the risk of COVID-19 in nursing home residents, various restrictions, including limiting visits of relatives and friends in addition to less frequent recreational activities, have been enforced after the onset of COVID-19 [8].

In addition to residents, nursing home employees have been required to follow thorough control measures to prevent the spread of infection in the event of an outbreak. Oral care procedures are considered high risk for COVID-19 spread due to the direct contact of the operator with the inside of the mouth and the oral secretions that spread outside the mouth during care. Indeed, all related staff have had to be more careful while providing oral health care for residents, with the provision of oral care with adequate infection control measures being recommended by the Ministry of Health, Labour and Welfare of Japan on 30 July 2021 [9]. However, a lack of masks and additional medical equipment hindered the proper implementation of oral care [10].

Since the spread of severe acute respiratory syndrome coronavirus 2 (SARS-CoV-2), the circumstances of residents and employees in nursing care facilities have dramatically changed, which may have exacerbated mental stress and increased duties and burden, respectively. Such alterations may also differ between urban, suburban, and rural areas since larger cities suffered higher numbers of infection, and so the atmospheres of care facilities in the face of COVID-19 might have varied. Therefore, we conducted a questionnaire survey of nursing care facility staff in different areas of Japan to clarify the changes in environments and infection control, including oral health care procedures, among residents and staff caused by the spread of SARS-CoV-2.

2. Methods

2.1. Study Design and Participants

A questionnaire survey was sent to staff working at 40 long-term nursing homes in Tokyo, Aichi and Kagoshima prefectures as representatives of urban, suburban, and rural areas of Japan, respectively, in September and October 2021 following study protocol approval by the ethics committee of Tokyo Medical and Dental University (D2021-038). The survey was administered by mail as a self-administered, unsigned questionnaire, an explanatory document describing the purpose of the study, and a consent form. Respondents were regarded as agreeing with participation in the study by submitting their answers. The survey was administered both on paper and online, giving respondents options on the mode of questionnaire completion. Completed questionnaires were returned using an enclosed return envelope or via the Internet.

2.2. Questionnaire

We asked staff about the environment at nursing homes following the spread of SARS-CoV-2 up to October 2021. The questionnaire was developed based on the Guideline for Infection Control in Nursing Care Settings from the Ministry of Health, Labour and Welfare of Japan (second edition, revised 30 July 2021) [9,11] (Figure 1). The survey included items related to changes in (1) the surrounding environment of nursing home residents, (2) awareness and attitudes towards daily work among staff, and (3) attitudes and procedures of oral health care among staff after the spread of SARS-CoV-2. More specifically, the questionnaire aimed to clarify the following items:

(1) Surrounding environments of nursing home residents: items included the frequency of family visits, staff communication, and rehabilitation and recreation, as well as quality of life and activities of daily living.

(2) Awareness and attitudes towards daily work among staff: items included changes in workload before and after the spread of infection, work precautions, and concerns.

(3) Attitudes and procedures of oral health care: items included changes in infection control, equipment, and time and frequency of performing oral care.

(1) Circumstances of nursing home residents		
Q1	Did the frequency of family visits to residents change after the start of the pandemic?	
	(1) increased (2) no change (3) decreased slightly (4) decreased substantially	
Q2	Did the frequency of rehabilitation or recreational activities of residents change after the start of the pandemic?	
	(1) increased (2) no change (3) decreased slightly (4) decreased substantially	
Q3	Do you think the quality of life of residents changed after the start of the pandemic?	
	(1) increased (2) no change (3) decreased slightly (4) decreased substantially	
Q4	What resident behaviors changed after the start of the pandemic? (multiple answers acceptable)	
	(1) expression became dull (2) speaking fewer words (3) slower walking speed (4) increased forgetfulness	
	(5) less going out (6) less appetite (7) less motivation to do things (8) easily depressed	
(2) Attitudes and procedures towards daily work among staff		
Q5	Did you feel more anxious after the start of the pandemic?	
	(1) not at all (2) no change (3) a little (4) very much	
Q6	Have you felt an increase in workload after the start of the pandemic? (yes/no)	
Q7	What work environment factors have changed after the start of the pandemic? (multiple answers acceptable)	
	(1) number of staff decreased (2) working hours increased (3) online work increased (4) telecommuting work increased	
Q8	What infection control measures have you paid more attention to in your daily work after the start of the pandemic? (multiple answers acceptable)	
	(1) using hand sanitizer before meal service (2) wearing protective clothing when handling excreta	
	(3) using hand sanitizer after toilet care (4) cleaning bathrooms more frequently after bathing	
	(5) disinfecting handrails (6) using disposable tools during dressing care	
(3) Attitudes and procedures towards oral health care among staff		
Q9	Do you normally provide oral health care for residents? (yes/no)	
Q10	Did the frequency of oral health care change after the start of the pandemic?	
	(1) increased (2) no change (3) decreased slightly (4) decreased substantially	
Q11	Did the time spent on oral care for residents change after the start of the pandemic?	
	(1) increased (2) no change (3) decreased slightly (4) decreased substantially	
Q12	Has oral care equipment changed after the start of the pandemic?	
	(1) decreased (2) no change (3) increased slightly (4) increased substantially	
Q13	For responses including "increased" in Q12, please select the additional equipment. (multiple answers acceptable)	
	(1) medical gloves (2) medical mask (3) goggles (4) face shield (5) eye guard (6) disposable plastic apron	
	(7) disposable gown (8) cap	
Q14	What infection control measures did you pay more attention to in oral care after the start of the pandemic? (multiple answers acceptable)	
	(1) hand sanitizing before oral care (2) hand sanitizing after oral care	
	(3) distance from residents (4) cleaning oral care products	

Figure 1. Questionnaire (translated from Japanese).

2.3. Statistical Analysis

Each survey item was summarized by region using descriptive statistics. Regional differences were examined by means of the χ^2 test, and significance levels were adjusted using the Bonferroni method. All statistical analyses were performed using SPSS 25.0 software (IBM Corp., Armonk, NY, USA). A *p*-value of <0.05 was considered statistically significant.

3. Results

3.1. Participant Characteristics

Completed questionnaires were returned from 929 nursing care staff (313 men [33.7%]) of 40 nursing homes. By region, 200 respondents (21.5%) were from urban areas, 547 (58.9%) were from suburban areas, and 182 (19.6%) were from rural areas. By age group, respondents in their forties accounted for the largest number (280, 30.4%), followed next by those in their thirties (205, 22.1%) and in their fifties (195, 21.0%). The most common respondent job position was 'nursing care worker' (618, 66.5%), followed next by 'nurse' (134, 14.4%) and 'care manager' (38, 4.1%).

3.2. Surrounding Environment of Nursing Home Residents

More than 70% of respondents reported that the frequency of family involvement with facility residents had decreased, which tended to be more prevalent in urban areas than in suburban areas (Q1; $p = 0.052$ for urban vs. suburban in multiple comparison testing) (Table 1). Approximately 60% of respondents answered that the frequency of recreation and rehabilitation activities decreased after the spread of SARS-CoV-2, which was significantly higher in urban and rural areas than in suburban areas (Q2; $p < 0.01$ in multiple comparison testing). A similar trend was observed for changes in the quality of life of residents in that 69.5% of staff in urban, 52.7% in suburban, and 61.5% in rural areas reported diminished quality of life among residents. This finding was significantly higher in urban and rural areas than in suburban areas (Q3; $p < 0.05$ in multiple comparison testing).

Table 1. Proportion of answers described as "decreased slightly" or "decreased substantially" in frequency of family visits, rehabilitation and recreation, and resident QOL after the start of the pandemic (N, %) (Q1–Q3).

	Total	Urban	Suburban	Rural	*p*-Value
Frequency of family visits	702 (87.2)	167 (83.5)	392 (71.7)	143 (78.6)	0.027 [b]
Frequency of rehabilitation and recreation	575 (67.9)	144 (76.1)	311 (56.9)	120 (65.9)	0.002 [ac]
Resident QOL	539 (63.6)	139 (73.5)	288 (58.3)	112 (67.9)	0.002 [ac]

a, urban vs. suburban; b, urban vs. rural; c, suburban vs. rural. QOL, quality of life.

Table 2 shows the changes in resident behavior after the spread of the pandemic (Q4). More than 60% of respondents reported that facility residents no longer went out. Approximately 25% responded that residents showed a lack of facial expression, increased time in bed, and increased forgetfulness, although the response rates exhibited regional differences.

3.3. Awareness and Attitudes towards Daily Work among Staff

For Q5, about anxiety in their lives, more than 60% of respondents reported that their sense of anxiety 'increased' after the spread of SARS-CoV-2, with no significant regional differences ($p = 0.219$). We observed that 62.5% of respondents described an overall increase in workload after the onset of COVID-19 (Q6). Twenty-nine percent of staff reported more online work, the percentage of which was particularly high in rural areas (Q7) (Table 3). Approximately 15% responded that the number of staff decreased, particularly in urban areas (26.9%) over other areas ($p < 0.001$ for urban vs. suburban and $p < 0.001$ for urban vs. rural). Telecommuting work did not increase remarkably in any region.

Table 2. Changes in resident behavior after the start of the pandemic (N, %) (Q4).

	Total (881)	Urban (191)	Suburban (517)	Rural (172)	p-Value
Physical factors					
Less going out	562 (63.8)	130 (68.0)	319 (61.7)	113 (65.7)	0.252
Slower walking speed	67 (7.6)	24 (12.6)	33 (6.3)	10 (5.8)	0.014 [ab]
Psychological factors					
Expression became dull	243 (27.5)	67 (35.0)	116 (22.4)	60 (34.9)	<0.001 [a]
Less motivation to do things	217 (24.6)	55 (28.8)	118 (22.8)	44 (25.6)	0.244
Speaking fewer words	221 (25.1)	49 (25.6)	124 (24.0)	48 (27.9)	0.570
Increased forgetfulness	180 (20.4)	58 (30.4)	96 (18.6)	26 (15.1)	<0.001 [ab]
Easily depressed	89 (10.1)	29 (15.2)	46 (8.9)	14 (8.1)	0.030 [ab]
Nutritional factors					
Less appetite	96 (10.8)	23 (12.0)	44 (8.5)	29 (16.8)	0.008 [c]

a, urban vs. suburban; b, urban vs. rural; c, suburban vs. rural.

Table 3. Changes in work environment after the start of the pandemic (N, %) (Q7).

	Total (871)	Urban (156)	Suburban (535)	Rural (180)	p-Value
Online work increased	250 (28.7)	37 (23.7)	146 (27.3)	67 (37.2)	0.010 [c]
Number of staff decreased	120 (14.8)	42 (26.9)	68 (12.7)	19 (10.5)	<0.001 [ab]
Working hours increased	111 (12.7)	29 (18.6)	57 (10.7)	25 (13.9)	0.029 [a]
Telecommuting work increased	1 (0.1)	0 (0)	1 (0.2)	0 (0)	0.730

a, urban vs. suburban; b, urban vs. rural; c, suburban vs. rural.

Items related to infection control, such as sanitizing hands and wearing masks, were cited as receiving increased awareness in daily work (Q8) (Table 4). Attention to infection control increased significantly more in rural areas than other areas after the start of the pandemic.

Table 4. Increased attention to infection control measures after the start of the pandemic (N, %) (Q8).

	Total (925)	Urban (196)	Suburban (547)	Rural (182)	p-Value
Using hand sanitizer after toilet care	657 (71.0)	129 (65.8)	383 (70.0)	145 (79.6)	0.010 [bc]
Disinfecting handrails	607 (65.6)	129 (65.8)	348 (63.6)	130 (71.4)	0.156
Using hand sanitizer before meal service	579 (62.6)	118 (60.2)	327 (59.8)	134 (73.6)	0.003 [bc]
Wearing protective clothing when handling excreta	149 (16.1)	42 (21.4)	56 (10.2)	51 (28.0)	<0.001 [ac]
Frequent cleaning of bathrooms after bathing	138 (14.9)	50 (25.5)	53 (9.7)	35 (19.2)	<0.001 [ac]
Using disposable tools during dressing care	80 (8.6)	16 (8.1)	36 (6.6)	28 (15.4)	0.001 [bc]

a, urban vs. suburban; b, urban vs. rural; c, suburban vs. rural.

3.4. Attitudes and Procedures of Oral Health Care

A total of 744 respondents (80.1%) answered to be involved in oral health care work in Q9. We witnessed that 95.9% and 95.2% reported 'no change' in the frequency and time spent on oral health care procedures (Q10 and Q11, respectively). More than 70% of participants cited 'no change' in the equipment used for oral health care after the infection spread in Q12. Approximately 10% described the addition of equipment, including face shields, medical gloves, and medical masks (Q13). Regarding infection control for oral health care procedures, hand sanitizing 'before' and 'after' oral health care tended to be selected most frequently by roughly 60% of respondents each, especially in rural areas (roughly 80%). This was followed next by 'cleaning oral care products (42.3%)' and 'distance from the patient (23.9%)' (Q14) (Table 5).

Table 5. Increased infection control measures in oral health care after the start of the pandemic (N, %) (Q14).

	Total (829)	Urban (163)	Suburban (500)	Rural (166)	p-Value
Hand sanitizing after oral care	519 (62.6)	106 (65.0)	278 (55.6)	135 (81.7)	<0.001 [bc]
Hand sanitizing before oral care	470 (56.7)	53 (32.5)	248 (49.6)	129 (77.7)	<0.001 [bc]
Cleaning oral care products	351 (42.3)	75 (46.0)	194 (38.8)	82 (49.3)	0.039 [bc]
Distance from the patient	198 (23.9)	52 (31.9)	102 (20.4)	44 (26.5)	0.007 [a]

a, urban vs. suburban; b, urban vs. rural; c, suburban vs. rural.

4. Discussion

In this study, answers from staff members suggested several significant changes in the surrounding environment of nursing home residents as well as in the working environment, including oral health care, of nursing home staff after the spread of SARS-CoV-2. Many of these alterations differed among urban, sub-urban, and rural settings. Our findings showed that many staff recognized a negative impact of COVID-19 on the activities of daily life of facility residents. However, there was also a possible positive influence on the awareness and attitudes towards infection control in oral health care and other daily work among staff, as significant increases in attention to infection control measures in daily work and oral health care were observed.

4.1. Differences in the Changes in Attitudes of Nurisng Care Staff in Different Areas of Japan

We observed significant differences in survey answers among urban, suburban, and rural areas. Our findings suggested that nursing care staff perceived that the residents' living environments deteriorated significantly, and more so in urban centers than in other locations. However, attention to infection control at work, including oral health care, changed significantly more in rural areas than elsewhere. Since April 2020, a state of emergency has been declared multiple times in Japan, but many restrictions depended on the area and circumstances of COVID-19 spread. According to a survey by the Cabinet Office of Japan [12], there has been an increased desire to move to rural areas among urbanites after the spread of infection and a change in commuting time with the introduction of remote work. Urban residents have reported greater anxiety and poorer mental health related to COVID-19, which may have influenced regional differences [13–15].

4.2. Surrounding Environments of Nursing Home Residents

Many staff cited that the surrounding environments of nursing home residents became restricted after the spread of SARS-CoV-2. The decreased access to residents' family visits and recreation activities may have impacted them both psychosocially and physically. A longer bedridden status may have increased the risk of frailty and sarcopenia [16,17]. In addition to physical frailty, the prohibition of family visits and reduced group recreation at institutions could have reduced psychosocial functioning [18–20]. Our findings suggest that the reduced activity levels caused by the COVID-19 pandemic had a strong impact on the activities of daily living and quality of life of institution residents.

4.3. Awarenesss and Attitudes towards Daily Work among Staff

Many respondents reported an overall increase in workload. Nursing care facilities are chronically understaffed [21]. In addition to a rise in COVID-19-related work, absenteeism due to coronavirus infection may have caused work to be transferred to the remaining staff members [22]. A recent study revealed that nursing home staff were more likely to leave their jobs under the complex and stressful circumstances of prolonged SARS-CoV-2 infections [23]. Indeed, the pandemic significantly influenced the working situation in nursing care facilities.

Respondents replied that online communication increased significantly, especially in rural areas, which indicated that the nature of their work had changed. Since restricting interactions with the outside world was described as effective in preventing SARS-CoV-2 transmission [24], many nursing care facilities shifted to online interaction tools for residents to see their families instead of face-to-face contact after the start of the pandemic. Our findings suggested that many facilities in rural areas adopted online tools after the pandemic onset.

Institutional attitudes towards infection control have dramatically changed since the start of COVID-19 [25]. Our findings showed that a high percentage of respondents paid more attention to infection control in their daily work. Since the transmission of COVID-19 is often asymptomatic, the difficulty of infection control measures raised anxiety levels among staff [26]. The rapid spread of SARS-CoV-2 infection may have augmented the awareness and attitudes towards disinfection in all areas of Japan as compared with beforehand.

4.4. Attitudes and Procedures of Oral Health Care

Our findings indicated that the awareness and attitudes towards infection control in oral health care procedures significantly increased after the onset of the pandemic. Approximately 60% of respondents reported sanitizing their hands before and after oral health care, with the higher percentage of these being significantly higher in rural areas. As with other domains of infection control, attitudes to oral health care were also heightened in all areas of Japan. The number of deaths from pneumonia significantly decreased during the pandemic [27]. The commitment to thorough infection control in older adults as well as among nursing care and hospital staff may have contributed to reducing mortality by respiratory infection diseases [28–30].

Our survey indicated that the procedures of oral health care themselves were not remarkably changed after the spread of SARS-CoV-2. However, staff awareness towards oral health care equipment has changed during the pandemic. Goggles and face shields have been reported to be preferentially worn over eyeglasses since oral health care can increase the risk of droplets entering into the eyes [31,32]. The increased frequency of protective equipment use might have been driven by improvements in knowledge and attitudes towards infection control.

This study had several limitations. First, the findings were based on the responses of staff members belonging to each facility rather than on a facility-by-facility basis. The answers may therefore have been influenced by the subjectivity of individual respondents. Also, we did not identify the total number of employees of each facility; thus the result may be limited to the opinions of certain employees. Second, due to the need for quickly assessing the influence of COVID-19 in nursing homes, the reliability and validity of the questionnaire may not have been sufficiently evaluated. Third, the risk of confounding factors, selection bias, and recall bias needs to be considered when interpreting the results. Lastly, due to the large number of categorical variables, the possibility of type II error cannot be ruled out. However, this study was conducted swiftly during a pandemic and was therefore considered important in capturing the real-life impact of COVID-19. Future studies should examine the reliability and validity of the questionnaire, increase the number of facilities surveyed, and examine the long-term effects of the changing situation.

5. Conclusions

This questionnaire survey of staff in nursing homes across Japan revealed a decline in physical and psychological function of the residents, and an increased awareness of infection control among facility staff members, especially in rural areas. Efforts to maintain good oral hygiene and persistent attention to other infection control measures are being implemented on an ongoing basis.

Author Contributions: Conceptualization, K.M.; Data curation, T.M. and K.K.; Investigation, R.H., I.T., M.A., S.S., K.H., E.J. and T.Y.; Methodology, R.H.; Resources, M.A., S.S., K.H., E.J. and T.Y.; Supervision, K.M. and S.M.; Writing—original draft, R.H.; Writing—review & editing, K.M. All authors have read and agreed to the published version of the manuscript.

Funding: This work was supported by a grant-in-aid MEXT KAKENHI from the Ministry of Education, Culture, Sports, and Science of Japan and the Japan Science (grant number 21H03154) and Technology Agency (JST) program SICORP (grant number JPMJSC1813).

Institutional Review Board Statement: The study was conducted in accordance with the Declaration of Helsinki, and approved by the ethics committee of Tokyo Medical and Dental University (D2021-038).

Informed Consent Statement: Informed consent was obtained from all subjects involved in the study.

Data Availability Statement: The data presented in this study are available on request from the corresponding author. The data are not publicly available due to the protection of personal data.

Acknowledgments: The authors would like to thank all of the respondents who completed the survey.

Conflicts of Interest: The authors have no financial or other kinds of personal conflicts to declare in relation to this work.

References

1. Abe, T.; Nofuji, Y.; Seino, S.; Hata, T.; Narita, M.; Yokoyama, Y.; Amano, H.; Kitamura, A.; Shinkai, S.; Fujiwara, Y. Physical, social, and dietary behavioral changes during the COVID-19 crisis and their effects on functional capacity in older adults. *Arch. Gerontol. Geriatr.* **2022**, *101*, 104708. [CrossRef] [PubMed]
2. Ataka, T.; Kimura, N.; Eguchi, A.; Matsubara, E. Changes in objectively measured lifestyle factors during the COVID-19 pandemic in community-dwelling older adults. *BMC Geriatr.* **2022**, *22*, 326. [CrossRef] [PubMed]
3. Kyan, A.; Takakura, M. Socio-economic inequalities in physical activity among Japanese adults during the COVID-19 pandemic. *Public Health* **2022**, *207*, 7–13. [CrossRef] [PubMed]
4. Grasselli, G.; Zangrillo, A.; Zanella, A.; Antonelli, M.; Cabrini, L.; Castelli, A.; Cereda, D.; Coluccello, A.; Foti, G.; Fumagalli, R.; et al. COVID-19 Lombardy ICU Network. Baseline characteristics and outcomes of 1591 patients infected with SARS-CoV-2 admitted to ICUs of the Lombardy region, Italy. *JAMA* **2020**, *323*, 1574–1581. [CrossRef]
5. Verity, R.; Okell, L.C.; Dorigatti, I.; Winskill, P.; Whittaker, C.; Imai, N.; Cuomo-Dannenburg, G.; Thompson, H.; Walker, P.G.T.; Fu, H.; et al. Estimates of the severity of coronavirus disease 2019: A model-based analysis. *Lancet Infect. Dis.* **2020**, *20*, 669–677. [CrossRef] [PubMed]
6. Matsunaga, N.; Hayakawa, K.; Terada, M.; Ohtsu, H.; Asai, Y.; Tsuzuki, S.; Suzuki, S.; Toyoda, A.; Suzuki, K.; Endo, M.; et al. Clinical epidemiology of hospitalized patients with coronavirus disease 2019 (COVID-19) in Japan: Report of the COVID-19 Registry Japan. *Clin. Infect. Dis.* **2021**, *73*, e3677–e3689. [CrossRef]
7. Tanaka, C.; Tagami, T.; Nakayama, F.; Kudo, S.; Takehara, A.; Fukuda, R.; Kaneko, J.; Ishiki, Y.; Sato, S.; Shibata, A.; et al. Association between mortality and age among mechanically ventilated COVID-19 patients: A Japanese nationwide COVID-19 database study. *Ann. Intensive Care* **2021**, *11*, 171. [CrossRef]
8. Eriksson, E.; Hjelm, K. Residents' experiences of encounters with staff and communication in nursing homes during the COVID-19 pandemic: A qualitative interview study. *BMC Geriatr.* **2022**, *22*, 957. [CrossRef] [PubMed]
9. Ministry of Health, Labour and Welfare. Kaigogenba ni Okeru Kannsenntaisaku no Tebiki. (A Guide to Infection Control in Nursing Homes). Available online: https://www.mhlw.go.jp/content/12300000/000814179.pdf (accessed on 30 May 2022). (In Japanese)
10. Zhang, Y.; Li, Z.; Zhao, Y. Multi-mitigation strategies in medical supplies for epidemic outbreaks. *Socioecon. Plann. Sci.* **2023**, 101516. [CrossRef] [PubMed]
11. Wammes, J.D.; Kolk, D.; Besselaar, J.H.; MacNeli-Vroomen, J.L.; Buurman-van, B.M.; Rijin, M. Evaluating Perspectives of Relatives of Nursing Home Residents on the Nursing Home Visiting Restrictions during the COVID-19 Crisis: A Dutch Cross-Sectional Survey Study. *J. Am. Med. Dir. Assoc.* **2020**, *21*, 1746–1750. [CrossRef]
12. Cabinet Office, Shingatakorona Virus No Eikyokaniokeru Seikatsuisiki Koudou No Henka Ni Kannsuru Tyousa (Survey on Changes in Lifestyle Awareness and Behavior under the Influence of New Coronavirus Infection). Available online: https://www5.cao.go.jp/keizai2/wellbeing/covid/pdf/result5_covid.pdf (accessed on 31 October 2022). (In Japanese)
13. Willberg, E.; Järv, O.; Väisänen, T.; Toivonen, T. Escaping from Cities during the COVID-19 Crisis: Using Mobile Phone Data to Trace Mobility in Finland. *ISPRS Int. J. Geo. Inf.* **2022**, *10*, 103. [CrossRef]
14. Khavarian-Garmsira, A.R.; Sharifibcd, A.; Moradpoure, N. Are high-density districts more vulnerable to the COVID-19 pandemic? *Sustain. Cities Soc.* **2021**, *70*, 102911. [CrossRef] [PubMed]
15. Okubo, R.; Yoshioka, T.; Nakaya, T.; Hanibuchi, T.; Okano, H.; Ikezawa, S.; Tsuno, K.; Murayama, H.; Tabuchi, T. Urbanization level and neighborhood deprivation, not COVID-19 case numbers by residence area, are associated with severe psychological distress and new-onset suicidal ideation during the COVID-19 pandemic. *J. Affect. Disord.* **2021**, *287*, 89–95. [CrossRef] [PubMed]
16. Kilroe, S.P.; Fulford, J.; Jackman, S.R. Temporal muscle-specific disuse atrophy during one week of leg immobilization. *Med. Sci. Sport. Exerc.* **2020**, *52*, 944–954. [CrossRef] [PubMed]
17. Kirwan, R.; McCullough, D.; Butler, T.; Perez de Heredia, F.; Davies, I.G.; Stewart, C. Sarcopenia during COVID-19 lockdown restrictions: Long-term health effects of short-term muscle loss. *Geroscience* **2020**, *42*, 1547–1578. [CrossRef]

18. Hayashi, T.; Umegaki, H.; Makino, T. Association between sarcopenia and depressive mood in urban-dwelling older adults: A cross-sectional study. *Geriatr. Gerontol. Int.* **2019**, *19*, 508–512. [CrossRef]
19. Kimura, Y.; Akasaka, H.; Takahashi, T.; Yasumoto, S.; Kamide, K.; Ikebe, K.; Kabayama, M.; Kasuga, A.; Rakugi, H.; Gondo, Y. Factors related to preventive behaviors against a decline in physical fitness among community-dwelling older adults during the COVID-19 pandemic: A qualitative study. *Int. J. Environ. Res. Public Health* **2022**, *19*, 6008. [CrossRef] [PubMed]
20. McArthur, C.; Turcotte, L.A.; Sinn, C.J.; Berg, K.; Morris, J.N.; Hirdes, J.P. Social engagement and distress among home care recipients during the COVID-19 pandemic in Ontario, Canada: A retrospective cohort study. *J. Am. Med. Dir. Assoc.* **2022**, *23*, 1101–1108. [CrossRef]
21. Zarei, H.R.; Bart, Y.; Ergun, O. Impact of using a centralized matching process on nursing home staffing. *Front. Digit. Health Geriatr. Nurs.* **2023**, *49*, 89–93. [CrossRef]
22. Ministry of Health, Labour and Welfare. Kaigojinzai no Kakuho Nitsuite (Securing Caregivers). Available online: https://www.mhlw.go.jp/file/05-Shingikai-12201000-Shakaiengokyokushougaihokenfukushibu-Kikakuka/0000047617.pdf (accessed on 30 May 2022). (In Japanese)
23. White, E.M.; Wetle, T.F.; Reddy, A.; Baier, R.R. Front-line nursing home staff experiences during the COVID-19 pandemic. *J. Am. Med. Dir. Assoc.* **2021**, *22*, 199–203. [CrossRef]
24. Yen, M.Y.; Schwartz, J.; King, C.C.; Lee, C.-M.; Hsueh, P.-R. Society of Taiwan Long-term Care Infection Prevention and Control. Recommendations for protecting against and mitigating the COVID-19 pandemic in long-term care facilities. *J. Microbiol. Immunol. Infect.* **2020**, *53*, 447–453. [CrossRef]
25. Siddiquea, B.N.; Shetty, A.; Bhattacharya, O.; Afroz, A.; Billah, B. Global epidemiology of COVID-19 knowledge, attitude and practice: A systematic review and meta-analysis. *BMJ Open* **2021**, *11*, e051447. [CrossRef]
26. Bai, Y.; Yao, L.; Wei, T.; Tian, F.; Jin, D.-Y.; Chen, L.; Wang, M. Presumed asymptomatic carrier transmission of COVID-19. *JAMA* **2020**, *323*, 1406–1407. [CrossRef]
27. Ministry of Health, Labour and Welfare. Zinkodoutaitoukei. 2020. Available online: https://www.mhlw.go.jp/toukei/saikin/hw/jinkou/kakutei20/index.html (accessed on 31 August 2022). (In Japanese)
28. Wee, L.E.I.; Conceicao, E.P.; Tan, J.Y.; Magesparan, K.D.; Amin, I.B.M.; Ismail, B.B.S.; Toh, H.X.; Jin, P.; Zhang, J.; Wee, E.G.L.; et al. Unintended consequences of infection prevention and control measures during COVID-19 pandemic. *Am. J. Infect. Control* **2021**, *49*, 469–477. [CrossRef]
29. Wee, L.E.; Venkatachalam, I.; Sim, X.Y.J.; Tan, K.B.; Wen, R.; Tham, C.K.; Gan, W.H.; Ko, K.K.K.; Ho, W.Q.; Kwek, G.T.C.; et al. Containment of COVID-19 and reduction in healthcare-associated respiratory viral infections through a multi-tiered infection control strategy. *Infect. Dis. Health* **2021**, *26*, 123–131. [CrossRef]
30. Lotfinejad, N.; Peters, A.; Tartari, E.; Fankhauser-Rodriguez, C.; Pires, D.; Pittet, D. Hand hygiene in health care: 20 years of ongoing advances and perspectives. *Lancet Infect. Dis.* **2021**, *21*, e209–e221. [CrossRef] [PubMed]
31. Lammers, M.J.W.; Lea, J.; Westerberg, B.D. Guidance for otolaryngology health care workers performing aerosol generating medical procedures during the COVID-19 pandemic. *J. Otolaryngol. Head Neck Surg.* **2020**, *49*, 36. [CrossRef] [PubMed]
32. Volgenant, C.M.C.; Persoon, I.F.; de Ruijter, R.A.G.; de Soet, J.J.H. Infection control in dental health care during and after the SARS-CoV-2 outbreak. *Oral Dis.* **2021**, *3*, 674–683. [CrossRef] [PubMed]

Disclaimer/Publisher's Note: The statements, opinions and data contained in all publications are solely those of the individual author(s) and contributor(s) and not of MDPI and/or the editor(s). MDPI and/or the editor(s) disclaim responsibility for any injury to people or property resulting from any ideas, methods, instructions or products referred to in the content.

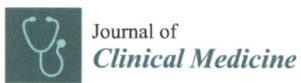

Review

Rapid Oral Health Deterioration in Older People—A Narrative Review from a Socio-Economic Perspective

Linda Slack-Smith [1,*], Gina Arena [1] and Lydia See [2,3]

[1] School of Population and Global Health M431, The University of Western Australia, 35 Stirling Highway, Crawley, WA 6009, Australia
[2] School of Dentistry, The University of Queensland, 288 Herston Road, Herston, QLD 4006, Australia
[3] School of Dentistry, The University of Western Australia, 35 Stirling Highway, Crawley, WA 6009, Australia
* Correspondence: linda.slack-smith@uwa.edu.au; Tel.: +61-8-6488-4505

Abstract: Poor oral health is a common morbidity in old age with older adults less likely to attend dental care and more likely to have dental disease; this situation is exacerbated by older adults retaining more teeth often with complex restorations. Evidence suggests that some older adults experience rapid oral health deterioration (ROHD). While more clinical and population level evidence is needed, current evidence suggests upstream changes addressing disadvantage through the social determinants of health (SDH) may impact broader disorders such as ROHD, often occurring as older adults become dependent. The aim of this paper is to conduct a narrative review to explore the social determinants of ROHD in older adults. The social determinants of health are important in understanding oral health including ROHD. This includes the important influence of the economic determinants. We explored the SDH as relevant to oral health and ROHD including using a framework based on that of the Fisher-Owens conceptual model (for children) but adapted for older adults. Better understanding of these relationships is likely to assist in future prevention and care.

Keywords: oral disease; older adults; rapid oral health deterioration; social determinants of health

1. Introduction

"No one should be denied access to life-saving or health promoting interventions for unfair reasons, including those with economic or social causes. These are some of the issues being addressed by the Commission on Social Determinants of Health. When health is concerned, equity really is a matter of life and death." (the then Director-General World Health Organization, Dr Margaret Chan, 2007) [1].

Oral disease is one of the most common health conditions globally with a substantial burden across the life-course including older adults [2,3]. Oral disease in older adults comprises a number of conditions including dental caries, periodontitis, xerostomia and a range of other conditions [4]. Studies consistently show a decline in dental service attendance and poorer oral health as older adults age [2,5]. While the number and proportion of older adults is increasing globally, the decrease in edentulism along with substantial numbers of complex restorations means not only a high demand for geriatric dental care but also the need for more complex dental care in this cohort [6]. Beliefs are changing with less acceptance that tooth loss and poor oral health are a natural consequence of normal ageing [7,8]. Evidence suggests that poor oral hygiene and poor diet are strong predictors of dental caries and periodontal disease—both of which are often considered preventable [9]. In addition, periodontal disease (and tooth loss) has been associated with significant co-morbidities such as cardiovascular disease, diabetes and respiratory disease [9]. We know from the current literature that some medications can influence oral health in older adults, probably through impacts on saliva [10].

Rapid oral health deterioration (ROHD) occurs when oral health declines more rapidly than expected [11]; the concept was developed to describe and deal with those older adults

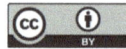

Citation: Slack-Smith, L.; Arena, G.; See, L. Rapid Oral Health Deterioration in Older People—A Narrative Review from a Socio-Economic Perspective. *J. Clin. Med.* **2023**, *12*, 2396. https://doi.org/10.3390/jcm12062396

Academic Editors: Takahiro Ono, Leonardo Marchini and Anastassia E. Kossioni

Received: 11 February 2023
Revised: 13 March 2023
Accepted: 17 March 2023
Published: 20 March 2023

Copyright: © 2023 by the authors. Licensee MDPI, Basel, Switzerland. This article is an open access article distributed under the terms and conditions of the Creative Commons Attribution (CC BY) license (https://creativecommons.org/licenses/by/4.0/).

who have a substantial decline in health followed by a decline in oral health [11]. We also know that oral disease is related to our patterns of life and particularly social determinants of health (SDH) and that individuals who are disadvantaged and have a lower socio-economic status are disproportionally affected [12]. There is a dearth of longitudinal total population or large population level cohort data in older adults so it is difficult to follow trajectories of oral health in this age group as have been explored in other age groups [13]. It is also difficult to look at associations with SDH at the population level [14]. However, we do know consistently from the literature that older adults often reach a point where many health and social issues are impacted as they lose capacity to care for themselves [15]. This is often the point where people enter aged care or receive in-home care [16]. There are two potential scenarios for ROHD: one where an older adult faces general decline (aligning with the definition given above) and another where it is particularly a dental problem without obvious general decline. There are a dearth of data on such nuances of the problem and as noted above, the term has primarily been used to understand oral health decline associated with general health decline [11].

Oral health is influenced by factors across the life-course and while key factors such as sugar in diet and fluoride in water and toothpaste are of central importance, there are many social and medical factors that are likely to be important [3,17]. The social determinants of health (SDH) influence the health and oral health of a population across the life-course [18], and are important to consider in terms of oral health for older adults. The SDH include various social, economic and environmental factors that shape health outcomes, including education, employment, access to healthcare, income and the physical environment [18]. Social determinants of health that are reflected in smoking, high alcohol consumption and the inability to access good quality food and nutrition over time are also predictors of poor oral health in older adults [19]. Other factors associated with social determinants include costs of dental treatment and access to transport, social isolation and lack of role models for good oral health and hygiene [16]. It has previously been reported that oral morbidity often occurs earlier in life for individuals with less financial security [20]. However, these poor outcomes may be exacerbated in older adults with reduced mobility and cognitive function, along with financial barriers, poorer access to healthy nutrition and difficulties accessing transport which may impact dental services [12].

Older adults may become frail although this should not be assumed for all older adults. Hakeem and colleagues conducted a systematic review to investigate frailty and oral health. They concluded that there were strong longitudinal associations between oral health and frailty with oral health being a potential predictor of frailty and with nutrition as a potential mediator [21]. Similarly, Kimble and colleagues identified an association between the decline in muscle strength and oral health using data from two cohort studies [22]. Often at a point where things deteriorate, there are multiple co-morbidities and social issues to address, yet a lack of interdisciplinary primary care means this trend is often only noted at the stage when things start to go very wrong [23]. One outcome that may occur in an older person is ROHD. The literature is limited regarding ROHD in older adults, even more limited when it comes to exploring associated factors such as social determinants of health.

In addition to individual level pathology, it is also important to acknowledge the context where broader socioeconomic factors can also undermine oral health in older adults. This would include factors that can impact macro level changes such as health policies and other interagency collaboration and initiatives that have a direct impact on oral health by addressing root causes and having long-term outcomes. As recognized by Watt, it is at this level where we might need effective upstream prevention [24,25]. Understanding what matters to participants in relation to oral health as they age is also important [26]. Current evidence of what is supposedly preventable oral disease in older adults suggests that upstream factors such as a siloed approach to oral health care and a focus on treatment rather than prevention is clearly not adequate to meet the changing needs of the current ageing population [17]. This includes increasing numbers of older adults with full or partial dentition [16,18].

A recent systematic review on oral health in older adults found that an important component of socioeconomic status was the educational attainment of individuals [27]. Individuals with a higher level of education had better oral health prevention practices and more access to healthcare services. Being able to identify oral health conditions, monitoring and implementing oral health plans can help to reduce the burden of oral health disease in this population [27].

One of the ways we can consider factors associated with ROHD is via the Fisher-Owens' conceptual model, developed to understand children's oral health and the complex interplay of risk factors [28]. The model includes five key components related to the SDH: genetic and biological factors, the social environment, the physical environment, health behaviors and dental and medical care. These components influence oral health outcomes and contribute to the dialogue surrounding oral health at a population level and can be adapted to suit older adults by reflecting on oral health influences across the life-course. A key aspect of the SDH is that they do not act in isolation of each other but instead through multiple and complex interactions [29].

The Seattle Care Pathway offers important guidance re care in this age group [30] Yeung [19] suggests that oral health care systems require an inter-sectoral and interprofessional approach to adapt to oral health in older adults that includes dental professionals; policymakers; health, medical professionals and public health professionals; and researchers. Yeung also suggests a plan of action that integrates oral care into primary health care, promotes oral health across the life-course and informs evidence-based oral health policies. Given the target group is the ageing population, many of whom are retired, Yeung [19] also suggests removing financial and physical barriers to accessing oral care and engaging and training appropriate stakeholders to provide oral health care to maintain the oral health of older adults.

The aim of this paper is to explore the SDH as potentially associated with ROHD in older adults. This will comprise consideration of the concept and evidence for ROHD in the context of poor oral health in older adults, exploration of the potential influence of social determinants with a focus on economic factors and consideration of potential future approaches.

2. Methods

This is a narrative review focusing on peer-reviewed literature and using appropriate grey literature when required.

3. Results

We will consider the issue of poor oral health in older adults, the more specific issue of ROHD, potential associations with factors with a focus on the SDH and potential strategies for prevention and care with ROHD.

3.1. Poor Oral Health of Older Adults

Poor oral health in older adults is a neglected and intractable problem, impacting on overall health and wellbeing of the older adults. It can affect their quality of life in many ways, including limiting the pleasure of eating, because of reduced chewing capacity with resultant malnutrition, feeling ashamed of dentures, and association with diabetes and mental health [2–4]. It can increase hospital admissions related to poor dental care such as aspiration pneumonia and dental care under general anesthetic as well as the broader impact of dental problems including malnutrition and falls [31,32]. Additionally, there is an increase in polypharmacy and medications' use with side effects of xerostomia resulting in an increased risk of oral diseases such as dental caries [33].

There is also the impact on dental treatment required. Barriers to optimal care include lack of specific training for dental professionals and aged care staff [19–21], overcoming patient fears related to past experiences of oral care [22], family attitudes to oral care [23] and lack of understanding of the importance of oral care and cost of and access to dental services [24,25].

3.2. The Concept of Rapid Oral Health Deterioration

Firstly, it is important to explore the concept of ROHD in older adults [11,34]. It is important both dental professions and other relevant professions and carers understand and can identify ROHD. There is limited but important work in the literature looking at measures of ROHD in older adults [11,35]. Meanwhile, the term "rapid deterioration of oral health" or "rapid oral health deterioration" has been used in various research articles—some of that work is not relevant here—such as when used in another age group or a particular context.

Prior to examining the factors associated with poor oral health, particularly ROHD, it is important to consider what is happening in older adults at a more systemic level. Whether oral health is impacted or not is associated with the individual's ability to care for themselves and their mobility to access oral health care. The physiology of ageing can be characterized by the progressive loss of physiological integrity, resulting in impaired function and increased vulnerability [36]. All of these can result in the development of a set of unifying pathological conditions of geriatric syndrome [37,38]. This syndrome is a complex relationship between multimorbidity, polypharmacy and frailty that can contribute to poorer oral health outcomes [33]. It can be used as a framework for addressing the complex oral health needs of older adults and the presentation of common geriatric oral syndromes [33,39]. A complex array of shared risk factors (e.g., increased age, cognitive impairment, functional impairment and impaired mobility) can result in the traditional geriatric syndrome (incontinence, falls, pressure ulcers, delirium and functional decline) and may be influenced by multi-morbidities (e.g., diabetes, neurodegenerative disorders, Alzheimer's/dementia and cardiovascular disease), polypharmacy and resultant frailty [33,39]. All of which have an impact on oral health with the presentation of a common set of symptoms (geriatric oral syndrome) such as burning mouth syndrome, xerostomia, dental caries, periodontitis, dysgeusia, dysphagia and dyskinesia/dystonia [33,39]. Ní Chróinín and colleagues found that poor oral health in older adults was associated with Alzheimer's disease and kidney failure—even when adjusted for medication and salivary pH [6]. Therefore, in addressing the oral health of an older adult, it will mean developing a preventive and management strategy that takes into consideration the impacts of the presence of geriatric syndrome as well as in the broader context of SDH. So, in understanding ROHD, geriatric syndrome may be part of the pathway in which SDH can influence ROHD.

There are at least two ways we could explore this topic. Firstly, we could determine changes in oral health (with appropriate measure for dental caries, periodontitis, tooth loss, etc.) in older adults with longitudinal studies of older adults (potentially concurrent with regular dental appointments) with associated data on SDH. Unfortunately, there are limited cohort data on older adults and a dearth of dental data. Collecting such data may be costly (without good administrative systems) and require some time, however this would be valuable longer term, especially if population-based and linkable with broader administrative data to help identify SDH [14]. Thus, it is more feasible that we could consider likely pathways for ROHD in older adults by reviewing the existing literature on oral health determinants more broadly. Consideration of the social gradient and inequalities in oral health may help further determine the specific factors disadvantaging older adults to target preventative oral health measures including policies and practices.

Frailty is an important consideration in terms of risk for ROHD, although with varied definitions, and work on frailty and oral health is still very much in progress [40]. One group at particular risk of ROHD are older adults with dementia [41]. We know generally that people with dementia have poorer access to dental services and poorer oral health outcomes than other older adults [42].

It is important that both dental professions and other relevant professions understand and can identify ROHD as a precursor to understanding the influence of social determinants. There is limited but important work in the literature looking at measures of ROHD in older adults [11,35]. Marchini and colleagues have developed a teaching tool to establish risk of ROHD in older adults and this was found useful in teaching geriatric oral health for dental students over a number of years [11,35]. It would be useful if such tools were considered for wider use in dental teaching.

3.3. Factors Associated with Poor Oral Health and Rapid Oral Heath Deterioration

Influences on oral health in older adults, including ROHD, are complex and affected by a range of social, heath and clinical factors. We will focus here on the social determinants. If we consider the impact of SDH on oral health, their importance is evident, although substantial work remains before obtaining a full understanding of the relationships between SDH and oral health in older adults and a translation of the findings. The SDH are underpinned by social justice. There is a substantial social justice issue when our older adults are impacted in terms of pain, poor ability to eat properly with reduced pleasure in eating and subsequent effects on wellbeing (including social isolation due to reduced social interactions because of embarrassment, shame, reluctance to smile because of their oral health status) because they are not receiving adequate dental care, this being worst in the more marginalized groups [1]. There are a number of pathways through which disadvantage in terms of social determinants impacts on oral health outcomes. Dental attendance is often affected and our own work using population level data from a national survey, shows that lower dental attendance is strongly associated with older age, less schooling, lower wealth and higher measures of disadvantage [5].

While Fisher-Owens et al. developed a model regarding oral health in children (with influences from Bronfenbrenner's work) some of the principles could be applied here [28,43]. Adapting Fisher-Owens, we could have the following categories of influences (see Table 1) [28].

Table 1. Influences on oral health in older adults-adapted from Fisher-Owens [28].

(Individual) Older adult influences: These influences would include the biology and genetics, the current state of dental care, behaviors and practices, the role of dental insurance and other financial support influencing oral health.
Family, care and care facility influences: The ongoing relation to socio-economic status, ability to access dental care, other interdisciplinary care, communication, decision making, safety, family function, culture, social practices and social support.
Community level influences: The type of dental services (systems), social environment, dental care system characteristics, social capital, physical environment and community oral health environment.

These influences do not fully address what occurred at different points during the life-course but instead largely reflect the current situation in relation to older age and ROHD. There also may be several overlaps between the different influences such as health behaviors that are part of both older adult and family as these key influences are linked to the environment and characteristics.

3.4. Potential Strategies for Dealing with Rapid Deterioration of Oral Health

The problem of ROHD is complex and it is likely that multiple approaches will be required to deal with the problem. Watt has identified the importance of upstream action in oral health [25]. Successful prevention could potentially mean more people with intact teeth and limited restorations, but this may take generations. Broader upstream actions include addressing social determinants more broadly. Education has strong socio-economic impacts on oral health outcomes. This would likely also apply in terms of impacts on ROHD. In addition, developing better integrated primary care for older adults, ideally with inclusion of a dental professional but also with skills in non-dental professionals to identify and predict this disorder. This is important as many older adults do not see a dental professional regularly [5].

We have limited dental professionals with appropriate training in dental care for older adults; in fact, in many countries we still have limited training in geriatrics for dental students. Slack-Smith et al. have noted the limited emphasis on geriatric dentistry in dental courses in Australia and others similarly overseas [44]. The current model of dental care, which largely depends on ad hoc access to a limited supply of public and private dentists working in residential aged care sector is clearly not adequately addressing this problem in Australia.

Due to such complexity of the interplay of risk factors, comorbidities, polypharmacy and frailty, the complexity of oral health management for these individuals increases. The health outcomes of frailty come with increased risk of falls, disability, dependency and death [45]. Therefore, it will be important to identify any determinants that could indicate that the individual is at the precipice of decline so that oral health interventions can occur with adequate timing and prior to any occurrence of ROHD. This is particularly important in the case of older adults in high-dependency residential facilities as these individuals are at the greatest risk of rapid health decline and by extension oral health decline. It is this identification of the window of opportunity that is currently elusive to dentistry.

One way of identifying the time frame in which oral health assessment, prevention and intervention can occur is utilizing the tools that consider factors of SDH. These are factors that can be assessed by non-dental professionals. As such, they can then give a quantifiable indication in which these determinants can then trigger a referral to an oral health care professional for further oral health assessments that may be required in the context of an expected deterioration in health as well as the level of oral health care intervention that is most suitable for the expected trajectory of the individual. This modality of assessment and care intervention looks at oral health in terms of not a disease but as a form of holistic care that puts the patient at the center of care.

Additionally, the concept of the Geriatric 5Ms of: mind, mobility, medications, multi-complexity and matters most can be used as a framework in the oral health management plans of older adults [46]. These 5Ms are domains in which they allow the consideration of functional status, medication reviews, careful evaluation of risks and benefits of treatment, assessment of goals of care as well as prognosis of the patient's condition to be incorporated into the overall management and comprehensive treatment planning of the older adult [46]. They consider the patient in a holistic manner and put the patient's beliefs and values at the center of care. Thus, the 5Ms allow management to be patient centered and not disease centered.

4. Discussion

This paper has focused on consideration of the issue of ROHD and the potential role of various factors focusing on SDH, including economic determinants. While clinical and public health evidence in this area is very limited, our growing knowledge of SDH and oral health is valuable in considering likely factors and pathways. There is no simple way of looking at ROHD or fixing it, it is a complex and multilayered problem [47]. However, we will probably never have adequate individual care systems to provide adequate care to resolve the problem of ROHD at a population level. If using a population health framework, it may help turn the perspective from treating oral disease to preventing oral disease, in this case ROHD. Fisher-Owens' adapted model provides this framework for understanding the complex interplay between various social determinants and the impact on ROHD for older adults. We argue that we need quality clinical knowledge and an understanding of associated factors and an improved understanding of causal pathways. MacEntee noted the need for better models in this area, noting many current health promotion models are not adequate for looking at the oral health of older adults [48]. This model offers a tool for healthcare professionals, policymakers and researchers to address health disparities among older adults that are not solely determined by medical interventions but also shaped by broader societal and environmental factors.

The consideration of ensuring the latest research data can be translated into action at a policy and clinical level will allow for the effective and efficient address of oral diseases. There needs to be a process in which evidence-based data can be readily and rapidly applied to clinical practice. It may mean simplifying bureaucratic processes to allow for more efficient and effective policy changes for such translatability to occur. Over the last 30 years, there has been an observed rise (as seen in the WHO's recent global oral health status report 2022) in estimated case numbers of oral diseases, growing by more than 1 billion [49]. There was a 50% increase in oral disease case-numbers, which is higher than the population increase of about 45% during the same period [49]. What is more concerning is the rate of increase in case numbers of oral diseases is higher than the demographic growth across countries of varying degrees of socio-economic status [49]. Therefore, it can be argued that the increasing prevalence of oral diseases is a cause for concern and may even indicate a silent crisis that could result in increased public expenditure in dealing with the individual and systemic repercussions of untreated oral diseases. The COVID-19 pandemic demonstrates at a global scale, in times of crisis, the ability to rapidly and efficiently expedite regulatory processes to allow for the development of vaccines and medications which would otherwise have taken years to occur. In this context can this not be applied to addressing the state of global oral health? This is particularly crucial in the context of ROHD in the elderly. ROHD, if left untreated, can have a downstream effect of poor health, and quality of life and in extreme cases, systemic infections resulting in increased hospitalizations and potential death from infection. Therefore, it becomes imperative that research should be undertaken in such a way that new data are readily translatable with concurrent influences on public policy such that it allows for the rapid dissemination of information and applications into clinical practice.

The strengths of the study include a novel approach and the application of the Fisher-Owens' model in older adults. There are limitations with a narrative review but it is an appropriate step for understanding the issue. A narrative review was provided as a first step in the exploration of this area as it helped us to identify gaps in the literature and highlight the areas requiring further investigation. As we develop our understanding and body of evidence, a systematic review would then be useful to help provide a more systematic and rigorous search process. This information can help to inform the development of search strategies, potential biases or limitations in the existing evidence and assist with a design that addresses these issues.

ROHD is likely to be a more extreme manifestation of normal dental disease. We need to better understand the clinical characteristics while exploring associated determinants in terms of the SDH. An adapted Fisher-Owens' model offers a potential framework to explore influences. Reducing serious poor health outcomes in older adults and supporting those who do experience RODH is important. Looking at our systems in terms of structures such as interdisciplinary care can be very powerful. We need to broadly disseminate information about this disorder not only to dental professionals, but all professionals and families engaged in elder adult care and consider most effective research questions and approaches to improve outcomes.

Author Contributions: L.S.-S. conceived the initial paper and led the process; all authors (G.A., L.S. and L.S.-S.) developed the paper, helped with writing and authorized the final version. All authors have read and agreed to the published version of the manuscript.

Funding: This research received no external funding.

Institutional Review Board Statement: No ethics issues as this was a narrative literature review.

Informed Consent Statement: Not applicable.

Data Availability Statement: Data sharing not applicable to this article as no datasets were generated or analyzed during the current study.

Conflicts of Interest: The authors declare no conflict of interest.

References

1. Chan, M. Address to the Eleventh Global Forum for Health Research. 2007. Available online: https://www.who.int/director-general/speeches/detail/address-to-the-eleventh-global-forum-for-health-research (accessed on 26 January 2023).
2. Collaborators, G.O.D.; Bernabe, E.; Marcenes, W.; Hernandez, C.; Bailey, J.; Abreu, L.; Alipour, V.; Amini, S.; Arabloo, J.; Arefi, Z. Global, regional, and national levels and trends in burden of oral conditions from 1990 to 2017: A systematic analysis for the global burden of disease 2017 study. *J. Dent. Res.* **2020**, *99*, 362–373. [CrossRef]
3. Heilmann, A.; Tsakos, G.; Watt, R.G. Oral health over the life course. In *A Life Course Perspective on Health Trajectories and Transitions*; Springer: Cham, Switzerland, 2015; Chapter 3; pp. 39–59.
4. Thomson, W.M. Epidemiology of oral health conditions in older people. *Gerodontology* **2014**, *31*, 9–16. [CrossRef] [PubMed]
5. Slack-Smith, L.; Hyndman, J. The relationship between demographic and health-related factors on dental service attendance by older Australians. *Br. Dent. J.* **2004**, *197*, 193–199. [CrossRef] [PubMed]
6. Ní Chróinín, D.; Montalto, A.; Jahromi, S.; Ingham, N.; Beveridge, A.; Foltyn, P. Oral health status is associated with common medical comorbidities in older hospital inpatients. *J. Am. Geriatr. Soc.* **2016**, *64*, 1696–1700. [CrossRef] [PubMed]
7. Bassim, C.W. Oral Health in Healthy Aging. *J. Am. Geriatr. Soc.* **2018**, *66*, 439–440. [CrossRef] [PubMed]
8. Slade, G.D.; Akinkugbe, A.A.; Sanders, A.E. Projections of U.S. Edentulism prevalence following 5 decades of decline. *J. Dent. Res.* **2014**, *93*, 959–965. [CrossRef]
9. Kossioni, A.E.; Hajto-Bryk, J.; Maggi, S.; McKenna, G.; Petrovic, M.; Roller-Wirnsberger, R.E.; Schimmel, M.; Tamulaitiene, M.; Vanobbergen, J.; Muller, F. An Expert Opinion from the European College of Gerodontology and the European Geriatric Medicine Society: European Policy Recommendations on Oral Health in Older Adults. *J. Am. Geriatr. Soc.* **2018**, *66*, 609–613. [CrossRef]
10. Deutsch, A.; Jay, E. Optimising oral health in frail older people. *Aust. Prescr.* **2021**, *44*, 153–160. [CrossRef]
11. Marchini, L.; Hartshorn, J.E.; Cowen, H.; Dawson, D.V.; Johnsen, D.C. A Teaching Tool for Establishing Risk of Oral Health Deterioration in Elderly Patients: Development, Implementation, and Evaluation at a U.S. Dental School. *J. Dent. Educ.* **2017**, *81*, 1283–1290. [CrossRef]
12. Hobdell, M.H.; Oliveira, E.R.; Bautista, R.; Myburgh, N.G.; Lalloo, R.; Narendran, S.; Johnson, N.W. Oral diseases and socio-economic status (SES). *Br. Dent. J.* **2003**, *194*, 91–96. [CrossRef]
13. Broadbent, J.M.; Thomson, W.M.; Poulton, R. Trajectory patterns of dental caries experience in the permanent dentition to the fourth decade of life. *J. Dent. Res.* **2008**, *87*, 69–72. [CrossRef] [PubMed]
14. Slack-Smith, L. How population-level data linkage might impact on dental research. *Community Dent. Oral Epidemiol.* **2012**, *40* (Suppl. S2), 90–94. [CrossRef] [PubMed]
15. Abdi, S.; Spann, A.; Borilovic, J.; de Witte, L.; Hawley, M. Understanding the care and support needs of older people: A scoping review and categorisation using the WHO international classification of functioning, disability and health framework (ICF). *BMC Geriatr.* **2019**, *19*, 195. [CrossRef]
16. McGilton, K.S.; Vellani, S.; Yeung, L.; Chishtie, J.; Commisso, E.; Ploeg, J.; Andrew, M.K.; Ayala, A.P.; Gray, M.; Morgan, D.; et al. Identifying and understanding the health and social care needs of older adults with multiple chronic conditions and their caregivers: A scoping review. *BMC Geriatr.* **2018**, *18*, 231. [CrossRef]
17. Nicolau, B.; Marcenes, W.; Bartley, M.; Sheiham, A. A life course approach to assessing causes of dental caries experience: The relationship between biological, behavioural, socio-economic and psychological conditions and caries in adolescents. *Caries Res.* **2003**, *37*, 319–326. [CrossRef]
18. Marmot, M. *Fair Society, Healthy Lives*; Institute of Health Equity: London, UK, 2013; 74p.
19. Kotronia, E.; Brown, H.; Papacosta, A.O.; Lennon, L.T.; Weyant, R.J.; Whincup, P.H.; Wannamethee, S.G.; Ramsay, S.E. Poor oral health and the association with diet quality and intake in older people in two studies in the UK and USA. *Br. J. Nutr.* **2021**, *126*, 118–130. [CrossRef]
20. Sanders, A. *Social Determinants of Oral Health: Conditions Linked to Socioeconomic Inequalities in Oral Health in the Australian Population*; Australian Institute of Health and Welfare: Canberra, Australia, 2008.
21. Hakeem, F.F.; Bernabe, E.; Sabbah, W. Association between oral health and frailty: A systematic review of longitudinal studies. *Gerodontology* **2019**, *36*, 205–215. [CrossRef] [PubMed]
22. Kimble, R.; McLellan, G.; Lennon, L.T.; Papacosta, A.O.; Weyant, R.J.; Kapila, Y.; Mathers, J.C.; Wannamethee, S.G.; Whincup, P.H.; Ramsay, S.E. Association between oral health markers and decline in muscle strength and physical performance in later life: Longitudinal analyses of two prospective cohorts from the UK and the USA. *Lancet Healthy Longev.* **2022**, *3*, e777–e788. [CrossRef]
23. Young, H.M.; Siegel, E.O.; McCormick, W.C.; Fulmer, T.; Harootyan, L.K.; Dorr, D.A. Interdisciplinary collaboration in geriatrics: Advancing health for older adults. *Nurs. Outlook* **2011**, *59*, 243–250. [CrossRef]
24. Watt, R.; Listl, S.; Peres, M.; Heilman, A. *Social Inequalities in Oral Health: From Evidence to Action*; International Centre for Oral Health Inequalities Research & Policy, University College London: London, UK, 2015.

25. Watt, R.G. From victim blaming to upstream action: Tackling the social determinants of oral health inequalities. *Community Dent. Oral Epidemiol.* **2007**, *35*, 1–11. [CrossRef]
26. Koistinen, S.; Stahlnacke, K.; Olai, L.; Ehrenberg, A.; Carlsson, E. Older people's experiences of oral health and assisted daily oral care in short-term facilities. *BMC Geriatr.* **2021**, *21*, 388. [CrossRef] [PubMed]
27. Baniasadi, K.; Armoon, B.; Higgs, P.; Bayat, A.-H.; Gharehghani, M.; Ali, M.; Hemmat, M.; Fakhri, Y.; Mohammadi, R.; Fattah Moghaddam, L.; et al. The Association of Oral Health Status and socio-economic determinants with Oral Health-Related Quality of Life among the elderly: A systematic review and meta-analysis. *Int. J. Dent. Hyg.* **2021**, *19*, 153–165. [CrossRef] [PubMed]
28. Fisher-Owens, S.A.; Gansky, S.A.; Platt, L.J.; Weintraub, J.A.; Soobader, M.J.; Bramlett, M.D.; Newacheck, P.W. Influences on children's oral health: A conceptual model. *Pediatrics* **2007**, *120*, e510–e520. [CrossRef] [PubMed]
29. Catalyst, N. Social determinants of health (SDOH). *NEJM Catal.* **2017**, *3*. Available online: https://catalyst.nejm.org/doi/full/10.1056/CAT.17.0312?targetBtn=articleToolSaveBtn (accessed on 26 January 2023).
30. Pretty, I.A.; Ellwood, R.P.; Lo, E.C.; MacEntee, M.I.; Müller, F.; Rooney, E.; Murray Thomson, W.; Van der Putten, G.J.; Ghezzi, E.M.; Walls, A. The Seattle Care Pathway for securing oral health in older patients. *Gerodontology* **2014**, *31*, 77–87. [CrossRef]
31. Van der Maarel-Wierink, C.D.; Vanobbergen, J.N.O.; Bronkhorst, E.M.; Schols, J.M.G.A.; de Baat, C. Oral health care and aspiration pneumonia in frail older people: A systematic literature review. *Gerodontology* **2013**, *30*, 3–9. [CrossRef] [PubMed]
32. Mochida, Y.; Yamamoto, T.; Fuchida, S.; Aida, J.; Kondo, K. Does poor oral health status increase the risk of falls? The JAGES Project Longitudinal Study. *PLoS ONE* **2018**, *13*, e0192251. [CrossRef]
33. Halpern, L.R. The Geriatric Syndrome and Oral Health: Navigating Oral Disease Treatment Strategies in the Elderly. *Dent. Clin. N. Am.* **2020**, *64*, 209–228. [CrossRef]
34. Ettinger, R.L.; Beck, J.D. Geriatric dental curriculum and the needs of the elderly. *Spec. Care Dentist.* **1984**, *4*, 207–213. [CrossRef]
35. Craig, T.; Johnsen, D.C.; Hartshorn, J.E.; Cowen, H.; Ashida, S.; Thompson, L.; Pendleton, C.; Xie, X.J.; Marchini, L. Teaching rapid oral health deterioration risk assessment: A 5-year report. *J. Dent. Educ.* **2020**, *84*, 1159–1165. [CrossRef]
36. López-Otín, C.; Blasco, M.A.; Partridge, L.; Serrano, M.; Kroemer, G. The hallmarks of aging. *Cell* **2013**, *153*, 1194–1217. [CrossRef]
37. Inouye, S.K.; Studenski, S.; Tinetti, M.E.; Kuchel, G.A. Geriatric Syndromes: Clinical, Research, and Policy Implications of a Core Geriatric Concept: (See Editorial Comments by Dr. William Hazzard on pp. 794–796). *J. Am. Geriatr. Soc.* **2007**, *55*, 780–791. [CrossRef]
38. Carlson, C.; Merel, S.E.; Yukawa, M. Geriatric syndromes and geriatric assessment for the generalist. *Med. Clin.* **2015**, *99*, 263–279. [CrossRef] [PubMed]
39. Nam, Y.; Kim, N.H.; Kho, H.S. Geriatric oral and maxillofacial dysfunctions in the context of geriatric syndrome. *Oral Dis.* **2018**, *24*, 317–324. [CrossRef] [PubMed]
40. Tôrres, L.H.d.N.; Tellez, M.; Hilgert, J.B.; Hugo, F.N.; de Sousa, M.d.L.R.; Ismail, A.I. Frailty, frailty components, and oral health: A systematic review. *J. Am. Geriatr. Soc.* **2015**, *63*, 2555–2562. [CrossRef]
41. Marchini, L.; Ettinger, R.; Caprio, T.; Jucan, A. Oral health care for patients with Alzheimer's disease: An update. *Spec. Care Dent.* **2019**, *39*, 262–273. [CrossRef]
42. Foley, N.C.; Affoo, R.H.; Siqueira, W.L.; Martin, R.E. A Systematic Review Examining the Oral Health Status of Persons with Dementia. *JDR Clin. Trans. Res.* **2017**, *2*, 330–342. [CrossRef]
43. Bronfenbrenner, U.; Ceci, S.J. Nature-nurture reconceptualized in developmental perspective: A bioecological model. *Psychol. Rev.* **1994**, *101*, 568. [CrossRef] [PubMed]
44. Slack-Smith, L.M.; Hearn, L.; Wilson, D.F.; Wright, F. Geriatric dentistry, teaching and future directions. *Aust. Dent. J.* **2015**, *60* (Suppl. 1), 125–130. [CrossRef]
45. Chen, X.; Mao, G.; Leng, S.X. Frailty syndrome: An overview. *Clin. Interv. Aging* **2014**, *9*, 433.
46. Tinetti, M.; Huang, A.; Molnar, F. The geriatrics 5M's: A new way of communicating what we do. *J. Am. Geriatr. Soc.* **2017**, *65*, 2115. [CrossRef] [PubMed]
47. Rittel, H.; Webber, M. Dilemmas in a general theory of planning. *Policy Sci.* **1973**, *4*, 155. [CrossRef]
48. MacEntee, M.I.; Hole, R.; Stolar, E. The significance of the mouth in old age. *Soc. Sci. Med.* **1997**, *45*, 1449–1458. [CrossRef] [PubMed]
49. World Health Organization. *Global Oral Health Status Report: Towards Universal Health Coverage for Oral Health by 2030*; World Health Organization: Geneva, Switzerland, 2022.

Disclaimer/Publisher's Note: The statements, opinions and data contained in all publications are solely those of the individual author(s) and contributor(s) and not of MDPI and/or the editor(s). MDPI and/or the editor(s) disclaim responsibility for any injury to people or property resulting from any ideas, methods, instructions or products referred to in the content.

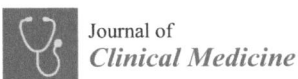

Essay

The Prevention, Diagnosis, and Treatment of Rapid Oral Health Deterioration (ROHD) among Older Adults

Leonardo Marchini [1,*] and Ronald L. Ettinger [2]

[1] Department of Comprehensive Care, Case Western Reserve University School of Dental Medicine, 9601 Chester Ave, Cleveland, OH 44106, USA
[2] Department of Prosthodontics, The University of Iowa College of Dentistry and Dental Clinics, Iowa City, IA 52242, USA
* Correspondence: leonardo.marchini@case.edu

Abstract: The world's population is aging. Older adults are at risk for multiple chronic medical problems as they age. The management of these diseases requires these people to take a variety of medications, which may have undesired side effects. These medical issues can impact oral healthcare and result in a precipitous decline in oral health. A standardized teaching model has been developed to help novice dental practitioners learn how to access and treat oral health problems in older adults. This model is called rapid oral health deterioration (ROHD) risk assessment. The model has four steps for assessment and four categories of risk. This paper describes the components of the ROHD risk assessment, and how it can be used to prevent, diagnose and treat ROHD among older adults.

Keywords: aged; frail elderly; risk assessment; geriatric dentistry

Citation: Marchini, L.; Ettinger, R.L. The Prevention, Diagnosis, and Treatment of Rapid Oral Health Deterioration (ROHD) among Older Adults. *J. Clin. Med.* **2023**, *12*, 2559. https://doi.org/10.3390/jcm12072559

Academic Editor: Denis Bourgeois

Received: 13 February 2023
Revised: 27 March 2023
Accepted: 28 March 2023
Published: 28 March 2023

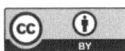

Copyright: © 2023 by the authors. Licensee MDPI, Basel, Switzerland. This article is an open access article distributed under the terms and conditions of the Creative Commons Attribution (CC BY) license (https://creativecommons.org/licenses/by/4.0/).

1. Introduction

Population aging is a well-described demographic fact that is reshaping societies across the globe, especially regarding the way healthcare systems are developed and implemented [1]. These systems have been influenced by an increase in chronic diseases that accompanies aging, resulting in older adults using a disproportional share of the healthcare system [2,3]. The high number of chronic illnesses associated with aging, the social repercussions of aging and retirement, as well as the cumulative nature of the most prevalent oral diseases result in an increased risk for rapid oral health deterioration (ROHD) among older adults. The ROHD concept was developed to identify older patients who experienced a decline in general health as they aged, with a concurrent precipitous decline in their oral health [4]. The increased risk of ROHD might help to explain why so many oral health indicators are poorer among older adults when compared to younger cohorts in most countries [5–8]. This is especially prevalent among the most vulnerable groups, such as institutionalized and homebound older adults [9–12]. Although the consequences of inadequate oral healthcare can be incapacitating, resulting in localized pain and infection, there are circumstances where more serious oral infections can spread and impact systemic health [13,14].

The evidence-based risk factors for ROHD among older adults can be categorized into three main groups, i.e., systemic health conditions, social aspects, and oral health conditions. Among the most prevalent chronic systemic diseases diagnosed in older adults are arthritis [15], hypertension and diabetes [15–17], depression [18,19], neuro-degenerative conditions and dementia [19–21], and stroke [15,22]. Older adults usually need to take many medications to treat their multiple chronic diseases, which results in a condition often referred to as polypharmacy [17,23,24].

Aging does not only consist of the biological processes related to senescence because it is influenced by social conditions and how society reacts to aging. These factors will help to determine how a person ages. Often appropriate social support is lacking [25]. The lack of adequate social support also constitutes an important set of risk factors for ROHD. For instance, the inability to afford oral health care and/or the lack of dental insurance after retirement can be an important access-to-care barrier for older adults. In the US, dental insurance is linked to employment. Consequently, it is lost when a person retires, unless he/she can afford to buy private insurance, or is eligible for Medicaid, whose dental benefits vary by state [5,26,27]. Another important barrier is linked to institutionalization since appropriate oral hygiene routines have consistently been reported to be lacking in long-term care institutions [10,12,28].

As the prevalence of tooth loss has declined globally [29–31], more and more older adults are able to keep their teeth into old age, which is an important positive achievement of both preventive and restorative dentistry programs. As a consequence, oral health conditions also play an important role in the risk of ROHD. Oral health conditions that increase the risk of ROHD include but are not limited to poor oral hygiene, xerostomia, prosthetic status, heavily restored dentitions, and the presence of gingival recession and root exposure [6,23,32]. These oral health problems also play an important role in treatment planning, as they will impact necessary recall schedules and dental treatment outcomes [33].

Geriatric dental medicine programs have focused on teaching the symbiotic relationship among existing systemic health issues, socio-economic problems, and oral conditions, and how they impact treatment planning for older adults [34,35]. However, the concept of ROHD risk assessment has only been introduced recently [36]. The ROHD risk assessment tool simplifies the teaching of treatment planning, as it can be used by students as a standardized model for caring for their older patients. This risk assessment model is also familiar to students, as it was borrowed and modified from one developed for caries risk assessment [37,38].

When treatment planning using the ROHD risk assessment tool, there are primarily four steps to consider [39]:

(1) Data gathering for evidence-based ROHD risk factors;
(2) Data assessment and prioritization (what matters most?);
(3) ROHD risk categorization;
(4) Identifying viable treatment alternatives.

The data for evidence-based risk factors for ROHD are gathered by taking health histories and medication lists during the patient interview. Other evaluations include an extra-oral and intra-oral examination of the patient, as well as complementary examinations, such as radiographs and other imagery, as well as laboratory examinations, pulp tests, and also mounted dental casts. This process will usually result in a sizeable amount of information, and some items are likely to be more significant for oral disease progression and treatment planning than others. It is important for the practitioner to be able to weigh the importance of specific problems in order to appropriately address them during treatment planning.

The third step is to categorize the risk of ROHD, which is a function of the risk factors and disease progression, which can be divided into four risk categories [39]:

(1) Risk factors are not present, and there is no ROHD occurring (Figure 1);
(2) Risk factors are present; ROHD has not started (Figure 2);
(3) Risk factors are present; ROHD is happening (Figure 3);
(4) Risk factors are present; ROHD has already happened (Figure 4).

This step-by-step assessment helps the provider to understand the current influence of risk factors on disease progression in order to evaluate what might happen if no intervention takes place, as well as the possible impact of different types of intervention. As a consequence, it helps the practitioner to choose among different treatment options, such as between more preventive or more invasive options. The treatment of older adults can change with time; therefore, the use of ROHD helps the dentist to be aware of changes in the patient's condition and react appropriately. This step naturally leads to the fourth step, which consists of providing viable treatment alternatives. This includes recommending a specific option and providing the patient and/or caregiver with the rationale for your choice. This will require developing an appropriate communication strategy to address the patient's needs and to be able to explain it to all involved parties, such as family members, caregivers, or person(s) who have the power of attorney, and other healthcare team members.

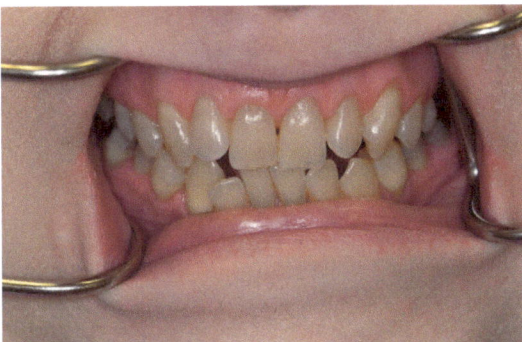

Figure 1. A 62-year-old female has moved to the region recently and seeks treatment. Apart from hypertension, which she controls through diet, medication (thiazide diuretic), and exercise, she has no other systemic diseases. She has all of her dentition, except for the third molar. There is some anterior crowding in the mandible, with minimal bone loss. She has no other important risk factors, and her daily oral hygiene is excellent. This patient represents a person who has no important risk factors, and therefore rapid oral health deterioration is not occurring.

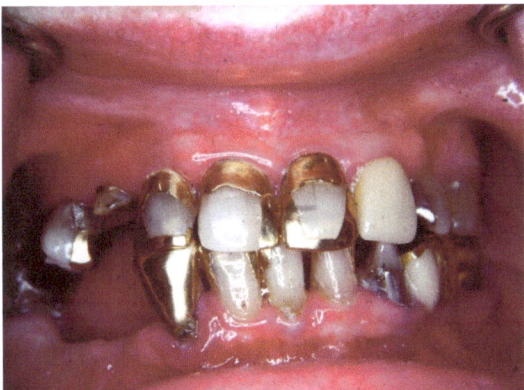

Figure 2. An 82-year-old female is referred for care by her daughter, as the dentist she used to go to has retired. She has a history of allergy to penicillin and sulfa drugs and has been diagnosed with hypertension and coronary artery disease. She also has arthritis in her hips and her hands. She is taking a calcium channel blocker, an ACE inhibitor, and a thiazide diuretic. For her arthritis, she is taking slow-release acetaminophen three times a day. Her chief complaint is that she is beginning to have difficulty eating some of the foods that require more chewing. Her oral examination shows extensive restorative work, which includes several gold inlays. Her periodontal examination revealed no probing depths beyond 3mm and mild bone loss. Although she has a lot of margins at risk, there was no evidence of recurrent caries or root caries. Her treatment will require maintenance care and the addition of a mandibular partial denture. Although the maxillary right lateral incisor is broken down, it was asymptomatic, has no caries or periapical pathology, and she was not concerned with the esthetic correction of this tooth. This patient represents a person who has several important risk factors but does not show any signs of rapid oral health deterioration.

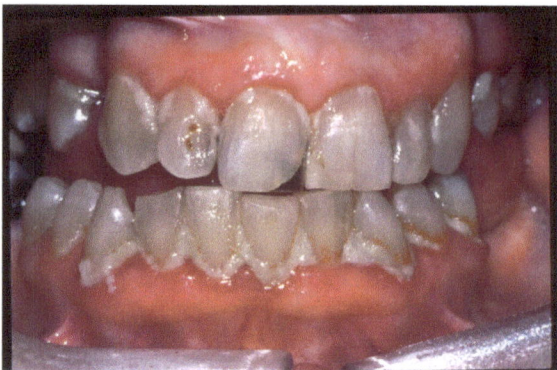

Figure 3. A 75-year-old male was brought to the clinic by his daughter and his wife. The patient has not seen a dentist regularly for the last five years. His wife complains that he is having difficulty eating hard foods. About six months ago, he suffered a cerebral vascular accident that affected the left side of his brain and left him with some weakness in his right side, including aphasia and difficulty walking. Since that time, he also has had difficulty with being able to brush his teeth independently. His other medical problems include hypertension, hypercholesterolemia, arthritis, and type II diabetes. His medications include clopidogrel, metformin, furosemide, potassium, simvastatin, and a calcium channel blocker. An intra-oral examination revealed a dry mouth, heavy plaque, and calculus, especially on the right side of his mouth, accompanied by multiple cervical and coronal carious lesions and marginal gingivitis. His treatment will require significant changes in his daily oral hygiene, which will require his wife to help him. This patient represents a person who has many important risk factors and shows multiple signs that he is developing rapid oral health deterioration.

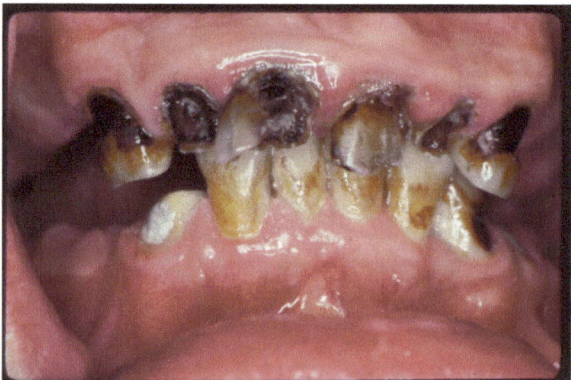

Figure 4. A 65-year-old male is brought for treatment by a social worker as he is in pain. The patient is currently being treated for alcoholism and drug misuse in a hospital setting. He has no family members with whom he is in contact and has been homeless for the last five years. His health history includes smoking a pack of cigarettes a day, hypertension, type II diabetes, osteoporosis, and osteoarthritis. He had not been medicated before hospitalization and is currently receiving naltrexone to help him manage his alcoholism. He is also currently taking an oral antidiabetic, a calcium channel blocker, a thiazide diuretic, and a non-steroidal anti-inflammatory agent. An oral examination revealed multiple carious lesions and root tips, with a sinus tract associated with a mandibular left second premolar root tip, which is the probable cause of his oral pain. The prognosis for his remaining teeth is very poor, and he will need help to find funding for his oral treatment needs. His immediate treatment is the extraction of the infected root tip. This patient represents a person who has many important risk factors, and to whom rapid oral health deterioration has already occurred.

This paper aims to provide some examples of how to use the evidence-based risk factors for ROHD to prevent, diagnose, and treat the consequences of ROHD among the growing population of older adults.

2. Preventing ROHD among Older Adults

Prevention should be part of any treatment planning strategy for all four ROHD categories. For those patients who are not currently experiencing ROHD, a plan to promote a preventive program should be instituted, so that these patients are less likely to ever experience ROHD. For patients who are currently experiencing ROHD, prevention is key to avoiding further progression of ROHD, such as tooth loss, which is an irreversible consequence of ROHD. When ROHD has already occurred, and there are still some teeth remaining that are healthy enough to be used as abutments for a prosthesis, the long-term survival of these abutments relies on preventive measures [39].

Frequent plaque removal is important to reduce plaque accumulation and therefore control the oral bacterial load. However, if people do not brush their teeth frequently, they have more plaque-related issues, which include gingivitis and caries [40]. Unfortunately, frail older adults are often unable to brush their own teeth. This can occur due to cognitive deficits; some of these patients/residents may only need to be reminded to brush their teeth, and some may need to be supervised while brushing so that they brush appropriately. Nevertheless, some patients/residents will need to have their teeth brushed by their caregivers. Another impediment for patients/residents to be able to brush their own teeth may be physical and not cognitive, such as those who do not have the manual dexterity to brush, or whose vision is so poor that they cannot see what they are doing. Patients/residents in this group may be able to brush their teeth if they have larger toothbrush handles and/or power toothbrushes, while others may still need to be helped by a caregiver. Many techniques have been reported for customizing toothbrush handles to allow older adults with impaired manual dexterity to brush their own teeth [41]. Electric toothbrushes usually have larger handles and have been reported to remove plaque more efficiently than conventional toothbrushes when used by patients/residents or a caregiver [42–44].

Increasing exposure to topical fluoride can help reduce caries incidence, arrest existing carious lesions, and prevent new lesions among older adults [45]. A frequently recommended regimen is using 5000 ppm fluoride toothpaste twice a day and having fluoride varnish applied every three to six months. Rising daily with a 0.09% fluoride solution and applying 1.23% fluoride gel every three to six months has also been suggested. This approach, however, presents some challenges, e.g., as the rinse can be easily swallowed by patients with cognitive deficits, and it is difficult for some patients with physical deficits to swish and spit a rinse. In addition, the gel needs to stay in the patient's mouth for four minutes, which can also be difficult for frail older adults [45].

Silver diamine fluoride (SDF) is a topical fluoride agent that has been used for a long time in many countries to arrest and prevent caries and was introduced to the US market in 2014. The active ingredients in SDF are silver, ammonia, and fluoride [46]. Silver ions inhibit bacterial DNA replication, denaturize bacterial cytoplasmic enzymes, and destroy the cell wall, thus reducing the bacterial load. Fluoride and ammonia improve remineralization and induce the formation of fluorapatite [47].

SDF application is simple and cheap. The technique only requires isolating the tooth with cotton rolls, drying it with an air syringe or a cotton pellet, and then applying SDF using a microbrush for about a minute. The excess can be removed using a cotton pellet [48]. SDF has been reported to be safe [48]. and effective for caries prevention, as well as for arresting caries among frail older adults [49,50]. A contraindication to the use of SDF is an allergy to silver. In addition, SDF stains the carious lesion black, and this needs to be carefully discussed with patients and caregivers before applying the SDF [48].

Xerostomia, or dry mouth, is a very common consequence of polypharmacy, which is frequently observed among older adults [51]. Dry mouth is an important risk factor for ROHD, especially because there is a reduction in the protective mechanisms of saliva, which include its buffer capacity, calcium and phosphate replenishment, and antimicrobial activity [52]. Dentists should always consider some important issues when planning dental treatment for patients with dry mouth or xerostomia. This management includes overall hydration, as patients presenting with dehydration produce less saliva. It also includes the relief of discomfort caused by the absence of saliva, which results in a lack of moisture and lubrication. It is also important to take the necessary measures to prevent dental caries and soft tissue trauma. Saliva also plays an important role in retaining and being able to comfortably wear removable dentures; therefore, the dentist should be aware of the role that saliva plays in denture-wearing [53]. Medications play an important role in the genesis of xerostomia. Consequently, dentists should understand the undesirable side effects of their patient's medications, and work with other healthcare team members, notably pharmacists and medical prescribers, to evaluate the patient's medication list in an attempt to reduce their xerostomic effects [53].

After evaluating the patient's hydration level and evaluating their medications to attempt to reduce their xerostomic effect, the dentist can prescribe saliva stimulants or saliva substitutes to reduce the patient's discomfort caused by xerostomia and improve their quality of life [39]. Dehydration is a prevalent issue among older adults. However, patients and caregivers are frequently unaware of this condition, as the feeling of thirst declines with age [54]. One way to combat dry mouth, or xerostomia, is to sip liquids regularly. It is not uncommon for older patients/residents to drink juices or liquids rich in sugar as their beverage of choice, thus increasing their risk of developing caries [39]. Consequently, dentists should inform patients and caregivers about the importance of drinking water. Drinking water helps reduce dehydration, as well as the dry mouth sensation, and does not increase caries risk [54].

Some patients may present with drastically reduced salivary secretory capacity, a condition called hyposalivation [53]. For this group of patients, two approaches can be taken. The first one is trying to increase their salivary output by using saliva stimulants, such as lozenges or chewing non-sugared chewing gums. The other approach is to prescribe drugs that induce increased salivary flow, such as bethanechol, anethole trithione, and pilocarpine [52]. Saliva substitutes are not aimed at inducing salivary flow, but instead serve as a replacement for natural saliva. Common forms of saliva substitutes include sprays, oral rinses, and oral gels. By providing moisture and lubrication, saliva substitutes help reduce the sensation of dry mouth and provide some relief for the patients' discomfort [55]. Dietary changes are another option to reduce the discomfort caused by xerostomia. A less acidic and spicy diet can help to avoid a burning mouth sensation. In addition, there are oral hygiene products specifically formulated for patients with dry mouth, which usually have fewer flavoring agents, such as menthol, and do not use SLS (sodium lauryl sulfate) in their composition [56].

Polypharmacy is a common finding among older adults [17,23,24], and a strong association has been reported between polypharmacy and xerostomia in this age group [51,52]. It has also been reported that medication list reconciliation can help improve patients' overall health outcomes and reduce adverse drug reactions and healthcare costs [57]. The dentist should work with other healthcare team members, especially pharmacists and medical prescribers, to emphasize the deleterious effects of xerostomia on a patient's quality of life and evaluate the patient's medication list in an attempt to reduce the xerostomic effects of the drugs [39].

Xerostomia is an important risk factor for caries among older adults [39]. Therefore, it is important to discuss some strategies which are designed to reduce the risk of developing caries for patients with xerostomia. The dentist should consider customizing these strategies to each individual according to the patient's ability to manage a preventive therapy and reduce their specific risk factors. The main products that can be used to reduce caries risk are products that induce remineralization of the tooth structure, as well as the use of some other topical antimicrobial agents, such as chlorhexidine [39].

A casein phosphopeptide-stabilized–amorphous calcium phosphate nanocomplex, CPP–ACP, which commercially is called Recaldent, was developed and is the active ingredient of a toothpaste: MI Paste (GC America, Alsip, IL, USA), which can be used as a remineralizing product. This product has been used in clinical trials, which have shown it to be beneficial for patients with xerostomia [58]. It acts by helping to increase the availability of calcium and phosphate in saliva, which induces remineralization [59]. This product can be directly applied to the tooth surface; and, when used at bedtime, can also provide some relief from dry mouth [60]. Regular MI Paste does not contain fluoride, but a newer version, MI Paste Plus (GC America, Alsip, IL, USA), does [61].

Fluoride is another product that can be used to reduce caries risk for patients with xerostomia. An approach that has been used consists of a combination of a high-concentration fluoride toothpaste (5000 ppm) to be used twice a day and the application of a fluoride varnish every 3 months [52]. To maximize the benefit of high-fluoride toothpaste, it is important to explain to patients and caregivers they should not rinse their mouth with water after brushing, and only spit after brushing.

Maintaining an appropriate diet that meets the nutritional requirements is indispensable for the overall health and quality of life among older adults [62]. However, the consumption of sugar is a causative factor for caries, and appropriate control of sugar consumption can help reduce the risk of caries [63–65]. Improving diet quality by increasing vegetables and total grains intake has been shown to reduce root surface caries. The consequences of an increased intake of sugar-rich beverages, favored by many older adults, can cause the development of root surface caries [65]. Therefore, it seems important that health practitioners inform patients and caregivers about the importance of having an adequate diet and reducing their consumption of sugar.

3. Diagnosing ROHD among Older Adults

When new patients schedule their first appointment in a typical dental office, they need to fill out some forms about their systemic health and dental histories, and personal and insurance information. In order to fill out these forms, patients need to be cognitively intact, literate and have a reasonable understanding of the information being asked. Unfortunately, this assumption is not true for about 59% of American older adults, who have just a basic or below-proficiency level in health literacy [66]. In addition, slower cognitive processing and visual impairments can also make it more difficult for older adults to process the forms [66].

The forms completed by patients should be used as a means to begin a dialogue with the patients and/or their caregivers, in order to expand the interview, so that the clinician may be aware of all the other possible risk factors influencing the patient's oral health. Empathetic listening is very important to fully investigate the social context, the extent of medical conditions, including the medication list, and to better understand the patient's complaints [33].

When assessing a patient's health history, the clinician should proceed with focused follow-up questions. For instance, if a patient reports a history of *diabetes mellitus type 2*, how does this information influence dental treatment? How is the patient controlling his/her diabetes, and how stable is his/her HbA1c? Did he/she achieve stability through diet and exercise, or is he/she taking an oral antiglycemic medication? Is he/she utilizing insulin, and does he/she have an electronic real-time blood glucose monitor? Unless the patient has had a recent medical appointment or monitors their blood sugar levels on a daily basis, it may be necessary to contact their physician or, if available, to measure their blood glucose level. Prior to treatment, it is also important to investigate if the patient had a meal prior to using their anti-diabetic medication, in order to prevent hypoglycemic episodes. If the patient is stable, then his/her oral health outcomes are less likely to be impacted by the delayed healing or infection related to diabetes. If a surgical procedure is required in an unstable patient with diabetes, it may be necessary to prescribe antibiotics prior to treatment.

Clinical geriatric dental medicine requires data-gathering, in order to problem-solve and make decisions to present patient-centered treatment plans. The factors that influence decision-making and treatment planning for younger adults are relatively simple and are associated with four main factors: first, the patient's willingness to accept the care; second, the patient being able to schedule time for the delivery of the necessary treatment; third, does the patient have the will and the means to pay for the required care? Finally, does their dentist have the skills, the will, and the resources to carry out the planned care or should the patient be referred?

However, when caring for older adults, the problems tend to become much more complex. Consequently, the oral health care provider should possess more experience and skills in decision-making in order to present the patient with an age-appropriate treatment plan. Age-appropriate care should consider the wide range of modifying factors that older persons are subjected to. These factors can be categorized into socioeconomic factors, systemic health problems, pharmacotherapies, and oral health conditions. Socioeconomic factors include barriers and enablers to accessing dental care, such as transportation issues, lack of dental insurance, and being institutionalized. Systemic health problems include their multimorbidities and the side effects of their medications. Their oral health conditions may reflect the cumulative effects of previous and current dental diseases, as well as any iatrogenic effects caused by previous dental care [67,68].

Planning age-appropriate dental treatments for older adults does not require the development of new technical skills. It does require more in-depth knowledge about the physiological, psychological, and pathological changes associated with aging, as well as its socio-economic consequences. This will allow the dentist to understand how the patient functions in their environment, influenced by their modifying factors so that a dental treatment plan can be developed that fits into their way of living. It is imperative that the benefits of treatment must outweigh any risks or problems related to possible adverse events. Ettinger and Beck have developed a concept of treatment planning for older adults named "rational treatment planning" [69].

As stated earlier, diagnosis and treatment planning for older adults require the gathering of information from and about the patient. A tool to help practitioners process the large amount of information gathered from the patient and make these decisions is known as ROHD risk assessment. By analyzing the ROHD risk assessment, the provider should be able to develop rational treatment plans.

4. Treating ROHD among Older Adults

Treatment plans for older patients can vary depending on the severity of their modifying factors. The treatment can generally be divided into four broad groups, listed below.

4.1. Comprehensive Care

To develop an appropriate treatment plan in geriatric dental medicine, the dentist needs to develop skills in problem-solving and decision-making. A treatment plan for older patients should consider all of the modifying factors. These might need to include the patient's medical problems, the side effects of their medications, their socioeconomic status, and any psychological problems they may have. One must also include the iatrogenic effects of previous dental care, which results in cumulative damage to the dentition [67,68].

Treatment planning for older adults does not require the dentist to learn new technical skills. However, the dentist needs to develop new thought processes in order to understand the more complex modifying factors presented by older adults, as well as how these factors influence treatment. The dentist needs to assess and understand how the patients are functioning in their environments and, consequently, assess how their dental treatment impinges on their lifestyle. Therefore, the dentist should also consider if the benefits of the proposed dental care outweigh the inherent risks of adverse events. Ettinger and Beck have developed a concept of decision-making, which they called "rational treatment planning". This concept proposes that the dentist needs to evaluate the patient's modifying factors and develop a treatment plan which is individualized for a patient's needs; this could be no treatment at all, or the most sophisticated treatment dentistry has available [69]. For instance, if a patient has a limited number of treatable risk factors and can tolerate dental treatment, then comprehensive care is possible [33].

Initially, the dentist would scale and clean the teeth and assess the patient's ability to maintain oral hygiene independently. If periodontal pockets exist that are deeper than 3mm, non-surgical periodontal therapy, such as deep scaling and curettage, should be considered. If carious lesions are present, excavating the lesions to determine their depth is important. If the lesion is shallow, it may be possible to remove all the caries and restore the tooth. If the lesion is deep, there is data to support partial caries removal, placement of glass ionomers in the deepest areas, and immediate final restoration with a composite, which has been described as the closed sandwich technique [70]. However, if the lesion is very large or very deep, root canal therapy may be required, followed by crowning the tooth. If there are missing teeth, different prosthetic options will need to be discussed with the patient, which might include removable, fixed, or implant options [33,70].

4.2. Limited Care

If the patient is frail and cannot tolerate long periods in the dental chair, the treatment may need to be modified. It is essential after scaling and cleaning to establish who is responsible for the patient's daily oral hygiene routine because the outcome of treatment is dependent on the quality of the oral hygiene [39].

Among frail older adults, there is a high prevalence of cognitive impairment, multimorbidity, polypharmacy, and inadequate ability to maintain daily oral hygiene. This combination puts the patient at risk for aspiration pneumonia if their plaque is not disturbed every five days [71–73]. Therefore, it is important to improve oral hygiene routines for frail older adults [74]. For frail older adults who need assistance with daily oral hygiene, the dentist needs to help caregivers with overcoming the barriers in order to provide appropriate care for the patient [75].

If the patient has carious lesions, and it is not possible to use a handpiece, atraumatic restorative techniques (ART) are useful. Traditionally, the ART hand excavates the carious lesions and restores them with glass ionomer [76]. It should also include domiciliary preventive measures, such as the use of high-concentration (5000 ppm) fluoride toothpaste, and 6-month recalls [39]. Another option to treat carious lesions, if esthetics is not an issue, is the use of silver diamine fluoride (SDF) to arrest caries, which is associated with regular 6-month recalls and the reapplication of SDF [50]. All of these patients should have fluoride varnish applied to their remaining teeth during the regular recalls [77]. All prostheses can be considered added risk factors for caries and periodontal disease [78]; therefore, not all missing teeth should be replaced unless they are necessary for chewing and eating, or if the patient requests them for esthetic purposes [79].

4.3. Emergency Care (Pain and Infection Control)

The first step in any comprehensive care plan is the treatment of pain and/or infection [80]. For the small group of patients who resist care, it may be the treatment of choice if he or she only seeks care for his/her emergency problem. However, if the patient presents with odontogenic pain and has a dental abscess, the source of the pain needs to be identified and treated. The treatment of the dental abscess will depend upon the size of the lesion and the patient's will and ability to tolerate root canal therapy. Otherwise, the tooth will need to be extracted. The use of oral antibiotics should be limited to patients where there is an increased risk of spread of the infection [81]. If the clinician diagnoses that pain is from a non-odontogenic source, the cause should be identified and treated appropriately [82]. However, referral of the patient to an appropriate medical or dental specialist may be necessary.

4.4. No Treatment

There are circumstances in which a frail older patient presents for dental treatment but has systemic conditions that preclude visits to a dental office, or any invasive procedures in their oral cavity, for example, a patient in the severe stage of Alzheimer's disease who resists care and also has unstable angina, where stress caused by the patient's resistance to care could trigger an adverse cardiovascular event. In such a situation, the family and/or caretaker should be encouraged to daily spray chlorhexidine into the patient's mouth in order to reduce the microbial burden [83].

Occasionally, a patient may seek oral healthcare but, when offered various options for their dental treatment, decides that they do not which to proceed with any of these options. When this happens, the dentist needs to document the refusal in detail in order to avoid any legal consequences. Table 1 summarizes ROHD risk factors, risk categories, and potential treatment modes.

Table 1. Summary of ROHD risk factors, its risk categories, and potential treatment modes.

ROHD risk factors (based on research evidence)
1. General health conditions   -Cognitive deficits   *Alzheimer's, other dementias*   -Functional deficits   *Stroke, osteoarthritis, Parkinson's, etc.*   -Sensory loss   *Speech, sight, hearing, taste*   -Medications   *Oral and systemic side-effects, drug interactions*   -Manageable chronic diseases   *Hypertension, diabetes, osteoporosis, etc.*   -Degree of dependence/autonomy   *Institutionalization, home care, dependence on caregivers, etc.*   -Terminal diseases/palliative care   -Life expectancy   **2. Social support**   -Institutional support   -Family/social support   -Financial issues   *Insurance, Medicaid, Social Security, etc.*   -Expectations   **3. Oral conditions**   -Oral hygiene   -Periodontal condition   -Number of teeth/restorations   -Prosthetic status   *Fixed, removable, implants*   -Oral lesions   *Inflammation, oral cancer*   -Stopped seeing the dentist
Assessment of the Risk for ROHD (based on risk factors and disease progression)
1. Risk factors for ROHD are not present.   2. Patient has risk factors for ROHD but is not currently experiencing ROHD.   3. Patient has risk factors for ROHD and is currently experiencing ROHD.   4. ROHD has occurred.

Table 1. *Cont.*

Treatment alternatives
Comprehensive Care
Limited Care
Emergency Care only
No treatment

5. Conclusions

As older adults age, their risk for multiple chronic medical problems increases. The care and management of these diseases require their physician to prescribe multiple medications, leading to polypharmacy. These medical issues and the side effects of the medications can impact an older adult's oral health and result in rampant caries and severe periodontal disease. For a novice oral health practitioner, understanding the complexities and interrelation of systemic health issues and dental treatment planning is very difficult. Consequently, to guide novices in decision-making, a standardized teaching model was developed. This concept is named the rapid oral health deterioration (ROHD) risk assessment. There are four steps for assessment in the model, as well as four categories of risk. The four steps are (1) data gathering for evidence-based ROHD risk factors, (2) data assessment and prioritization (what matters most?), (3) ROHD risk categorization, and (4) identifying viable treatment alternatives. The four risk categories are (1) risk factors are not present, and there is no ROHD occurring, (2) risk factors are present, ROHD has not started, (3) risk factors are present, and ROHD is happening, and (4) risk factors are present, and ROHD has already happened.

This paper described in detail how to use the ROHD teaching model to develop appropriate/rational treatment plans for frail older adults who have both systemic and oral health problems. If a patient has no risk factors and ROHD is not occurring, the dental treatment for this patient will depend upon the time they have available and their financial resources. If a patient has risk factors, but ROHD has not begun, then it is imperative to focus on preventive measures to avoid severe oral health problems. However, if the patient has risk factors and ROHD has started, it is important, as soon as possible, to restore the oral cavity to health within the constraints of the systemic condition, followed by aggressive preventive procedures. Lastly, if the patient has risk factors and ROHD has occurred, the remaining dentition needs to be evaluated to determine which teeth need to be extracted and which key teeth can be maintained to help support a prosthesis if it is required for appropriate function. In certain circumstances, the risk of oral healthcare is too great, and the only treatment is to try to reduce the microbial burden by the use of chlorhexidine.

Author Contributions: Conceptualization, methodology, formal analysis, data curation, writing—original draft preparation, writing—review and editing, and visualization were all performed together by L.M. and R.L.E. All authors have read and agreed to the published version of the manuscript.

Funding: This research received no external funding.

Informed Consent Statement: Not applicable.

Data Availability Statement: No new data were created or analyzed in this study. Data sharing is not applicable to this article.

Conflicts of Interest: The authors declare no conflict of interest.

References

1. WHO. *World Report on Ageing and Health*; Wolrd Health Organization: Geneva, Switzerland, 2015; p. 260.
2. Prince, M.J.; Wu, F.; Guo, Y.; Gutierrez Robledo, L.M.; O'Donnell, M.; Sullivan, R.; Yusuf, S. The burden of disease in older people and implications for health policy and practice. *Lancet* **2015**, *385*, 549–562. [CrossRef] [PubMed]
3. Banerjee, S. Multimorbidity—Older adults need health care that can count past one. *Lancet* **2015**, *385*, 587–589. [CrossRef]

4. Marchini, L.; Hartshorn, J.E.; Cowen, H.; Dawson, D.V.; Johnsen, D.C. A Teaching Tool for Establishing Risk of Oral Health Deterioration in Elderly Patients: Development, Implementation, and Evaluation at a U.S. Dental School. *J. Dent. Educ.* **2017**, *81*, 1283–1290. [CrossRef] [PubMed]
5. Friedman, P.K.; Kaufman, L.B.; Karpas, S.L. Oral health disparity in older adults: Dental decay and tooth loss. *Dent. Clin. N. Am.* **2014**, *58*, 757–770. [CrossRef] [PubMed]
6. Jablonski, R.Y.; Barber, M.W. Restorative dentistry for the older patient cohort. *Br. Dent. J.* **2015**, *218*, 337–342. [CrossRef] [PubMed]
7. Gil-Montoya, J.A.; de Mello, A.L.; Barrios, R.; Gonzalez-Moles, M.A.; Bravo, M. Oral health in the elderly patient and its impact on general well-being: A nonsystematic review. *Clin. Interv. Aging* **2015**, *10*, 461–467. [CrossRef]
8. Thomson, W.M. Dental caries experience in older people over time: What can the large cohort studies tell us? *Br. Dent. J.* **2004**, *196*, 89–92, discussion 87. [CrossRef]
9. Ornstein, K.; DeCherrie, L.; Gluzman, R.; Scott, E.; Kansal, J.; Shah, T.; Katz, R.; Soriano, T.A. Significant Unmet Oral Health Needs of Homebound Elderly Adults. *J. Am. Geriatr. Soc.* **2015**, *63*, 151–157. [CrossRef]
10. Marchini, L.; Recker, E.; Hartshorn, J.; Cowen, H.; Lynch, D.; Drake, D.; Blanchette, D.R.; Dawson, D.V.; Kanellis, M.; Caplan, D. Iowa nursing facility oral hygiene (INFOH) intervention: A clinical and microbiological pilot randomized trial. *Spec. Care Dent.* **2018**, *38*, 345–355. [CrossRef]
11. Mendes, M.S.S.; Chester, L.N.; Fernandes Dos Santos, J.F.; Chen, X.; Caplan, D.J.; Marchini, L. Self-perceived oral health among institutionalized older adults in Taubate, Brazil. *Spec. Care Dent.* **2020**, *40*, 49–54. [CrossRef]
12. De Visschere, L.M.; Grooten, L.; Theuniers, G.; Vanobbergen, J.N. Oral hygiene of elderly people in long-term care institutions–a cross-sectional study. *Gerodontology* **2006**, *23*, 195–204. [CrossRef]
13. Scannapieco, F.A.; Cantos, A. Oral inflammation and infection, and chronic medical diseases: Implications for the elderly. *Periodontol. 2000* **2016**, *72*, 153–175. [CrossRef] [PubMed]
14. Ramsay, S.E.; Whincup, P.H.; Watt, R.G.; Tsakos, G.; Papacosta, A.O.; Lennon, L.T.; Wannamethee, S.G. Burden of poor oral health in older age: Findings from a population-based study of older British men. *BMJ Open* **2015**, *5*, e009476. [CrossRef]
15. Tavares, M.; Lindefjeld Calabi, K.A.; San Martin, L. Systemic diseases and oral health. *Dent. Clin. N. Am.* **2014**, *58*, 797–814. [CrossRef]
16. Eke, P.I.; Wei, L.; Borgnakke, W.S.; Thornton-Evans, G.; Zhang, X.; Lu, H.; McGuire, L.C.; Genco, R.J. Periodontitis prevalence in adults $\geq$ 65 years of age, in the USA. *Periodontol. 2000* **2016**, *72*, 76–95. [CrossRef] [PubMed]
17. de Deco, C.P.; do Santos, J.F.; da Cunha, V.E.P.; Marchini, L. General health of elderly institutionalised and community-dwelling Brazilians. *Gerodontology* **2007**, *24*, 136–142. [CrossRef] [PubMed]
18. Hybels, C.F.; Bennett, J.M.; Landerman, L.R.; Liang, J.; Plassman, B.L.; Wu, B. Trajectories of depressive symptoms and oral health outcomes in a community sample of older adults. *Int. J. Geriatr. Psychiatry* **2016**, *31*, 83–91. [CrossRef]
19. Brennan, L.J.; Strauss, J. Cognitive impairment in older adults and oral health considerations: Treatment and management. *Dent. Clin. N. Am.* **2014**, *58*, 815–828. [CrossRef]
20. Machado, M.C.; Lopes, G.H.; Marchini, L. Oral health of Alzheimer's patients in Sao Jose dos Campos, Brazil. *Geriatr. Gerontol. Int.* **2012**, *12*, 265–270. [CrossRef]
21. Ni Chroinin, D.; Montalto, A.; Jahromi, S.; Ingham, N.; Beveridge, A.; Foltyn, P. Oral Health Status Is Associated with Common Medical Comorbidities in Older Hospital Inpatients. *J. Am. Geriatr. Soc.* **2016**, *64*, 1696–1700. [CrossRef]
22. Lam, O.L.; McMillan, A.S.; Samaranayake, L.P.; Li, L.S.; McGrath, C. Effect of oral hygiene interventions on opportunistic pathogens in patients after stroke. *Am. J. Infect. Control* **2013**, *41*, 149–154. [CrossRef]
23. Singh, M.L.; Papas, A. Oral implications of polypharmacy in the elderly. *Dent. Clin. N. Am.* **2014**, *58*, 783–796. [CrossRef] [PubMed]
24. de Deco, C.P.; Reis, M.R.V.S.; Marchini, A.M.P.S.; da Rocha, R.F.; dos Santos, M.B.F.; Marchini, L. Taste alteration, mouth dryness and teeth staining as side effects of medications taken by elderly. *Braz. J. Oral Sci.* **2014**, *13*, 257–260. [CrossRef]
25. World Health Organization. *Global Report on Ageims*; WHO: Geneva, Switzerland, 2021; 173 p.
26. Manski, R.J.; Moeller, J.F.; Chen, H.; Schimmel, J.; Pepper, J.V.; St Clair, P.A. Dental use and expenditures for older uninsured Americans: The simulated impact of expanded coverage. *Health Serv. Res.* **2015**, *50*, 117–135. [CrossRef]
27. Manski, R.J.; Cohen, L.A.; Brown, E.; Carper, K.V.; Vargas, C.; Macek, M.D. Dental service mix among older adults aged 65 and over, United States, 1999 and 2009. *J. Public Health Dent.* **2014**, *74*, 219–226. [CrossRef]
28. Marchini, L.; Vieira, P.C.; Bossan, T.P.; Montenegro, F.L.; Cunha, V.P. Self-reported oral hygiene habits among institutionalised elderly and their relationship to the condition of oral tissues in Taubaté, Brazil. *Gerodontology* **2006**, *23*, 33–37. [CrossRef] [PubMed]
29. Slade, G.D.; Akinkugbe, A.A.; Sanders, A.E. Projections of U.S. Edentulism prevalence following 5 decades of decline. *J. Dent. Res.* **2014**, *93*, 959–965. [CrossRef] [PubMed]
30. Dye, B.A.; Weatherspoon, D.J.; Lopez Mitnik, G. Tooth loss among older adults according to poverty status in the United States from 1999 through 2004 and 2009 through 2014. *J. Am. Dent. Assoc.* **2019**, *150*, 9–23.e3. [CrossRef] [PubMed]
31. Müller, F.; Naharro, M.; Carlsson, G.E. What are the prevalence and incidence of tooth loss in the adult and elderly population in Europe? *Clin. Oral Implants Res.* **2007**, *18* (Suppl. S3), 2–14. [CrossRef]
32. Hayes, M.; Da Mata, C.; Cole, M.; McKenna, G.; Burke, F.; Allen, P.F. Risk indicators associated with root caries in independently living older adults. *J. Dent.* **2016**, *51*, 8–14. [CrossRef]

33. Ettinger, R.L. Treatment planning concepts for the ageing patient. *Aust. Dent. J.* **2015**, *60* (Suppl. S1), 71–85. [CrossRef]
34. Ettinger, R.; Goettsche, Z.; Qian, F. Pre-doctoral Teaching of Geriatric Dentistry in US Dental Schools. *J. Dent. Educ.* **2017**, *81*, 921–928. [CrossRef]
35. Marchini, L.; Montenegro, F.R.E. Gerodontology as a dental specialty in Brazil: What has been accomplished after 15 years? *Braz. Dent. Sci.* **2016**, *19*, 10–17. [CrossRef]
36. Craig, T.; Johnsen, D.C.; Hartshorn, J.E.; Cowen, H.; Ashida, S.; Thompson, L.; Msc, C.P.; Xie, X.J.; Marchini, L. Teaching rapid oral health deterioration risk assessment: A 5-year report. *J. Dent. Educ.* **2020**, *84*, 1159–1165. [CrossRef]
37. Featherstone, J.D.; Adair, S.M.; Anderson, M.H.; Berkowitz, R.J.; Bird, W.F.; Crall, J.J.; Besten, P.K.D.; Donly, K.J.; Glassman, P.; Milgrom, P.; et al. Caries management by risk assessment: Consensus statement, April 2002. *J. Calif. Dent. Assoc.* **2003**, *31*, 257–269. [CrossRef] [PubMed]
38. Guzman-Armstrong, S.; Warren, J.J.; Cunningham-Ford, M.A.; von Bergmann, H.; Johnsen, D.C. Concepts in critical thinking applied to caries risk assessment in dental education. *J. Dent. Educ.* **2014**, *78*, 914–920. [CrossRef]
39. Marchini, L.; Ettinger, R.; Hartshorn, J. Personalized Dental Caries Management for Frail Older Adults and Persons with Special Needs. *Dent. Clin. N. Am.* **2019**, *63*, 631–651. [CrossRef]
40. Kumar, S.; Tadakamadla, J.; Johnson, N.W. Effect of Toothbrushing Frequency on Incidence and Increment of Dental Caries: A Systematic Review and Meta-Analysis. *J. Dent. Res.* **2016**, *95*, 1230–1236. [CrossRef] [PubMed]
41. Reeson, M.G.; Jepson, N.J. Customizing the size of toothbrush handles for patients with restricted hand and finger movement. *J. Prosthet. Dent.* **2002**, *87*, 700. [CrossRef] [PubMed]
42. Yaacob, M.; Worthington, H.V.; Deacon, S.A.; Deery, C.; Walmsley, A.D.; Robinson, P.G.; Glenny, A.-M. Powered versus manual toothbrushing for oral health. *Cochrane Database Syst. Rev.* **2014**, *2014*, Cd002281. [CrossRef]
43. De Visschere, L.M.; van der Putten, G.J.; Vanobbergen, J.N.; Schols, J.M.; de Baat, C. Dutch Association of Nursing Home Physicians. An oral health care guideline for institutionalised older people. *Gerodontology* **2011**, *28*, 307–310. [CrossRef]
44. Papas, A.S.; Singh, M.; Harrington, D.; Ortblad, K.; de Jager, M.; Nunn, M. Reduction in caries rate among patients with xerostomia using a power toothbrush. *Spec. Care Dent.* **2007**, *27*, 46–51. [CrossRef]
45. Weyant, R.J.; Tracy, S.L.; Anselmo, T.T.; Beltran-Aguilar, E.D.; Donly, K.J.; Frese, W.A.; Hujoel, P.P.; Iafolla, T.; Kohn, W.; Kumar, J.; et al. Topical fluoride for caries prevention: Executive summary of the updated clinical recommendations and supporting systematic review. *J. Am. Dent. Assoc.* **2013**, *144*, 1279–1291. [CrossRef]
46. Crystal, Y.O.; Niederman, R. Evidence-Based Dentistry Update on Silver Diamine Fluoride. *Dent. Clin. N. Am.* **2019**, *63*, 45–68. [CrossRef] [PubMed]
47. Peng, J.J.; Botelho, M.G.; Matinlinna, J.P. Silver compounds used in dentistry for caries management: A review. *J. Dent.* **2012**, *40*, 531–541. [CrossRef]
48. Horst, J.A.; Ellenikiotis, H.; Milgrom, P.L. UCSF Protocol for Caries Arrest Using Silver Diamine Fluoride: Rationale, Indications and Consent. *J. Calif. Dent. Assoc.* **2016**, *44*, 16–28. [CrossRef]
49. Oliveira, B.H.; Cunha-Cruz, J.; Rajendra, A.; Niederman, R. Controlling caries in exposed root surfaces with silver diamine fluoride: A systematic review with meta-analysis. *J. Am. Dent. Assoc.* **2018**, *149*, 671–679.e1. [CrossRef] [PubMed]
50. Hendre, A.D.; Taylor, G.W.; Chavez, E.M.; Hyde, S. A systematic review of silver diamine fluoride: Effectiveness and application in older adults. *Gerodontology* **2017**, *34*, 411–419. [CrossRef] [PubMed]
51. Storbeck, T.; Qian, F.; Marek, C.; Caplan, D.; Marchini, L. Dose-dependent association between xerostomia and number of medications among older adults. *Spec. Care Dent.* **2022**, *42*, 225–231. [CrossRef] [PubMed]
52. Su, N.; Marek, C.L.; Ching, V.; Grushka, M. Caries prevention for patients with dry mouth. *J. Can. Dent. Assoc.* **2011**, *77*, b85.
53. Thomson, W.M. Dry mouth and older people. *Aust. Dent. J.* **2015**, *60* (Suppl. S1), 54–63. [CrossRef] [PubMed]
54. Abdallah, L.; Remington, R.; Houde, S.; Zhan, L.; Melillo, K.D. Dehydration reduction in community-dwelling older adults: Perspectives of community health care providers. *Res. Gerontol. Nurs.* **2009**, *2*, 49–57. [CrossRef] [PubMed]
55. Jose, A.; Atassi, M.; Shneyer, L.; Cronin, M. A Randomized Clinical Trial to Measure Mouth Moisturization and Dry Mouth Relief in Dry Mouth Subjects Using Dry Mouth Products. *J. Clin. Dent.* **2017**, *28*, 32–38.
56. Hitz Lindenmuller, I.; Lambrecht, J.T. Oral care. *Curr. Probl. Dermatol.* **2011**, *40*, 107–115.
57. Rose, A.J.; Fischer, S.H.; Paasche-Orlow, M.K. Beyond Medication Reconciliation: The Correct Medication List. *Jama* **2017**, *317*, 2057–2058. [CrossRef]
58. Cochrane, N.J.; Cai, F.; Huq, N.L.; Burrow, M.F.; Reynolds, E.C. New approaches to enhanced remineralization of tooth enamel. *J. Dent. Res.* **2010**, *89*, 1187–1197. [CrossRef] [PubMed]
59. Huq, N.L.; Myroforidis, H.; Cross, K.J.; Stanton, D.P.; Veith, P.D.; Ward, B.R.; Reynolds, E.C. The Interactions of CPP-ACP with Saliva. *Int. J. Mol. Sci.* **2016**, *17*, 915. [CrossRef] [PubMed]
60. Sbaraini, A.; Adams, G.G.; Reynolds, E.C. Experiences of oral health: Before, during and after becoming a regular user of GC Tooth Mousse Plus(®). *BMC Oral Health* **2021**, *21*, 14. [CrossRef]
61. Raphael, S.; Blinkhorn, A. Is there a place for Tooth Mousse in the prevention and treatment of early dental caries? A systematic review. *BMC Oral Health* **2015**, *15*, 113. [CrossRef]
62. Leslie, W.; Hankey, C. Aging, Nutritional Status and Health. *Healthcare* **2015**, *3*, 648–658. [CrossRef]
63. Sheiham, A.; James, W.P. A reappraisal of the quantitative relationship between sugar intake and dental caries: The need for new criteria for developing goals for sugar intake. *BMC Public Health* **2014**, *14*, 863. [CrossRef]

64. Bailey, R.L.; Ledikwe, J.H.; Smiciklas-Wright, H.; Mitchell, D.C.; Jensen, G.L. Persistent oral health problems associated with comorbidity and impaired diet quality in older adults. *J. Am. Diet. Assoc.* **2004**, *104*, 1273–1276. [CrossRef] [PubMed]
65. Kaye, E.K.; Heaton, B.; Sohn, W.; Rich, S.E.; Spiro, A., 3rd; Garcia, R.I. The Dietary Approaches to Stop Hypertension Diet and New and Recurrent Root Caries Events in Men. *J. Am. Geriatr. Soc.* **2015**, *63*, 1812–1819. [CrossRef] [PubMed]
66. McGee, J. Things to know if your written material is for older adults. In *Toolkit for Making Written Material Clear and Effective*, 1st ed.; McGee, J., Ed.; Centers for Medicare & Medicaid Services: Washington, DC, USA, 2010; pp. 1–10.
67. Berkey, D.B. Clinical decision-making for the geriatric dental patient. *Gerodontics* **1988**, *4*, 321–326.
68. Ettinger, R.L. Rational dental care: Part 1. Has the concept changed in 20 years? *J. Can. Dent. Assoc.* **2006**, *72*, 441–445.
69. Ettinger, R.; Beck, J.D.; Jakobsen, J. The development of teaching programs in geriatric dentistry in the United States from 1974 to 1979. *Spec. Care Dent.* **1981**, *1*, 221–224. [CrossRef] [PubMed]
70. Ettinger, R.L.; Marchini, L.; Hartshorn, J. Consideration in Planning Dental Treatment for Older Adults. *Dent. Clin. N. Am.* **2020**, *65*, 361–376. [CrossRef]
71. Bassim, C.W.; Gibson, G.; Ward, T.; Paphides, B.M.; Denucci, D.J. Modification of the risk of mortality from pneumonia with oral hygiene care. *J. Am. Geriatr. Soc.* **2008**, *56*, 1601–1607. [CrossRef]
72. Quagliarello, V.; Ginter, S.; Han, L.; Van Ness, P.; Allore, H.; Tinetti, M. Modifiable risk factors for nursing home-acquired pneumonia. *Clin. Infect. Dis.* **2005**, *40*, 1–6. [CrossRef]
73. Tada, A.; Miura, H. Prevention of aspiration pneumonia (AP) with oral care. *Arch. Gerontol. Geriatr.* **2012**, *55*, 16–21. [CrossRef]
74. Coleman, P. Improving oral health care for the frail elderly: A review of widespread problems and best practices. *Geriatr. Nurs.* **2002**, *23*, 189–199. [CrossRef]
75. de Lugt-Lustig, K.H.; Vanobbergen, J.N.; van der Putten, G.J.; De Visschere, L.M.; Schols, J.M.; de Baat, C. Effect of oral healthcare education on knowledge, attitude and skills of care home nurses: A systematic literature review. *Community Dent. Oral Epidemiol.* **2014**, *42*, 88–96. [CrossRef] [PubMed]
76. da Mata, C.; Allen, P.F.; McKenna, G.; Cronin, M.; O'Mahony, D.; Woods, N. Two-year survival of ART restorations placed in elderly patients: A randomised controlled clinical trial. *J. Dent.* **2015**, *43*, 405–411. [CrossRef] [PubMed]
77. Gluzman, R.; Katz, R.V.; Frey, B.J.; McGowan, R. Prevention of root caries: A literature review of primary and secondary preventive agents. *Spec. Care Dent.* **2013**, *33*, 133–140. [CrossRef] [PubMed]
78. Mengatto, C.M.; Marchini, L.; Bernardes, L.A.; Gomes, S.C.; Silva, A.M.; Rizzatti-Barbosa, C.M. Partial denture metal framework may harbor potentially pathogenic bacteria. *J. Adv. Prosthodont.* **2015**, *7*, 468–474. [CrossRef] [PubMed]
79. McKenna, G.; Allen, F.; Woods, N.; O'Mahony, D.; Cronin, M.; DaMata, C.; Normand, C. Cost-effectiveness of tooth replacement strategies for partially dentate elderly: A randomized controlled clinical trial. *Community Dent. Oral Epidemiol.* **2014**, *42*, 366–374. [CrossRef] [PubMed]
80. Stefanac, S.J. Acute Phase of Treatmet. In *Diagnosis and Treatment Planning in Dentistry*, 3rd ed.; Stefanac, S.J., Nesbit, S.P., Eds.; Elsevier: St. Louis, MO, USA, 2017; pp. 173–190.
81. Fouad, A.F.; Rivera, E.M.; Walton, R.E. Penicillin as a supplement in resolving the localized acute apical abscess. *Oral Surg. Oral Med. Oral Pathol. Oral Radiol. Endod.* **1996**, *81*, 590–595. [CrossRef] [PubMed]
82. Renton, T. Chronic Pain and Overview or Differential Diagnoses of Non-odontogenic Orofacial Pain. *Prim. Dent. J.* **2019**, *7*, 71–86. [CrossRef]
83. Chalmers, J.; Pearson, A. Oral hygiene care for residents with dementia: A literature review. *J. Adv. Nurs.* **2005**, *52*, 410–419. [CrossRef]

Disclaimer/Publisher's Note: The statements, opinions and data contained in all publications are solely those of the individual author(s) and contributor(s) and not of MDPI and/or the editor(s). MDPI and/or the editor(s) disclaim responsibility for any injury to people or property resulting from any ideas, methods, instructions or products referred to in the content.

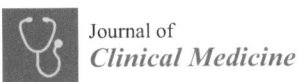

Article

Prevalence of Possible Dementia in Patients with Maxillofacial Defects and Difficulty of Inserting Obturator in Maxillectomy Patients: Toward Better Provision of Supportive Care

Hongli Yu, Haruka Fujita, Masako Akiyama, Yuka I. Sumita * and Noriyuki Wakabayashi

Department of Advanced Prosthodontics, Graduate School of Medical and Dental Sciences, Tokyo Medical and Dental University, Tokyo 113-8510, Japan
* Correspondence: yuka.mfp@tmd.ac.jp; Tel.: +81-3-5803-4757

Abstract: As society ages, it is important to understand the prevalence of dementia and the difficulties of inserting prostheses in patients with maxillofacial defects in order to clarify issues in supportive care. We screened 183 patients for dementia using the revised Hasegawa's dementia scale (HDS-R) at the Clinic for Maxillofacial prosthetics, Tokyo Medical and Dental University, and investigated age and sex differences in HDS-R score. We asked 47 of the 183 participants about the difficulty of inserting a maxillofacial obturator prosthesis and collected subjective comments, information about the prosthesis, and data from five assessments. Multiple regression analysis was used to reveal factors associated with insertion difficulty. Overall, 8.7% of the participants were judged to have possible dementia. Men were more likely than women to have possible dementia, and the risk increased with age. Of the 47 participants, 26 reported difficulty inserting their prosthesis, 12 of whom attributed it to their oral defect. Fourteen patients advised following doctor's instructions to practice insertion in order to become accustomed to it. A lower HDS-R score had a significant impact on insertion difficulty. Cognitive function and difficulty inserting maxillary obturator prostheses should be considered in the provision of continuous supportive care to patients with maxillary defects.

Keywords: dementia; Hasegawa's dementia scale; defect; maxillofacial prosthetics; difficulty of inserting maxillofacial prostheses

1. Introduction

Maxillofacial prosthodontics provides prosthetic rehabilitation for functions such as speech, swallowing, mastication, and esthetics and is a well-recognized subspecialty of prosthodontics [1–3]. In 2018, Yanagi et al. conducted a study at the Clinic for Maxillofacial Prosthetics, Tokyo Medical and Dental University, and found that the average age of patients had shown an increasing trend over the previous 35 years and that almost 80% of patients had developed tumors in Japan's now super-aging society [4], and we feel that this could be even higher now. Aging causes various problems, not only in oral function but also in manual dexterity, grip strength, cognition, and other areas [5]. In fact, the number of older adults with dementia in Japan was estimated to be 4.62 million in 2012 and is projected to reach about 7 million by 2025, affecting nearly 1 in 5 people over the age of 65 years [6]. People with dementia experience memory loss and poor judgment and may take longer to complete normal daily tasks. Thus, the providers of medical and dental care cannot ignore problems associated with dementia. In the field of maxillofacial prosthetic treatment in particular, the current status of the care system must be considered for several reasons. The patient population is elderly and aging [4]. In addition, the structure of maxillofacial prostheses is quite unique compared with general prostheses, and the oral cavity is sensitive and prone to bleeding, especially in maxillectomy patients. Sumita et al. reported a case in which a maxillectomy patient experienced difficulty inserting his maxillary obturator prosthesis after developing cerebrovascular disease and dementia [3]. However, there

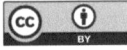

has been no report on the actual situation of patients who need maxillofacial prosthetic treatment from the perspective of dementia and patient-reported difficulty of inserting prostheses. To clarify the issues in providing supportive care, including terminal care, to patients with maxillofacial defects, it is important to determine the prevalence of dementia and the factors associated with patients' difficulties in inserting maxillofacial prostheses.

Many scales for dementia screening are available, including the clinical dementia rating (CDR), mini-mental state examination (MMSE), Montreal cognitive assessment (MoCA), Addenbrooke's cognitive examination-III (ACE-III), and the revised Hasegawa's dementia scale (HDS-R). The CDR has high validity and reliability for this purpose but requires a considerable amount of data from both the patient as well as an informant [7]. The MMSE is the most widely used screening method for cognitive impairment, including dementia, but its level of sensitivity and specificity for dementia has been criticized because it was originally developed to evaluate elderly psychiatric patients rather than people with dementia [8,9]. The MoCA-J is the Japanese translation of the original English version of the MoCA and was translated by a Japanese geriatrician and a Japanese psychologist. The MoCA-J was finalized after a pilot study involving 20 elderly volunteers. The diagnostic accuracy of the MoCA-J for detecting Alzheimer's disease in healthy individuals (100% sensitivity and 89% specificity) was found to be superior to that of the MMSE (97% and 89%, respectively) but slightly inferior to that of the HDS-R (97% and 97%, respectively) [10]. The ACE-III is a screening technique that can differentiate patients with and without cognitive impairment and shows high sensitivity for the early stages of dementia [11]. Its subdomains are significantly correlated with neuropsychological tests specific to the domains assessed [11]. However, ACE-III has 100 items and takes 20 min to complete [11]. The HDS-R is the revised version of the HDS, a brief cognitive scale developed by Hasegawa in 1974 to screen for dementia [12]. The HDS-R is widely used both in the clinical setting and in epidemiological research in Japan and was developed after considering its feasibility for worldwide use [12]. It examines the main areas of cognitive function, including orientation, attention, language, and memory. Studies have shown that the HDS-R has high sensitivity for detecting Alzheimer's disease in healthy individuals. The HDS-R is commonly used as a screening instrument in hospitals and welfare facilities for the elderly and in epidemiological surveys in Japan [13]. The scale can be completed in a short time (about 5 min) [14], has no movement-related or visual tasks, and is easy for healthy elderly people to complete. A study in the United Kingdom showed an increased incidence of dementia with age and the apparent influence of sex in Alzheimer's disease [15]. Another study showed that Alzheimer's disease and other dementias disproportionately affect women [16]. However, the applicability of these findings in elderly people with head and neck defects is not known.

Maxillofacial prostheses are an important tool in providing continuous supportive care to patients with maxillofacial defects, including in terminal care [1,2]. In other words, many patients would have difficulty surviving in daily life without their maxillofacial prosthesis [3]. Thus, ongoing care to enable their continuous use of the prosthesis is important. However, there has been no report focusing on patient-reported problems in inserting an obturator after maxillectomy. Additionally, patients' approaches for overcoming these problems have not been shared. Thus, it is necessary to collect patients' comments, opinions, and concerns about obturator insertion in order to provide a suitable clinical flow and effective care and to give appropriate advice to those who have difficulty inserting their obturator.

To provide supportive care for maxillectomy patients, it is necessary to analyze which factors may cause difficulty with inserting maxillary obturator prostheses. Insertion difficulty can be objectively reflected by the time taken to insert the prosthesis. The main factor expected to be related to insertion difficulty is the structure of the prosthesis and the cognitive and physical functioning of the patient. Structural factors for maxillary obturator prostheses include their weight, height, and clasps. We speculated that with increasing obturator height, the higher number of clasps would lead to greater weight and would increase the difficulties that patients experienced during prosthesis insertion. For patient factors, on the other hand, physical function, manual dexterity, coordination, strength, and cognitive function all decline with age [17], and we therefore speculated that these declines would increase the difficulties patients experience when inserting their prosthesis.

The aim of this study was to determine the prevalence of possible dementia at a maxillofacial prosthetic clinic in order to collect the patients' subjective comments about the difficulty of inserting their maxillofacial obturator prosthesis and to reveal the factors associated with such difficulty after maxillectomy.

2. Materials and Methods

Informed consent was obtained before participation in the study, which was approved by the Ethics Committee of the Faculty of Dentistry, Tokyo Medical and Dental University (approval number D2016-012).

2.1. Participants

In part I of this study, patients aged 65 years or older who attended the maxillofacial prosthetics clinic at the Tokyo Medical and Dental University Dental Hospital between 2016 and 2022 were recruited, and 183 patients (100 men, and 83 women) agreed to participate in our survey regarding the possible prevalence of dementia.

In part II, 56 of the 183 patients who participated in the survey on dementia who had a maxillary defect and used a maxilla obturator prosthesis after maxillectomy were recruited between October 2020 and November 2022. Nine of the participants discontinued treatment for personal reasons and were excluded from the analysis. The remaining 47 patients (23 men, 24 women) completed a questionnaire and five assessments: the HDS-R, the Purdue Pegboard Test (PPT), maxillary obturator prosthesis insertion time, grip strength, and the understanding of the intraoral surgical site. In some cases, tests were completed over two visits to minimize the burden on the patient and prevent fatigue from affecting the results.

2.2. Part I: Survey on the Prevalence of Possible Dementia

Participants completed the HDS-R in a face-to-face setting (Table 1). The nine items of the HDS-R are as follows: item 1 concerns age (1 point) and tests self-orientation; item 2 concerns the date (4 points) and tests the relationship to time; item 3 concerns the location (2 points) and tests orientation to place; item 4 is the repetition of three familiar words (3 points), which tests the immediate memory; item 5 involves the subtraction of 7s from 100 (2 points), which assesses computational ability, immediate memory, and working memory; item 6 involves the backward repetition of three and four digits (2 points), which tests working memory; item 7 involves the recall of the three words out of four (6 points), which tests recent memory; item 8 involves the immediate recall of five objects that are shown then hidden (5 points), which tests the immediate memory and visual memory; and item 9 involves the listing of 10 vegetable names (5 points) tests language fluency [12,18]. The maximum score on the HDS-R is 30 points. A score of 20 or less is indicative of possible dementia, and a score of 10 or less is indicative of severe dementia.

Table 1. The revised Hasegawa's dementia scale.

Item No.	Questions		Score
1	Age (1 point if correct within ±2 years)		0, 1
2	Year, month, date, day (1 point each)	Year	0, 1
		Month	0, 1
		Date	0, 1
		Day	0, 1
3	Current location (2 points for a correct answer given within 5 s; 1 point for correct choice between hospital and office)		0, 1, 2
4	Repeating 3 words (1 point each; use only one version per test) 1 (a) cherry blossom, (b) cat, (c) train; 2 (a) plum blossom, (b) dog, (c) car		0, 1 0, 1 0, 1
5	100 − 7 = ? (1 point for the correct answer; if not correct, skip to item 6) −7 again = ? (1 point for a correct answer)	(93) (86)	0, 1 0, 1
6	Repeating 6-8-2 backward (Skip to item 7 if not correct answer) Repeating 3-5-2-9 backward	2-8-6 9-2-5-3	0, 1 0, 1
7	Recalling 3 words from item 4. (2 points for spontaneous recall; 1 point for a correct recall after category cue) (a) plant, (b) animal, (c) transportation		a: 0, 1, 2 b: 0, 1, 2 c: 0, 1, 2
8	Recalling 5 unrelated common objects after they are shown and then covered (Scissors, mirror, battery, pen, coin, etc.)		0, 1, 2 3, 4, 5
9	Naming all vegetables that come to mind (Stop after a 10 s interval with no response) 0–5 = 0 points, 6 = 1 point, 7 = 2 points, 8 = 3 points, 9 = 4 points, 10 = 5 points		0, 1, 2 3, 4, 5
	Total score		

2.3. Part II: Difficulty Inserting a Maxillary Obturator Prosthesis after Maxillectomy

2.3.1. Questionnaire

Participants completed a three-part questionnaire. The first part was a subjective evaluation by the patients concerning the difficulties they experienced when inserting their maxillary obturator prosthesis, as measured on a visual analogue scale (VAS 0–100). The second part asked them for personal comments regarding the cause of the insertion problems. They were also asked to share any personal advice for inserting a maxillary obturator prosthesis. The third part asked whether they had worn normal dentures before the maxillectomy and for how long.

2.3.2. Basic Information on Intraoral Condition and Maxillary Obturator Prostheses

The intraoral data collected included whether there was communication between the oral and nasal cavities due to the surgical defect, the number of remaining teeth in the maxilla, and the degree of mouth opening. The information collected about the maxillary obturator prosthesis included the material, weight, obturator height, and number of clasps.

2.3.3. HDS-R

The HDS-R was used to assess cognitive function. A score of ≤20 was taken to indicate possible dementia [14].

2.3.4. PPT

The PPT was used to evaluate manual dexterity and coordination in both hands [19]. Participants were seated comfortably at the testing table with the pegboard on the table in front of them. The pegboard had 4 cups across the top and two vertical rows of 25 small holes down the center. The four cups contained 25 pins each. This test measured how many pins could be inserted into a row in 30 s with each hand. The test was performed twice for each hand and the highest score of the dominant hand was used for analysis.

2.3.5. Maxillary Obturator Prosthesis Insertion Time

As an outcome for assessing the difficulty of inserting a maxillary obturator prosthesis, the time required for insertion was measured from when participants picked up their prosthesis from the table to when they raised their hand after it was in place. After the test, we checked whether the prosthesis was fully and correctly in place and, if so, we recorded the insertion time.

2.3.6. Grip Strength Test

There is no internationally unified standard for grip strength testing, and opinions differ on whether the results are consistent between measurements taken in the standing and sitting positions [20]. Considering the ease of testing, grip strength was measured with an electronic hand dynamometer (N-FORCE, Wakayama, Japan) in the left and right hands while the participants were standing with the arms hanging down naturally. Data from the dominant hand were used.

2.3.7. Understanding of the Intraoral Surgical Site

Participants were asked to circle the surgical site on an intraoral schematic drawing of the upper and lower dentition.

2.4. Statistical Analysis

2.4.1. Part I: Prevalence of Possible Dementia

Because the total score on the HDS-R was not normally distributed (Shapiro–Wilk test, $p < 0.001$), a two-sided Mann–Whitney U test was used for comparisons by sex. Frequency analysis was performed using Fisher's exact test. A p-value of less than 0.05 was considered to indicate statistical significance. All statistical analyses were performed using SPSS statistics version 28 (IBM Corp., Armonk, NY, USA).

2.4.2. Part II: Difficulty Inserting the Maxillary Obturator Prosthesis after Maxillectomy

To reveal factors associated with the difficulty of inserting a maxillary obturator prosthesis, the insertion time was selected as an outcome measure for difficulty. Multiple regression analysis was used to identify factors associated with the insertion time. All variables were entered into the multiple regression model. A p value of less than 0.05 was considered to indicate statistical significance. Statistical analysis was performed using SPSS statistical ver. 28 (IBM Corp.).

3. Results

3.1. Part I: Prevalence of Possible Dementia

Among the 183 participants, HDS-R scores were ≤ 20 in 16 and ≤ 10 in 3, giving a prevalence of possible dementia of 8.7% (95% CI: 4.6–12.9%). The HDS-R score was ≤ 20 in 12% of the male participants but 4.8% of the female participants.

Median age was 78 (interquartile range [IQR]: 71–82) years in men and 77 (IQR: 72–84) years in women. HDS-R score between men and women showed a significant difference ($p < 0.05$, Mann–Whitney U test) (Figure 1).

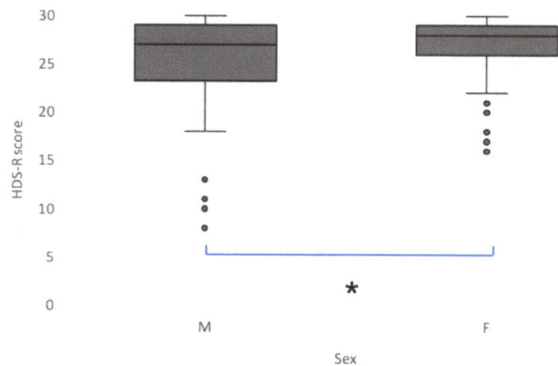

Figure 1. HDS-R scores by sex. Scores were significantly higher in women than in men (* $p = 0.037$, two-sided Mann–Whitney U test). The center line shows the mean, boxes show the IQR, and whiskers indicate the range. Dots indicate outliers.

In this study, following the definition of old age used by the United Nations and WHO (≥65 years), the 183 patients were divided into three age groups: 65–74 years (n = 71), 75–84 years (n = 80), and ≥85 years (n = 32). As shown in Table 2, there were significant differences in HDS-R total score between the 65–74-year age group and the 75–84-year age group and between the 65–74-year age group and the ≥85-year age group ($p < 0.05$, Fisher's exact test).

Table 2. Differences in total score on the HDS-R according to age group.

Age Group (Years)	HDS-R Score		Adjusted *p*-Value
	0–20 [#]	21–30	
65–74	0	71	65–74 vs. 75–84: 0.010 *
75–84	9	71	65–74 vs. ≥85: 0.001 *
≥85	7	25	75–84 vs. ≥85: 0.690
Total	16	167	

[#]: HDS-R score ≤ 20 indicates possible dementia. *: Significant difference between age groups (adjusted $p < 0.05$, Fisher's exact test with Bonferroni correction for multiple comparisons).

There was a significant difference in HDS-R total score between men and women in the 75–84-year age group according to the two-sided Mann–Whitney U test (Figure 2). HDS-R score decreased with age in men and in women.

Table 3 shows scores for each HDS-R item for men, women, and all participants. Sex differences were seen in the HDS-R item scores for working memory (item 6), recent memory (item 7), and language fluency (item 9). The complete accuracy rate was low for recent memory (item 7) at 41.5% (95% CI: 34.3–48.7%) compared with the other items.

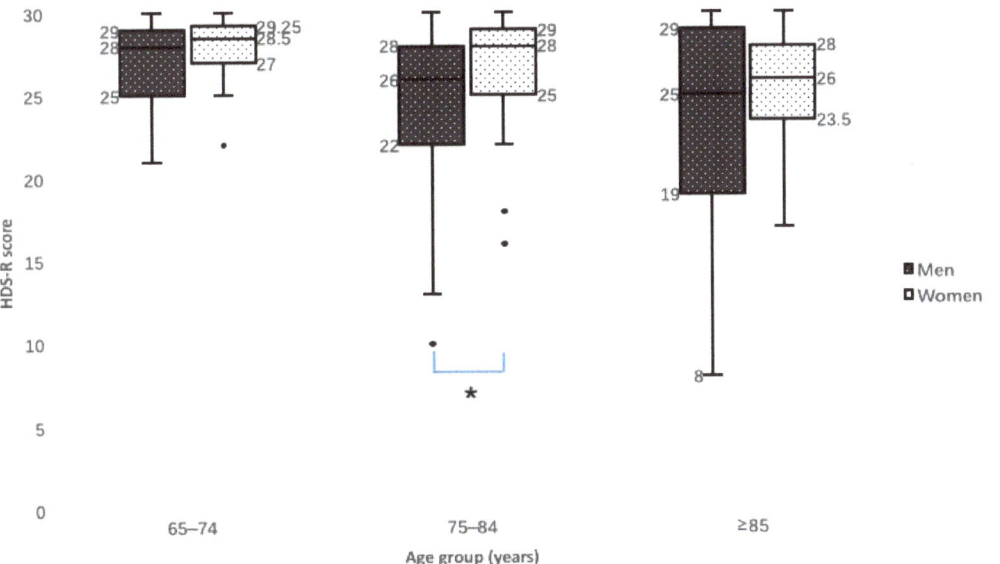

Figure 2. Relationship between HDS-R score and sex by age group. * $p = 0.044$, two-sided Mann–Whitney U test.

Table 3. Sex differences for total score and individual item score on the HDS-R.

Question	Score	Male, n (%)	Female, n (%)	Total, n (%)	p-Value
1 (Age)	0	2 (2)	0 (0)	2 (1.1)	0.502
	1	98 (98)	83 (100)	181 (98.9)	
2 (Date)	0–3	13 (13)	11 (13.3)	24 (13.1)	1
	4	87 (87)	72 (86.7)	159 (86.9)	
3 (Place)	0–1	2 (2)	0 (0)	2 (1.1)	0.502
	2	98 (98)	83 (100)	181 (98.9)	
4 (Repetition)	0–2	1 (1)	0 (0)	1 (0.5)	1
	3	99 (99)	83 (100)	182 (99.5)	
5 (Subtraction)	0–1	15 (15)	17 (20.5)	32 (17.5)	0.337
	2	85 (85)	66 (79.5)	151 (82.5)	
6 (Backward repetition)	0–1	23 (23)	32 (38.6)	55 (30.1)	0.024 *
	2	77 (77)	51 (61.4)	128 (69.9)	
7 (Recall)	0–5	66 (66)	41 (49.4)	107 (58.5)	0.025 *
	6	34 (34)	42 (50.6)	76 (41.5)	
8 (Naming objects)	0–4	44 (44)	28 (33.7)	72 (39.3)	0.174
	5	56 (56)	55 (66.3)	111 (60.7)	
9 (Naming vegetables)	0	14 (14)	0 (0)	14 (7.7)	<0.001 **
	1–2	17 (17)	5 (6)	22 (12)	
	3–4	9 (9)	13 (15.7)	22 (12)	
	5	60 (60)	65 (78.3)	125 (68.3)	
Total score	0–10	3 (3)	0 (0)	3 (1.6)	0.178
	11–20	9 (9)	4 (4.8)	13 (7.1)	
	21–30	88 (88)	79 (95.2)	167 (91.3)	

* Men vs. women: $p < 0.05$, ** $p < 0.01$, Fisher's exact test.

3.2. Part II: Difficulty Inserting a Maxillary Obturator Prosthesis after Maxillectomy

Of the 47 participants asked for subjective comments about insertion difficulties, 26 responded that they had such a difficulty. In particular, 12 indicated the difficulty was due to an oral defect, 5 due to limited mouth opening, and 4 due to hand coordination problems. Regarding the participants' advice for inserting maxillofacial obturator prostheses, 14 participants said to follow the doctor's instructions and practice repeatedly in order to gradually become accustomed to inserting the prosthesis. One participant responded that he used his tongue to assist with insertion. The other participants did not provide advice (Table 4).

Table 4. Comments from the participants.

Subjective Comments	(N = 47)
Visual analogue scale score	n (%)
<50	1 (2)
≥50, <70	4 (9)
≥70, <90	11 (23)
≥90, <100	31 (66)
Problems with inserting a maxillary obturator prosthesis	n (%)
No	21 (45)
Yes	26 (55)
Reasons for problems	
Defect	12 (26)
Hand coordination	4 (9)
Mouth opening	5 (10)
Other	5 (10)
Advice for inserting a maxillary obturator prosthesis	n (%)
Follow doctor's instructions and become accustomed to it	14 (30)
Use tongue to help	1 (2)
No advice provided	32 (68)

Table 5 shows the intraoral data, information about the maxillary obturator prostheses, and results of the five assessments for each participant.

Table 5. Characteristics of the participants.

Characteristics	(N = 47)
Age (years), (mean ± SD)	74 ± 8
Sex, n	
Men	23
Women	24
Duration of wearing dentures before maxillectomy (year), median (range, IQR)	0 (0–40, 7)
Communication between the oral cavity and nasal cavity, n	
Yes	31
No	16
Number of remaining teeth, median (range, IQR)	3 (0–10, 6)
Mouth opening (mm), median (range, IQR)	42 (11–70, 14)
Prosthesis material, n	
Resin base denture	43
Metal flame denture	4
Prosthesis weight (g) (mean ± SD)	25.8 ± 10.4
Obturator height (mm) (mean ± SD)	24.4 ± 11.2
Number of clasps, median (range, IQR)	2 (0–6, 3)
HDS-R total score, median (range, IQR)	27 (10–30, 5)
PPT score (mean ± SD)	13 ± 3
Insertion time, median (range, IQR)	5 (2–31, 3.39)
Grip strength (kg), median (range, IQR)	24.5 (13.9–48.2, 13)
Understanding of the surgical site, n	
Yes	39
No	8

Multiple regression analysis identified which of the factors we had hypothesized would affect prosthesis insertion time (Table 6). Not all of these factors had an impact on the insertion time. Age, number of remaining teeth, number of clasps, grip strength, and understanding of the intraoral surgical site showed higher VIF scores.

Table 6. Results of multiple regression analysis for all factors hypothesized to affect prosthesis insertion time in patients with maxillectomy.

Potential Affecting Factors	Regression Coefficient		Standardized Coefficients	p Value	VIF
	B	Std. Error			
Age	0.080	0.167	0.130	0.634	3.875
sex	−2.359	2.394	−0.244	0.332	3.255
Duration of wearing dentures before maxillectomy (years)	0.114	0.102	0.203	0.272	1.758
Communication between the oral and nasal cavities	0.923	1.555	0.090	0.557	1.234
Number of remaining teeth	0.048	0.387	0.034	0.901	3.992
Degree of mouth opening	−0.032	0.068	−0.077	0.643	1.458
Prosthesis materials	−1.356	2.916	−0.078	0.645	1.504
Prosthesis weight	−0.027	0.085	−0.057	0.755	1.745
Obturator height	−0.013	0.079	−0.030	0.870	1.718
Number of clasps	−0.328	0.820	−0.110	0.692	3.997
HDS-R total score	−0.394	0.251	−0.379	0.127	3.113
PPT score	−0.102	0.462	−0.054	0.827	3.213
Grip strength	−0.216	0.155	−0.383	0.174	4.036
Understanding the surgical site	−1.937	3.572	−0.150	0.591	4.095

Adjusted R^2: 0.136 ($p > 0.05$).

Communication between the oral and nasal cavities, number of remaining teeth, prothesis material, number of clasps, and obturator height can affect the weight of the maxillary obturator prosthesis. The HDS-R score was related to age and sex according to the results of part I in this study. The HDS-R item concerning the understanding of self-information and concerning understanding of intraoral surgical site were related. The correlation between HDS-R score and PPT score was significant ($p < 0.05$, Spearman's rank correlation test) (Figure 3). Grip strength was related to age and sex, as reported previously [17].

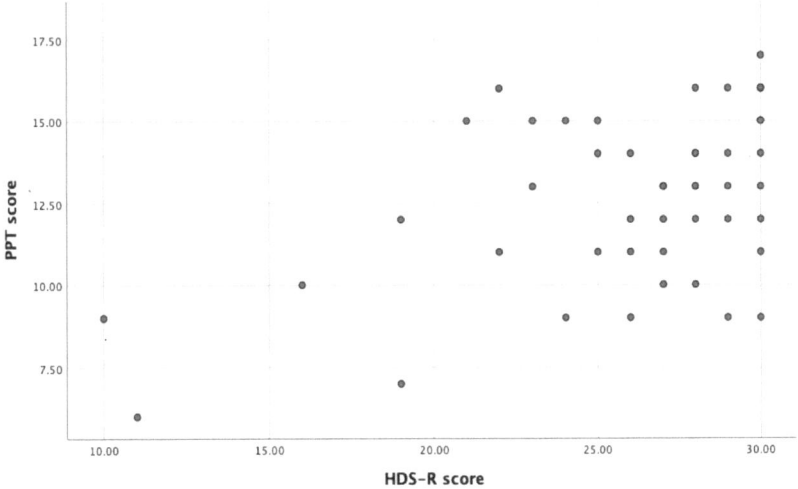

Figure 3. Correlation between HDS-R score and PPT score.

After trying different models and comparing the adjusted R^2 value among the models, multiple regression analysis identified the affecting factors of prosthesis insertion time (Table 7, Model 2). Multicollinearity was assessed using VIF scores. Because age was always considered as an affecting factor, it was added to Model 1. Without age, the VIF score was decreased when comparing Model 1 and Model 2. Both models showed that HDS-R score had a significant impact on the prosthesis insertion time in patients with maxillectomy. The p-values for duration of wearing dentures before maxillectomy and grip strength were close to 0.05 in the second model, so these two factors have an impact on the prosthesis insertion time in patients with maxillectomy.

Table 7. Affecting factors for prosthesis insertion time in patients with maxillectomy.

(a) Model 1					
Affecting Factors	Regression Coefficient		Standardized Coefficients	p Value	VIF
	B	Std. Error			
Age	0.112	0.105	0.182	0.289	1.79
Duration of wearing dentures before maxillectomy (years)	0.135	0.079	0.24	0.102	1.292
Prosthesis weight	−0.013	0.061	−0.029	0.828	1.06
HDS-R score	−0.357	0.157	−0.344	0.028	1.43
Grip strength	−0.110	0.092	−0.194	0.24	1.662
Adjusted R^2: 0.264					
(b) Model 2					
Affecting Factors	Regression Coefficient		Standardized Coefficients	p Value	VIF
	B	Std. Error			
Duration of wearing dentures before maxillectomy (years)	0.154	0.079	0.274	0.058	1.232
Prosthesis weight	−0.025	0.06	−0.053	0.68	1.026
HDS-R score	−0.437	0.139	−0.420	0.003	1.112
Grip strength	−0.154	0.082	−0.273	0.069	1.328
Adjusted R^2: 0.261					

4. Discussion

From our survey, 8.7% of patients who visited our maxillofacial prosthetics clinic at a university hospital between 2016 and 2022 were found to have possible dementia according to the HDS-R. This corresponds to about 1 in 12 elderly patients. After dividing the patients into three age groups, namely 65–74 years (n = 71), 75–84 years (n = 80), and ≥85 years (n = 32), significant differences in the HDS-R score were found between youngest age group and each of the two older age groups, indicating that the prevalence of possible dementia increased with age in our patients. However, there was no difference between the intermediate age group and the oldest group. This suggests that patients over 75 years old require more attention and their cognitive and physical condition should be monitored in order to detect changes in their status and to provide more support when needed.

There was a significant difference in the prevalence of possible dementia between men and women. Compared with female patients, more male patients had an HDS-R score of ≤20, particularly ≤10. This result is different from a previous study that found women are more likely to develop dementia [16]. These conflicting results might have arisen from a difference in the method for evaluating dementia. Another possibility is that the characteristics of patients with head and neck defects have some influence on the prevalence of dementia, and follow-up research is needed to focus on this aspect.

Sex differences were noted in the HDS-R total score and individual item scores (Table 3). In this study, men's scores for item 6 were higher than women's, but women's scores for items 7 and 9 were higher than men's. This could suggest that men's immediate memory and visual memory are better than women's, but women's recent memory and language fluency are better than men's. This might be related to men's and women's family life roles for this generation of patients in Japan, where men were more likely to take on a work role and women were more likely to take on a domestic role. This might account for women's better recent memory and the recall of vegetable names. This result suggests that when a high-frequency behavior occurs in life, the things involved in the behavior are easily recalled. The item 7 scores for recent memory were lower scores than the other item scores. This result is consistent with the fact that older people tend to easily forget recent events.

From the maxillectomy patients' subjective comments about difficulties inserting their maxillofacial obturator prosthesis (Table 4), it was revealed that 34% of them found insertion slightly difficult and 55% experienced clear problems when inserting them. According to the patients' comments regarding the reason for the difficulty, 26% attributed it to their intraoral defect, while 10% and 9% attributed it to a limitation of mouth opening and hand coordination problems, respectively. Thus, when providing continuous care for these patients, we should proactively ask patients about potential difficulties they might be experiencing, bearing in mind these three main reasons.

From the results of Table 7, we can see that the HDS-R score had a significant impact on difficulty inserting a maxillary obturator prosthesis. Moreover, age, the duration of wearing dentures before maxillectomy, the prosthesis weight, and grip strength were related to such difficulty. The duration of wearing dentures before maxillectomy was associated with increased difficulty, which may be related to the different ways that dentures and maxillary obturator prostheses are inserted and to the age of the patients. Because the duration of wearing dentures previously did not seem to help the patients with insertion, it seems that the oral defect itself also likely increased the difficulty. The weight of the maxillary obturator prosthesis depends on its structure, suggesting its structure could also have an impact on the difficulty experienced by patients. We initially thought that the weight was related to the defect area; however, it could also be related to many other factors, such as material differences and number of clasps. Thus, it is unclear which is the most important factor. The HDS-R score was related to the PPT score, indicating that cognitive decline was accompanied by declines in manual dexterity and coordination. In addition, age, HDS-R score, and grip strength were associated with increased insertion difficulty. Therefore, both cognitive and physical decline, but especially cognitive decline, can contribute to patients' difficulties inserting their maxillary obturator prosthesis.

When we combine the comments we collected from patients with the results of our analysis, we consistently find that prosthesis structure and decreased hand manual dexterity and coordination were related to increased insertion difficulty. When we combine the conclusions of the two parts of this study, we find that declines in cognitive function, manual dexterity, and grip strength were related to increased insertion difficulty, and these functional declines are related to age. Therefore, in the treatment of older patients, it is necessary to assess their cognitive ability and hand function in a timely manner. If functional decline is evident, the structure of the maxillary obturator prosthesis should be adjusted promptly to make it easier for them to wear, and more attention and support should be given. Then, when we combine the advice from patients with our two conclusions, it seems that things and events involving high-frequency behaviors earlier in life are relatively easily recalled by older people while recent events are more easily forgotten. To reduce the difficulty of inserting a maxillary obturator prosthesis, older patients may need repeated reminding and guidance as well as increased practice.

Based on the above conclusions, for maxillectomy patients who have difficulty inserting their maxillary obturator prosthesis, the first step is to communicate with the patients to understand the nature of the difficulty and to determine which part of the prosthesis design is connected with the problem. After addressing any design issues, in order to lessen the difficulty experienced by these patients, they need to regularly practice inserting their prosthesis to form a habit. If they wore dentures before the maxillectomy, it would be helpful to highlight the differences between wearing a maxillary obturator prosthesis and dentures for them and encourage them to practice insertion. In patients with severely impaired cognitive and hand functions, prompt communication with the patient's family members or caregivers is necessary, so that they can help the patient safely and correctly insert and use their maxillary obturator prosthesis.

A previous study found that implants with appropriate attachment systems dramatically improved the retention of the maxillary obturators [21], which may have an impact on patients' insertion of maxillary obturator prostheses. At present, there are not many elderly patients with implants in our clinic, and none of the participants in this study had implants. As the use of implants increases, we will pay attention to whether they increase the difficulty in prothesis insertion in follow-up studies.

There are some limitations to this study. The first is that the HDS-R was used for the screening of possible dementia. The HDS-R was developed after considering its feasibility for worldwide use [12], but it does not have a drawing and reading component, making it impossible to test these abilities in older adults with hearing impairments. Therefore, future research is needed to identify the clinical population with possible dementia by using other scales, such as the widely used MMSE. The second limitation is the small number of patients with dementia in this study. This may be due to the characteristics of our clinic, which belongs to a university hospital; is located in a bustling area of Tokyo, Japan; and has a large train station nearby. These may all be factors affecting the patients who visit our clinic. The third limitation is that maxillary obturator prosthesis insertion time was selected as an outcome measure for the difficulty of inserting the maxillary obturator. The insertion time may be affected by factors such as the patient's personality, so a better outcome measure for this is needed. Lastly, the structure of maxillary obturator prostheses is complicated and the information collected was not sufficient to analyze which part of the structure was connected with patients' difficulties with insertion. Future studies could investigate additional information, such as defect location and defect area, and then group and compare the prosthesis structures. In terms of patients practicing inserting their maxillary obturator prosthesis, virtual reality (VR) that gamifies practice could be one solution.

The results of this study indicate issues to consider for continuous medical and dental care in a super-aging society. The possibilities of patients having dementia and/or difficulties inserting their maxillofacial prosthesis should be kept in mind when providing supportive care, including terminal care, for patients with maxillary defects.

5. Conclusions

In this study, 8.7% of the participants were judged to have possible dementia, and a lower HDS-R score had a significant impact on insertion difficulty. Cognitive function and difficulty inserting maxillary obturator prostheses should be considered in the provision of continuous supportive care to patients with maxillary defects.

Author Contributions: Conceptualization, H.Y. and Y.I.S.; methodology, H.Y. and Y.I.S.; formal analysis, H.Y., M.A. and Y.I.S.; resources, H.F. and Y.I.S.; investigation, H.Y.; writing—original draft preparation, H.Y.; writing—review and editing, H.Y., H.F., M.A., Y.I.S. and N.W.; visualization, H.Y.; supervision, Y.I.S. and N.W. All authors have read and agreed to the published version of the manuscript.

Funding: This work was supported by JST SPRING, grant number JPMJSP2120. This research was supported in part by the Female Faculty Promotion Program (FFPP) of the Tokyo Medical and Dental University.

Institutional Review Board Statement: This study was approved by the Ethics Committee of the Faculty of Dentistry, Tokyo Medical and Dental University (approval number D2016-012).

Informed Consent Statement: Informed consent was obtained before participation in the study.

Data Availability Statement: Data sharing not applicable.

Acknowledgments: The author thanks Mariko Hatori, Mai Murase, Mihoko Haraguchi, and Wang Jiangyu for their help and support in the research. The author would like to say thank you to our patient especially to S.S. and his family.

Conflicts of Interest: The authors declare no conflict of interest.

References

1. Phasuk, K.; Haug, S.P. Maxillofacial prosthetics. *Oral Maxillofac. Surg. Clin. N. Am.* **2018**, *30*, 487–497. [CrossRef]
2. Rosen, E.B.; Palin, C.L.; Huryn, J.M.; Wong, R.J. The role of maxillofacial prosthetics for the surgically treated patient at National Cancer Institute-designated comprehensive cancer centers. *Laryngoscope* **2019**, *129*, 409–414. [CrossRef]
3. Sumita, Y.I.; Hattori, M.; Namba, T.; Ino, S. Obturators to facilitate speech and swallowing in a maxillectomy patient with dementia and cerebral infarction. *Int. J. Maxillofac. Prosthet.* **2019**, *2*, 33–35. [CrossRef]
4. Yanagi, A.; Sumita, Y.; Hattori, M.; Kamiyanagi, A.; Otomaru, T.; Kanazaki, A.; Haraguchi, M.; Murase, M.; Hatano, N.; Taniguchi, H. Clinical survey over the past 35 years at the clinic for maxillofacial prosthetics Tokyo Medical and Dental University. *J. Prosthodont. Res.* **2018**, *62*, 309–312. [CrossRef] [PubMed]
5. Jaul, E.; Barron, J. Age-related diseases and clinical and public health implications for the 85 years old and over population. *Front. Public Health* **2017**, *5*, 335. [CrossRef] [PubMed]
6. Kubota, K. Survival rate of patients with dementia. *Jpn. J. Insur. Med.* **2018**, *116*, 196–200, (Abstract in English).
7. Perneczky, R.; Wagenpfeil, S.; Komossa, K.; Grimmer, T.; Diehl, J.; Kurz, A. Mapping scores onto stages: Mini-Mental State Examination and Clinical Dementia Rating. *Am. J. Geriatr. Psychiatry* **2006**, *14*, 139–144. [CrossRef] [PubMed]
8. Galasko, D.; Klauber, M.R.; Hofstetter, C.R.; Salmon, D.P.; Lasker, B.; Thal, L.J. The Mini-Mental State Examination in the early diagnosis of Alzheimer's disease. *Arch. Neurol.* **1990**, *47*, 49–52. [CrossRef]
9. Hodges, J.R.; Salmon, D.P.; Butters, N. Differential impairment of semantic and episodic memory in Alzheimer's and Huntington's disease: A controlled prospective study. *J. Neurol. Neurosurg. Psychiatry* **1990**, *53*, 1089–1095. [CrossRef]
10. Fujiwara, Y.; Suzuki, H.; Yasunaga, M.; Sugiyama, M.; Ijuin, M.; Sakuma, N.; Inagaki, H.; Iwasa, H.; Ura, C.; Yatomi, N.; et al. Brief screening tool for mild cognitive impairment in older Japanese: Validation of the Japanese version of the Montreal Cognitive Assessment. *Geriatr. Gerontol. Int.* **2010**, *10*, 225–232. [CrossRef] [PubMed]
11. Bruno, D.; Schurmann Vignaga, S. Addenbrooke's cognitive examination III in the diagnosis of dementia: A critical review. *Neuropsychiatr. Dis. Treat.* **2019**, *15*, 441–447. [CrossRef]
12. Imai, Y.; Hasegawa, K. The Revised Hasegawa's Dementia Scale (HDS-R) evaluation of its usefulness as a screening test for dementia. *Hong Kong J. Psychiatry* **1994**, *4*, 20–24.
13. Jeong, J.W.; Kim, K.W.; Lee, D.Y.; Lee, S.B.; Park, J.H.; Choi, E.A.; Choe, J.Y.; Do, Y.J.; Ryang, J.S.; Roh, H.A.; et al. A normative study of the Revised Hasegawa Dementia Scale: Comparison of demographic influences between the Revised Hasegawa Dementia Scale and the Mini-Mental Status Examination. *Dement. Geriatr. Cogn. Disord.* **2007**, *24*, 288–293. [CrossRef]
14. Takiura, T. Dementia screening scales in Japan. *Bull. Hiroshima Shudo Univ. Stud. Humanit.* **2007**, *48*, 347–379, (Abstract in English).
15. Copeland, J.R.; McCracken, C.F.; Dewey, M.E.; Wilson, K.C.; Doran, M.; Gilmore, C.; Scott, A.; Larkin, B.A. Undifferentiated dementia, Alzheimer's disease, and vascular dementia: Age- and gender-related incidence in Liverpool. The MRC–ALPHA Study. *Br. J. Psychiatry* **1999**, *175*, 433–438. [CrossRef] [PubMed]
16. Mazure, C.M.; Swendsen, J. Sex differences in Alzheimer's disease and other dementias. *Lancet Neurol.* **2016**, *15*, 451–452. [CrossRef]
17. Furuna, T.; Nagasaki, H.; Nishizawa, S.; Sugiura, M.; Okuzumi, H.; Ito, H.; Kinugasa, T.; Hashizume, K.; Maruyama, H. Longitudinal change in the physical performance of older adults in the community. *J. Jpn. Phys. Ther. Assoc.* **1998**, *1*, 1–5. [CrossRef]
18. Kounnavong, S.; Ratsavong, K.; Soundavong, K.; Xayavong, S.; Kariya, T.; Saw, Y.M.; Yamamoto, E.; Horibe, K.; Toba, K.; Hamajima, N. Cognitive function measured with the Revised Hasegawa's Dementia Scale among elderly individuals in Lao PDR. *Nagoya J. Med. Sci.* **2019**, *81*, 281–290. [PubMed]
19. Irie, K.; Iseki, H.; Okamoto, K.; Nishimura, S.; Kagechika, K. Introduction of the Purdue Pegboard Test for fine assessment of severity of cervical myelopathy before and after surgery. *J. Phys. Ther. Sci.* **2020**, *32*, 210–214. [CrossRef]
20. Roberts, H.C.; Denison, H.J.; Martin, H.J.; Patel, H.P.; Syddall, H.; Cooper, C.; Sayer, A.A. A review of the measurement of grip strength in clinical and epidemiological studies: Towards a standardised approach. *Age Ageing* **2011**, *40*, 423–429. [CrossRef]
21. Alqutaibi, A.Y. Enhancing retention of maxillary obturators using dental implants. *Int. J. Contemp. Dent. Med. Rev.* **2015**, *2*, 010915.

Disclaimer/Publisher's Note: The statements, opinions and data contained in all publications are solely those of the individual author(s) and contributor(s) and not of MDPI and/or the editor(s). MDPI and/or the editor(s) disclaim responsibility for any injury to people or property resulting from any ideas, methods, instructions or products referred to in the content.

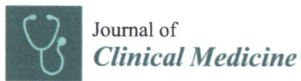 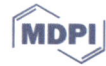

Systematic Review

The Effect of Domiciliary Professional Oral Care on Root Caries Progression in Care-Dependent Older Adults: A Systematic Review

Elisabeth Morén [1,2,3], Pia Skott [1,4,5], Kristina Edman [3,6,7], Nivetha Gavriilidou [1,4,5], Inger Wårdh [1,5,8,*] and Helena Domeij [9]

1. Department of Dental Medicine, Karolinska Institute, 141 04 Huddinge, Sweden
2. Public Dental Service, Folktandvården Region Dalarna, 791 29 Falun, Sweden
3. Centre for Clinical Research Dalarna, Uppsala University, 791 82 Falun, Sweden
4. Public Dental Services, Folktandvården Stockholm AB, 118 27 Stockholm, Sweden
5. Academic Centre for Geriatric Dentistry, 112 19 Stockholm, Sweden
6. Administrative Centre for Public Dental Service, 791 29 Falun, Sweden
7. Department of Surgical Sciences, Odontology & Maxillofacial Surgery, Uppsala University, 751 85 Uppsala, Sweden
8. Department of Health Sciences, Karlstad University, 651 88 Karlstad, Sweden
9. Health Technology Assessment—Odontology, Faculty of Odontology, Malmö University, 205 06 Malmö, Sweden
* Correspondence: inger.wardh@ki.se; Tel.: +46-8-524-882-26

Abstract: With care dependency, untreated root caries lesions (RCLs) and irregular dental visits are common. RCLs, if left untreated, could lead to pain, tooth loss, difficulties eating, and impact on general health. Therefore, there is a need for prevention and effective treatment for RCLs, and especially in those with care dependency. The aim of this systematic review was to investigate the effect of domiciliary professional oral care on root caries development and progression, in comparison with self-performed or nurse-assisted oral care. A literature search was conducted in four databases in November 2022. Two authors independently screened the literature throughout the review process. Five of the identified studies were found to be relevant. Four of these were assessed as having moderate risk of bias and were included in the review, while one study had high risk of bias and was excluded from further analyses. Due to heterogenicity of the included studies (and of the interventions and outcomes), no meta-analysis or synthesis without meta-analysis (SWiM) was performed. The participation of dental personnel performing mechanical plaque removal and fluoride, or chlorhexidine application seems beneficial for care-dependent older adults with risk of RCLs development and progression. However, future studies are needed.

Keywords: dental personnel; domiciliary; root caries; fluoride

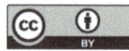

1. Introduction

Among care-dependent older adults living in nursing homes, the number of untreated root caries lesions (RCLs) is high [1,2]. A systematic review by Zhang et al. [3] discovered several risk predictors for developing RCLs. The risk predictors stated were the age of 60 years or older, having poor oral hygiene, smoking, gingival recession, low socioeconomic status, and previous dental caries experience [3]. The risk for developing RCLs increases with age due to gingival recession caused by age and/or periodontal disease leading to exposed root surfaces [4]. RCLs are located on exposed roots of teeth and are of two categories. The first category is shallow and saucer-shaped and can be healed mechanically by toothbrushing with fluoride toothpaste [5–7]. The second category has the same shape as the first but is deeper and should be restored because of the risk of pulp exposure [7]. Bashir [8] reports a prevalence of untreated root caries among independent adults aged

20 years and older of 10.1%, with the highest prevalence found in the age groups of 70 years and older (12.5%) [8]. In other reports, prevalence of RCLs among adults, and older adults, varied broadly between 3.7% and 100% [3,9,10]. The daily oral hygiene procedure recommended by the Swedish dental guidelines is to brush the teeth twice per day with toothpaste containing 1450 ppm sodium fluoride [11]. According to the guidelines, the recommendations for prevention of RCLs are toothbrushing with high fluoride toothpaste containing 5000 ppm sodium fluoride, rinsing with 0.2% sodium fluoride solution, fluoride gel administered in mouth guards, and fluoride varnish or fluoride topical agents applied by dental personnel [11]. Interventions such as fluoride varnish applied every third month by dental personnel or self-brushing with high fluoride toothpaste have been shown to have a positive effect on arresting and preventing RCLs in care-dependent older adults living in nursing homes [12,13]. The definition of "care dependency" is "dependence on care in those who are young, ill, elderly or disabled, and dependent on another" [14].

Care-dependent individuals may therefore need help with basic care in daily living, for example with eating, personal hygiene including oral hygiene, transport outside or inside the home, and intake of medicine. Individual requirement of assistance with basic care is often related to the need for assistance with daily oral care [15].

Domiciliary dental care (DDC) is a service provided by dental personnel offering dental care at home, such as check-ups, preventive care, uncomplicated tooth extractions, simple/provisional tooth restorations, and adjustments of removable dentures [16,17]. Discontinued dental care attendance generally increases with age [18] and with cognitive impairment [19]. Further, with untreated RCLs the risk of pain, tooth loss, and eating difficulties could impact on general health [20]. Also, the risk of poor oral hygiene increases with age because of disease and disability [21]. With today's high number of teeth with advanced prosthodontic reconstructions [21], performing nurse-assisted oral care for care facility/nursing home residents is challenging [22]. Therefore, there is a need for prevention and effective treatment of RCLs among older adults, and especially among those who are care-dependent [20,23]. Domiciliary dental care could therefore be beneficial for frail older adults wanting to stay at home. The effect of DDC, and especially the effect of dental professional oral care on root caries development, has, to our knowledge, not yet been explored in care dependent older adults.

The aim of the present systematic review was to investigate the effect of domiciliary professional oral care on root caries development and progression in care-dependent older adults, in comparison with self-performed or nurse-assisted oral care.

2. Materials and Methods

This systematic literature review was registered in the international prospective register of systematic reviews (PROSPERO). The protocol can be accessed at www.crd.york.ac.uk/PROSPERO/display_record.asp?ID=CRD42021274595 (accessed on 14 September 2021), see Supplementary Materials. All six authors (E.M., P.S., K.E., N.G., I.W., and H.D.) participated in the reviewing process.

2.1. Inclusion and Exclusion Criteria
2.1.1. Inclusion Criteria

The review question was: What effect does domiciliary professional oral care have on root caries development and progression compared with oral care as usual in care-dependent older adults? The information was sorted into the categories population (P), intervention (I), comparison (C), and outcome (O) [24], as follows:

P: Individuals aged 60 years and older with at least one natural tooth. In addition, subjects must be care-dependent and not affected by congenital and/or acquired psychiatric disease.

I: Mechanical plaque removal, interproximal measures, as well as fluoride agents, and other preventive measures performed outside a dental clinic by dental personnel (dental nurse, dental hygienist, dentist).

C: Oral care as usual (self-performed or nurse-assisted).

O: Root caries development and progression, expressed as a caries index, for example the decayed, missing, and filled teeth (DMFT) index [25], the root caries index (RCI) [26,27] or the RCI described by Fejerskov et al. [28].

Only peer-reviewed, controlled clinical trials performed in humans (randomized controlled trials (RCTs), non-randomized controlled trials, and systematic reviews) written in Swedish, Norwegian, Danish, English, French, or German were included, with no limitations regarding the year of publication.

2.1.2. Exclusion Criteria

Qualitative studies were not included in the review.

2.2. Search Strategy

The literature search was conducted by a librarian using four databases, PubMed, Cochrane Library, Cinahl, and MEDLINE via OVID. A search string was designed by a librarian with the support of the Library at Falun Hospital, Falun, Sweden.

The full search strategy can be found at: https://www.crd.york.ac.uk/PROSPEROFILES/274595_STRATEGY_20210913.pdf (accessed on 14 September 2021), see Supplementary Materials. A preliminary search was performed in June 2021 for testing and modifying the search string, followed by a discussion in the review group with the librarian. It was unanimously concluded that the search string was complete. Thereafter, the final searches were performed at the beginning of September 2021 and repeated in April 2022 and November 2022. Titles, abstracts, and full-text articles of the literature identified by the search strategy were screened independently by all the authors reading in pairs. The software Rayyan.ai [29] was used for the screening process. All studies of potential relevance according to the inclusion criteria were obtained in full text and the same author pairs independently assessed them for inclusion. Any disagreements were resolved by discussion.

2.3. Quality Assessment and Overall Risk of Bias

A Swedish version [30] of the Cochrane risk-of-bias (RoB) tool for non-randomized trials (ROBINS-I) and randomized trials, version 2 (RoB 2) [31] was used to assess the quality of the included studies. Using the RoB tools, the studies were classified as low, moderate, or high RoB. This part of the screening process was performed independently by all the reviewing authors reading in pairs and any disagreements were resolved through discussion.

2.4. Data Extraction and Data Analysis

Data extraction from the included studies was performed independently by two authors (E.M. and H.D.) and discussed in detail within the review group. Name(s) of the author(s), publication year, country, study design, participant characteristics such as age, gender, and number of teeth, number of participants, type of intervention, baseline measurements, and length of follow-up were extracted from each study. Due to heterogenicity of the studies included, in terms of both interventions and outcomes, no meta-analysis or synthesis without meta-analysis (SWiM) was performed.

3. Results

3.1. Search Results

Based on the designed search string, a total of 212 records were identified in the electronic databases. After screening of the titles and abstracts according to the inclusion and exclusion criteria, 190 records were excluded. The remaining 22 records were sought for retrieval and assessed for eligibility in full text. In addition, the reference lists of the included records were also screened. Two additional reports were identified through this process and included for full-text assessment. Out of these 24 records, five studies were found to be relevant (Figure 1) and were included for RoB assessment. The studies that were excluded are listed in Table 1. The main reason for exclusion was "wrong PICO".

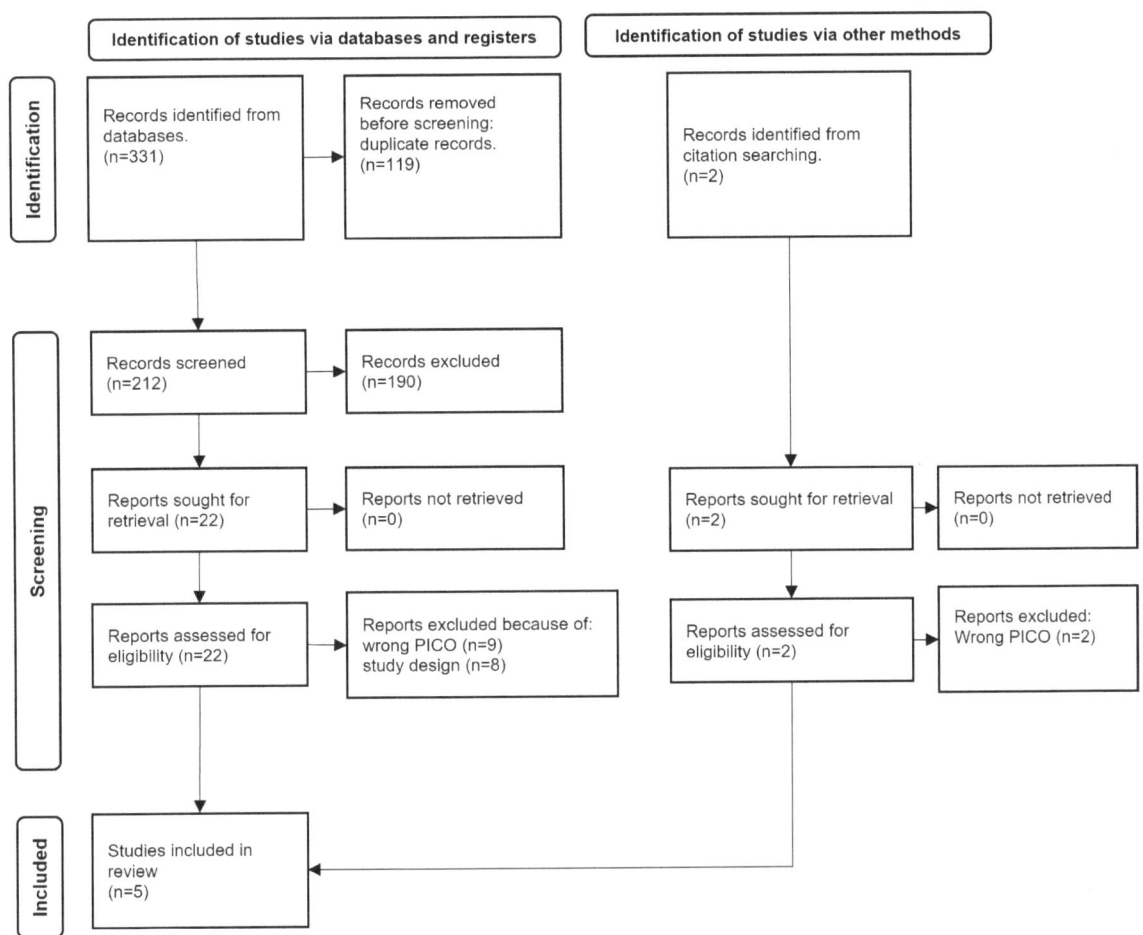

Figure 1. PRISMA flowchart of identification, screening, and inclusion of studies for the literature review [32].

Table 1. Excluded reports sought for retrieval and with reason for exclusion.

Author, Year	Title	Where Published	Reason for Exclusion
Wyatt, 2009, [33]	A 5-year follow-up of older adults residing in long-term care facilities: utilization of a comprehensive dental program	Gerodontology. 2009;26(4):282–90.	Wrong PICO
Wyatt and MacEntee, 2004, [34]	Caries management for institutionalized elders using fluoride and chlorhexidine mouth rinses	Community Dentistry & Oral Epidemiology. 2004;32(5):322–8.	Wrong PICO
Niessen, 2012, [35]	Chlorhexidine varnish, sodium fluoride varnish, and silver diamine fluoride solution can prevent the development of new root caries in elders living in senior homes in Hong Kong	Journal of Evidence-Based Dental Practice. 2012;12(2):95–6.	Wrong study design
López, Uribe, Rodríguez, and Casasempere, 2013, [36]	Comparison between amine fluoride and chlorhexidine with institutionalized elders: a pilot study	Gerodontology. 2013;30(2):112–8.	Wrong PICO

Table 1. Cont.

Author, Year	Title	Where Published	Reason for Exclusion
Yi Mohammadi, Franks, and Hines, 2015, [37]	Effectiveness of professional oral health care intervention on the oral health of residents with dementia in residential aged care facilities: a systematic review protocol	JBI Database System Rev Implement Rep. 2015;13(10):110–22. https://doi.org/10.11124/jbisrir-2015-2330.	Wrong study design
ClinicalTrials.gov, 2018, [38]	Effectiveness on SDF solution and PVP-I combined NaF varnish in preventing root caries in elders	Available online: https://clinicaltrials.gov/ct2/show/NCT03654820 (accessed on 10 September 2021)	Wrong study design
Mojon, Rentsch, Budtz-Jørgensen, and Baehni, 1998, [39]	Effects of an oral health program on selected clinical parameters and salivary bacteria in a long-term care facility	Eur J Oral Sci. 1998;106(4):827–34.	Wrong PICO
Ritter, 2013, [40]	The efficacy of fluoride on root caries progression may be dose-dependent	Journal of Evidence-Based Dental Practice. 2013;13(4):177–9.	Wrong study design
Marchesan, Byrd, Moss, Preisser, Morelli, Zandona et al., 2020, [41]	Flossing is associated with improved oral health in older adults	Journal of Dental Research. 2020;99(9):1047–53.	Wrong PICO
Barbe, Küpeli, Hamacher, and Noack, 2020, [42]	Impact of regular professional toothbrushing on oral health, related quality of life, and nutritional and cognitive status in nursing home residents	International Journal of Dental Hygiene. 2020;18(3):238–50.	Wrong study design
MacEntee, Silver, Gibson, and Weiss, 1985, [43]	Oral health in a long-term care institution equipped with a dental service	Community Dentistry & Oral Epidemiology. 1985;13(5):260–3.	Wrong study design
Pearson and Chalmers, 2004, [44]	Oral hygiene care for adults with dementia in residential aged care facilities	JBI Library of Systematic Reviews. 2004;2(3):65–113.	Wrong PICO
Al-Nasser and Lamster, 2020, [45]	Prevention and management of periodontal diseases and dental caries in the older adults	Periodontology 2000. 2020;84(1):69–83.	Wrong study design
Patel, Khan, Pennington, Pitts, Robertson, Gallagher, 2021, [46]	Protocol for a randomized feasibility trial comparing fluoride interventions to prevent dental decay in older people in care homes (FInCH trial)	BMC Oral Health. 2021;21(1):1–12.	Wrong PICO
TrialSearch.com, 2017, [47]	A randomized controlled trial to evaluate the cost effectiveness of prescribing high concentration fluoride toothpaste to prevent tooth decay in older adults	Available online: https://www.who.int/trialsearch/Trial2.aspx?TrialID=ISRCTN11992428. 2017. (accessed on 10 September 2021)	Wrong PICO
Ekstrand, Poulsen, Hede, Twetman, Qvist, and Ellwood, 2013, [13]	A randomized clinical trial of the anti-caries efficacy of 5000 compared to 1450 ppm fluoridated toothpaste on root caries lesions in elderly disabled nursing home residents	Caries Research. 2013;47(5):391–8.	Wrong PICO
Raghoonandan, Cobban, and Compton, 2011, [48]	A scoping review of the use of fluoride varnish in elderly people living in long term care facilities	Canadian Journal of Dental Hygiene. 2011;45(4):217–22.	Wrong study design
Wikstrom, Kareem, Almstahl, Palmgren, Lingstrom, and Wardh, 2017, [49]	Effect of 12-month weekly professional oral hygiene care on the composition of the oral flora in dentate, dependent elderly residents: a prospective study	Gerodontology. 2017;34(2):240–8.	Wrong PICO
Jabir, McGrade, Quinn, McGarry, Nic Iomhair, Kelly et al., 2022, [50]	Evaluating the effectiveness of fluoride varnish in preventing caries amongst long-term care facility residents	Gerodontology. 2022;39:250–6.	Wrong PICO
Ekstrand, Martignon, and Holm-Pedersen, 2008, [51]	Development and evaluation of two root caries controlling programmes for home-based frail people older than 75 years	Gerodontology. 2008;25(2):67–75.	High risk of bias (RoB)

3.2. Risk of Bias

The five included RCT studies were assessed using the RoB 2 tool [31]. Four out of five studies were conclusively deemed to have moderate RoB; the fifth study had high RoB (Table 2). Only the results from the studies with a moderate RoB were further analyzed. The characteristics of these four included studies are summarized in Table 3.

Table 2. Assessment of risk of bias (RoB), using the RoB tool, version 2 (RoB 2), of the five included studies, by domain and conclusive judgement.

RoB 2	Randomization process	Deviations from the intended interventions (effect of assignment to intervention)	Deviations from the intended interventions (effect of adhering to intervention)	Missing outcome data	Measurement of the outcome	Selection of the reported result	Conflict of interest	Conclusive judgment
Ekstrand et al., 2008 [51]	yellow	red	red	red	green	yellow	red	red
Barbe et al., 2019 [52]	yellow	yellow	yellow	green	red	green	green	yellow
Brailsford et al., 2002 [53]	red	yellow	yellow	yellow	green	green	red	yellow
Girestam Croonquist et al., 2020 [54]	green	red	red	green	yellow	yellow	yellow	yellow
Tan et al., 2010 [55]	green	yellow	yellow	red	yellow	yellow	yellow	yellow

Green = low RoB; yellow = moderate RoB; red = high RoB.

Table 3. Characteristics of the included studies.

Author(s)	Barbe, Kottmann, Derman, and Noack [52]	Brailsford, Fiske, Gilbert, Clark, and Beighton [53]	Girestam Croonquist, Dalum, Skott, Sjögren, Wårdh, and Morén [54]	Tan, Lo, Dyson, Luo, and Corbet [55]
Year	2019	2002	2020	2010
Country	Germany	Great Britain	Sweden	China
Title	Efficacy of regular professional brushing by a dental nurse for 3 months in nursing home residents—a randomized, controlled clinical trial.	The effects of the combination of chlorhexidine/thymol- and fluoride-containing varnishes on the severity of RCLs in frail institutionalized elderly people.	Effects of domiciliary professional oral care for care-dependent elderly in nursing homes—oral hygiene, gingival bleeding, root caries and nursing staff's oral health knowledge and attitudes.	A randomized trial on root caries prevention in elders.
Aim	To investigate the impact of professional brushing, performed every 2 weeks by a dental nurse, on the number of teeth, incidence of root caries, and further short-term oral health parameters, compared with residents whose oral hygiene was performed or supervised by staff according to standards of care corresponding to German law concerning the care for the elderly.	To determine the effect of a fluoride-containing varnish (Fluor protector) in combination with either Cervitec or a placebo varnish on the clinical characteristics of existing RCLs.	To describe the effects, for nursing home residents, of professional cleaning, and individual OHIs provided by registered dental hygienists, in comparison with daily oral care as usual.	To compare the effectiveness of the following four methods in preventing new root surface caries: (1) only OHIs every 3 months; (2) OHIs and applications of Cervitec varnish every 3 months; (3) OHIs and application of Duraphat every 3 months; (4) OHI and annual application of SDF solution.
Study design	RCT	Randomized double-blind longitudinal study	RCT	RCT
Primary outcome	Number of teeth	Root caries	Bleeding on probing (BoP), measured using the modified sulcus bleeding index (MSB)	Development of new caries on the exposed sound root surfaces of participants during the study period

Table 3. *Cont.*

Author(s)	Barbe, Kottmann, Derman, and Noack [52]	Brailsford, Fiske, Gilbert, Clark, and Beighton [53]	Girestam Croonquist, Dalum, Skott, Sjögren, Wårdh, and Morén [54]	Tan, Lo, Dyson, Luo, and Corbet [55]
Number (*n*) of participants at baseline	*n* = 50	*n* = 121	*n* = 146	*n* = 306
Mean age, yrs, ± standard deviation	83 ± 8	I = 85.6 ± 1.3 C = 79.8 ± 1.4	88.9 ± 4.1	78 ± 6.2
Gender	Female *n* = 34 Male *n* = 16	Female *n* = 65 Male *n* = 37	Female *n* = 108 Male *n* = 38	Female = 233 Male = 73
Mean number of teeth	17 ± 9	I = 13.73 ± 1.07 C = 15.50 ± 1.06	20.2 ± 3.0	14.3 ± 6.5
Study duration	3 mo	52 wks	6 mo	3 yrs
Number (*n*) of dropouts	*n* = 14	*n* = 19	*n* = 22	*n* = 103
Root caries index (RCI)	RCI (RCI1–RCI5), DMFT index	Length/distance from gingival margin, height, and width.	Fejerskov et al.'s five-level RCI [28]	RCI, DFS root score
Time of data examination	B + 3 mo	B + 13 wks + 26 wks + 1 yr	B + 3 mo + 6 mo	B + 1 yr + 2 yrs + 3 yrs
Intervention, and number (*n*) of participants at baseline	Professional brushing every second week by dental nurse, *n* = 25	Fluor protector varnish with Cervitec at baseline and at 6, 13, 26, and 39 wks, *n* = 52	Monthly professional cleaning, individual OHIs, and information, *n* = 72	(1) OHI + Cervitec every 3 mo, *n* = 71; (2) OHI + Duraphat every 3 mo, (3) OHI + SDF every 12 mo, *n* = 72
Intervention performed by	Dental nurse	Dentist	Dental hygienist	Dentist
Control and number (*n*) of participants at baseline	Oral care as usual or nurse-assisted, *n* = 25	Fluor protector varnish with placebo at baseline and at 6, 13, 26 and 39 wks, *n* = 50	Oral care as usual or nurse-assisted, *n* = 74	OHI—placebo (water) every 12 mo, *n* = 83
Risk of bias (RoB)	Moderate	Moderate	Moderate	Moderate

B = baseline; C = control group; Cervitec® = chlorhexidine (CHX) varnish; DFSs = decayed and filled surfaces; DMFT index = decayed, missing and filled teeth index; Duraphat® = sodium fluoride varnish; I = intervention group; mo = month (s); *n* = number of study subjects; OHI (s) = (individualized) oral hygiene instruction (s); RCI = root caries index; RCL = root caries lesion; RCT = randomized controlled trial; SDF = silver diamine fluoride; wk(s) = week(s); yr(s) = year(s).

3.3. Interventions

All four included studies [52–55] were RCTs studying the effect of various interventions for prevention and/or arrest of RCLs in care-dependent older adults. The study subjects were followed for different length study periods, from 3 months to 3 years. The interventions were: (1) professional tooth brushing every second week; (2) fluor protector varnish (Cervitec®) application at baseline and at 6, 13, 26, and 39 weeks; (3) professional cleaning with sodium fluoride varnish (Duraphat®), application, and oral hygiene instruction (OHI) once a month; and (4) OHI in combination with Cervitec or Duraphat application every 3 months, or application of silver diamine fluoride (SDF) every 12 months (Table 3).

3.4. Analysis

The four studies included in this systematic literature review all had different outcomes and different study population sizes, and further differed in the interventions administered, in data measurements, and study duration. Therefore, owing to the heterogenicity of the included studies, no meta-analysis or SWiM was performed. The findings for each study are therefore presented separately and in a narrative manner.

Root Caries Index

Barbe et al. [52] and Tan et al. [55] used the DMFT index and the five-level RCI, respectively. In addition, Tan et al. [55] also used the DFS root score. Girestam Croonquist et al. [54] used Fejerskov et al.'s five-level RCI [28], while Brailsford et al. [53] measured the length/distance from the gingival margin, the height, and width of the RCLs (Table 3).

3.5. Root Caries Development and Progression

Barbe et al. [52] found, in favor of the intervention group (professional brushing every second week by dental nurse), less development of RCLs at 3 months ($p = 0.002$). During the same period from baseline to 3 months, RCIs increased in the control group ($p = 0.006$) (Table 4).

Table 4. Results regarding root caries lesions (RCLs) in the included studies, from baseline to 3 years' follow-up.

Author(s), Year, Country	Results per Study							
Barbe et al., 2019 [52], Germany	Study groups		Baseline		3 mo		New RCLs	
	I^1 group mean (SD) for RCI		1.1 (1.2)		1.3 (1.3)		RCI increased in the control group between baseline and 3 months ($p = 0.006$).	
	C group mean (SD) for RCI		1.5 (1.8)		2.6 (1.3)			
	p-value		0.433		0.002 *			
Brailsford et al., 2002 [53], Great Britain	Baseline—1 yr							
	No new RCLs were detected in either the I^2 or the c/placebo group.							
Girestam Croonquist et al., 2020 [54], Sweden	RCI		Baseline—3 mo		Baseline—6 mo		3–6 mo	
			I^3	C	I^3	C	I^3	C
	Healthy *n* (%)	Deteriorated	20 (28.6)	24 (39.3)	22 (31.9)	15 (27.3)	15 (21.7)	9 (16.4)
		Unchanged	38 (54.3)	27 (44.3)	32 (46.4)	26 (47.3)	33 (47.8)	28 (50.9)
		Improved	12 (17.1)	10 (16.4)	15 (21.7)	14 (25.5)	21 (30.4)	18 (32.7)
		p-value	0.41		0.84		0.76	
	Initial caries *n* (%)	Deteriorated	15 (21.4)	18 (29.5)	20 (29.0)	14 (25.5)	20 (29.0)	10 (18.2)
		Unchanged	44 (62.9)	30 (49.2)	39 (56.5)	31 (56.4)	38 (55.1)	36 (65.5)
		Improved	11 (15.7)	13 (21.3)	10 (14.5)	10 (18.2)	11 (15.9)	9 (16.4)
		p-value	0.29		0.82		0.39	
	Active caries *n* (%)	Deteriorated	9 (12.9)	3 (4.9)	7 (10.1)	9 (16.4)	11 (15.9)	11 (20.0)
		Unchanged	40 (57.1)	37 (60.7)	41 (59.4)	32 (58.2)	46 (66.6)	42 (76.4)
		Improved	21 (30.0)	21 (34.4)	21 (30.4)	14 (25.5)	12 (17.4)	2 (3.6)
		p-value	0.28		0.55		0.05 *	
Tan et al., 2010 [55], China	Study groups	Mean number/SE of new active root caries or fillings in each study group						
		1 yr (*n* = 247)		2 yrs (*n* = 227)		3 yrs (*n* = 203)		
	OHI	1.5 (SE 0.2)		2.0 (SE 0.3)		2.5 (SE 0.5)		
	OHI + Cervitec	1.0 (SE 0.2)		1.0 (SE 0.3)		1.1 (SE 0.2)		
	OHI + Duraphat	0.8 (SE 0.2)		0.9 (SE 0.2)		0.9 (SE 0.3)		
	OHI + SDF	0.4 (SE 0.1)		0.7 (SE 0.2)		0.7 (SE 0.2)		
	All groups	0.9 (SE 0.1)		1.2 (SE 0.1)		1.3 (SE 0.2)		

C = control group; Cervitec® = chlorhexidine (CHX) varnish every 3 months; Duraphat® = sodium fluoride varnish every 3 months; I = intervention group; I^1 = professional brushing every second week by dental nurse; I^2 = Fluor protector varnish with Cervitec at baseline, and at 6, 13, 26, and 39 weeks; I^3 = monthly professional cleaning, individual oral hygiene instructions, and information; mo (s) = month (s); *n* = number of study subjects; OHI (s) = (individualized) oral hygiene instruction (s); RCI = root caries index; SD = standard deviation; SDF = silver diamine fluoride every 12 months; SE = standard error; yr(s) = year(s). * $p \leq 0.05$.

Girestam Croonquist et al. [54] used Fejerskov et al.'s five-level RCI for grouping root caries scores, namely: score 1—healthy root surface and/or no RCLs; scores 2 and

4—inactive initial and manifest RCLs; scores 3 and 5—active initial and manifest RCLs. For no RCLs and initial RCLs, improvements were seen for both groups throughout the study period. Between 3 and 6 months, improvement of active RCLs was reported for the intervention group ($p = 0.05$) (Table 4).

Brailsford et al. [53] detected no new RCLs from baseline to 52 weeks in either group and concluded that RCLs in both groups were unchanged or had improved (Table 4). Contrarily, regarding height and width, the RCLs in the control group had increased compared with the intervention group ($p < 0.001$).

Tan et al. [55] followed their study subjects for 3 years. After 3 years, the group with only OHIs had a higher mean number of root surfaces with new active root caries or fillings compared with those with OHIs in combination with Cervitec or Duraphat or SDF application (Table 4). The relative risk for developing new RCLs was lower in the intervention groups compared with the controls. Furthermore, no difference in prevention of new RCLs was found between applying chlorhexidine (CHX) (four times per year), sodium fluoride (four times per year), and 38% SDF annually for a 3-year period. Compared with only OHIs, the application groups had a lower risk of developing new RCLs. Also, groups with higher risk of developing root caries were detected among the study subjects. The groups with higher risk of developing root caries were denture users (denture type not specified, probably partial dentures or dentures in only one jaw) ($p = 0.021$), study subjects with higher visible plaque index (VPI) score and higher root caries experience at baseline ($p = 0.001$), and exposed root surfaces ($p = 0.001$).

4. Discussion

This systematic review aimed to investigate the effect of domiciliary professional oral care interventions on root caries development and progression, in comparison with self-performed or nurse-assisted oral care.

The four included studies investigated different intervention methods over a variety of intervals and study periods. However, all the studies showed a positive effect in reducing or arresting RCLs [52–55]. The parameters shared by all the studied interventions were participation of dental personnel in mechanical plaque removal combined with application of fluoride agents (varnish or toothpaste) or CHX. This combination may be beneficial for care-dependent older adults with risk of RCLs development and progression. The effectiveness of an intervention with fluoride varnish and topical agents for reduction of RCLs depends on the interval and the frequency of application. For example, sodium fluoride varnish (Duraphat) is recommended to be applied four times per year [11,12]; however, a frequency of twice a year has also been shown to be effective in reducing the number of RCLs in care-dependent older adults [50]. Tan et al. [55] performed an intervention using SDF only once a year; even at this relatively low rate of application, they were able to report greater effectiveness in reducing new RCLs incidence compared with the other substances (Duraphat or Cervitec) [55].

The successful use of SDF among children for preventing coronal caries [23] has led to increased interest in studies among the older population with annual application of 38% SDF [20,23,55]. Despite promising results for arresting RCLs, SDF is only approved for use in some countries [56]. After application, SDF leaves a dark discoloration of the caries lesions [57].

4.1. Active Participation of Dental Personnel

Professional dental hygiene interventions have shown advantageous effects on oral hygiene status and management of RCLs within a relatively short time interval such as 2 weeks [52] or 1 month [54]. Regular and effective oral hygiene routines are important for care-dependent older adults. In addition, despite the costs of the intervention, a visit by a dental nurse could serve as a reminder for oral self-care. Hesitation to spend more for oral hygiene services was observed among the study subjects and their relatives in Barbe et al. [52], who report that participation would have been compromised if it had not been free of charge.

4.2. Training Nursing Staff

Education and hands-on training for both care-dependent older adults and nursing staff could contribute to improving oral hygiene among those in need [17]. Nurse-assisted oral care, particularly oral hygiene, is tedious and requires meticulous attention [16,49,58], particularly in view of the higher tendency of older people to retain their own teeth in high ages, and in view of complex dental constructions [21]. Moreover, nurse-assisted oral care for nursing home residents with poor cognitive function and communication problems is challenging [22]. Therefore, training in oral health care skills may be more useful than theoretical education for health care personnel [59,60]. To our knowledge, improved oral hygiene and compliance to perform such oral care routines over time has not been noted. One possible reason could be the high turnover rate among nursing staff in care of care-dependent older adults [61].

4.3. Awareness and Information among the Older Adults

There is a lack of prioritization of oral health, both among care-dependent older adults and among the nursing staff [62]. This could be attributed to insufficient knowledge of the connection between poor oral health and systemic diseases [2]. It is an important task for the dental profession to provide this knowledge before or in the early stages of care dependency. Failing to do so could lead to problems and high costs for health and dental care at both individual and societal levels [21].

Even though we had fairly open inclusion criteria, it was hard to identify studies that matched these. We found great diversity in study design, choice of intervention, and reported outcomes in the included four studies. When outcomes and outcome measurements differ, making it impossible to perform a meta-analysis, it may not be possible to improve future patient care. For future studies in this field, one possible way of using similar outcome measurements is, for example, to use the Core Outcome Measures in Effectiveness Trials (COMET) database to improve the efficiency of clinical trials and outcome measures. This database can be used to develop core outcome sets (COSs) [63]. COSs allow us to compare and collate results from various studies so that the basis for decisions, for both patients and dentalcare personnel, could be strengthened. Additionally, international consensus on appropriate interventions and outcome measurements would increase the feasibility of performing a meta-analysis of selected RCT studies involving clinical management of RCLs in frail older adults. A meta-analysis is crucial for closing the knowledge gap and conducting a clinical protocol for managing RCLs in frail older adults.

5. Conclusions

Based on the available literature it is not possible to conclusively determine the effect of domiciliary professional oral care on root caries development and progression in care-dependent older adults. Future studies in this field should use a standardized protocol for RCT studies with similar study design, interventions, outcomes, and follow-up periods to enable comparison and meta-analysis.

6. Clinical Relevance

There is a need to investigate the current scientific knowledge of the effect of domiciliary professional oral care interventions to prevent and arrest progression of RCLs. A great proportion of care-dependent older adults are prone to this condition, which calls for identification of evidence-based strategies to address the issue among this population.

This review highlights the importance of dental personnel and optimal mechanical plaque removal with fluoride or CHX application in impeding or arresting RCLs. Adequate timely information and awareness about the risk of RCLs, prevention, and management methods are therefore crucial, ideally before the person enters the phase of care dependency.

7. Supporting Information

Contact was made with the author Anna-Grete Barbe regarding the number of participants included in her and her co-authors' study. The right number was 50 (25 in each group). They recruited one more person after randomization.

8. Difference between Protocol and Review

Root caries development and progression on buccal root surface were initially the primary outcome measures. This was changed to root caries development and progression measured by a caries index.

Supplementary Materials: Supporting information can be downloaded at: www.crd.york.ac.uk/PROSPERO/display_record.asp?ID=CRD42021274595 (accessed on 14 September 2021).

Author Contributions: E.M., P.S., K.E., N.G., I.W. and H.D. have all contributed equally to this review. All authors have read and agreed to the published version of the manuscript.

Funding: This research was funded by the Centre for Clinical Research Dalarna, Uppsala University: 975402, and the Kamprad Family Foundation for Entrepreneurship, Research & Charity: 20210055.

Institutional Review Board Statement: Not applicable.

Informed Consent Statement: Not applicable.

Data Availability Statement: Not applicable.

Acknowledgments: We would like to thank Daniel Sundgren, librarian at the Library Falu Hospital, Falun, for the work and effort with the literature search for our systematic review.

Conflicts of Interest: The authors declare no conflict of interest.

References

1. Silva, M.; Hopcraft, M.; Morgan, M. Dental caries in Victorian nursing homes. *Aust. Dent. J.* **2014**, *59*, 321–328. [CrossRef] [PubMed]
2. Rapp, L.; Maret, D.; Diemer, F.; Lacoste Ferré, M.H. Dental Caries in Geriatric Dentistry: An Update for Clinicians. *Int. J. Oral Dent. Health* **2019**, *5*, 1–6. [CrossRef]
3. Zhang, J.; Leung, K.C.M.; Sardana, D.; Wong, M.C.M.; Lo, E.C.M. Risk predictors of dental root caries: A systematic review. *J. Dent.* **2019**, *89*, 103166. [CrossRef] [PubMed]
4. Ritter, A.V.; Shugars, D.A.; Bader, J.D. Root caries risk indicators: A systematic review of risk models. *Community Dent. Oral Epidemiol.* **2010**, *38*, 383–397. [CrossRef]
5. Kumar, S.; Tadakamadla, J.; Johnson, N.W. Effect of Toothbrushing Frequency on Incidence and Increment of Dental Caries: A Systematic Review and Meta-Analysis. *J. Dent. Res.* **2016**, *95*, 1230–1236. [CrossRef]
6. Walsh, T.; Worthington, H.V.; Glenny, A.M.; Marinho, V.C.; Jeroncic, A. Fluoride toothpastes of different concentrations for preventing dental caries. *Cochrane Database Syst. Rev.* **2019**, *3*, CD007868. [CrossRef]
7. Burrow, M.F.; Stacey, M.A. Management of Cavitated Root Caries Lesions: Minimum Intervention and Alternatives. *Monogr. Oral Sci.* **2017**, *26*, 106–114. [CrossRef]
8. Bashir, N.Z. Update on the prevalence of untreated caries in the US adult population, 2017–2020. *J. Am. Dent. Assoc.* **2022**, *153*, 300–308. [CrossRef]
9. Gavriilidou, N.N.; Belibasakis, G.N. Root caries: The intersection between periodontal disease and dental caries in the course of ageing. *Br. Dent. J.* **2019**, *227*, 1063–1067. [CrossRef]
10. Pentapati, K.C.; Siddiq, H.; Yeturu, S.K. Global and regional estimates of the prevalence of root caries—Systematic review and meta-analysis. *Saudi Dent. J.* **2019**, *31*, 3–15. [CrossRef]
11. The Swedish National Board o Health and Welfare. "Nationella Riktlinjer för Tandvård—Stöd för Styrning Och Ledning". Socialstyrelsen. 2021. Available online: https://www.socialstyrelsen.se/globalassets/sharepoint-dokument/artikelkatalog/nationella-riktlinjer/2021-9-7549.pdf (accessed on 10 June 2022).
12. Meyer-Lueckel, H.; Machiulskiene, V.; Giacaman, R.A. How to Intervene in the Root Caries Process? Systematic Review and Meta-Analyses. *Caries Res.* **2019**, *53*, 599–608. [CrossRef]
13. Ekstrand, K.R.; Poulsen, J.E.; Hede, B.; Twetman, S.; Qvist, V.; Ellwood, R.P. A randomized clinical trial of the anti-caries efficacy of 5000 compared to 1450 ppm fluoridated toothpaste on root caries lesions in elderly disabled nursing home residents. *Caries Res.* **2013**, *47*, 391–398. [CrossRef]
14. European Commission. *One Hundred Words for Equality: A Glossary of Terms on Equality between Women and Men*; Office for Official Publications of the European Communities: Luxembourg, 1998.

15. Dixe, M.d.A.C.R.; Frontini, R.; Sousa, P.M.L.; Peralta, T.d.J.d.A.; Teixeira, L.F.d.C.; Querido, A.I.F. Dependent person in self-care: Analysis of care needs. *Scand. J. Caring Sci.* **2020**, *34*, 727–735. [CrossRef]
16. Wårdh, I.; Jonsson, M.; Wikstrom, M. Attitudes to and knowledge about oral health care among nursing home personnel—An area in need of improvement. *Gerodontology* **2012**, *29*, e787–e792. [CrossRef]
17. Sjögren, P.; Girestam, C.; Skott, P.; Marsson, N.; Nova, R.; Zimmerman, M.; Wårdh, I. Professional Domiciliary Oral Care for Elderly in Nursing Homes—A Randomized Controlled Pilot Trial. *Health* **2016**, *8*, 1112–1119. [CrossRef]
18. Gronbeck-Linden, I.; Hagglin, C.; Petersson, A.; Linander, P.O.; Gahnberg, L. Discontinued dental attendance among elderly people in Sweden. *J. Int. Soc. Prev. Community Dent.* **2016**, *6*, 224–229. [CrossRef]
19. Fereshtehnejad, S.M.; Garcia-Ptacek, S.; Religa, D.; Holmer, J.; Buhlin, K.; Eriksdotter, M.; Sandborgh-Englund, G. Dental care utilization in patients with different types of dementia: A longitudinal nationwide study of 58,037 individuals. *Alzheimers Dement.* **2018**, *14*, 10–19. [CrossRef]
20. Li, R.; Lo, E.C.; Liu, B.Y.; Wong, M.C.; Chu, C.H. Randomized clinical trial on arresting dental root caries through silver diammine fluoride applications in community-dwelling elders. *J. Dent.* **2016**, *51*, 15–20. [CrossRef]
21. Ástvaldsdóttir, Á.; Boström, A.M.; Davidson, T.; Gabre, P.; Gahnberg, L.; Sandborgh Englund, G.; Skott, P.; Ståhlnacke, K.; Tranaeus, S.; Wilhelmsson, H.; et al. Oral health and dental care of older persons-A systematic map of systematic reviews. *Gerodontology* **2018**, *35*, 290–304. [CrossRef]
22. Chalmers, J.; Pearson, A. Oral hygiene care for residents with dementia: A literature review. *J. Adv. Nurs.* **2005**, *52*, 410–419. [CrossRef]
23. Zhang, W.; McGrath, C.; Lo, E.C.; Li, J.Y. Silver diamine fluoride and education to prevent and arrest root caries among community-dwelling elders. *Caries Res.* **2013**, *47*, 284–290. [CrossRef] [PubMed]
24. Methley, A.M.; Campbell, S.; Chew-Graham, C.; McNally, R.; Cheraghi-Sohi, S. PICO, PICOS and SPIDER: A comparison study of specificity and sensitivity in three search tools for qualitative systematic reviews. *BMC Health Serv. Res.* **2014**, *14*, 579. [CrossRef] [PubMed]
25. World Health Organization. *Oral Health Surveys—Basic Methods*; WHO: Geneva, Switzerland, 2013; p. 125. ISBN 978-92-4-154864-9. Available online: https://www.who.int/oral_health/publications/9789241548649/en/ (accessed on 8 May 2020).
26. Katz, R.V. Assessing root caries in populations: The evolution of the root caries index. *J. Public Health Dent.* **1980**, *40*, 7–16. [CrossRef] [PubMed]
27. Hayes, M.; Burke, F.; Allen, P.F. Incidence, Prevalence and Global Distribution of Root Caries. *Monogr. Oral Sci.* **2017**, *26*, 1–8. [CrossRef] [PubMed]
28. Fejerskov, O.; Luan, W.M.; Nyvad, B.; Budtz-Jorgensen, E.; Holm-Pedersen, P. Active and inactive root surface caries lesions in a selected group of 60- to 80-year-old Danes. *Caries Res.* **1991**, *25*, 385–391. [CrossRef]
29. Mourad Ouzzani, H.H.; Fedorowicz, Z.; Elmagarmid, A. Rayyan—A web and mobile app for systematic reviews. *Syst. Rev.* **2016**, *5*, 210. Available online: https://www.rayyan.ai/ (accessed on 6 August 2021). [CrossRef]
30. Swedish Agency for Health Technology Assessment and Assessment of Social Service (SBU). Utvärdering av Metoder i Hälso-Och Sjukvården Och Insatser i Socialtjänsten: En Metodbok. 2020. Available online: https://www.sbu.se/metodbok (accessed on 24 May 2022).
31. Sterne, J.A.C.; Savović, J.; Page, M.J.; Elbers, R.G.; Blencowe, N.S.; Boutron, I.; Cates, C.J.; Cheng, H.Y.; Corbett, M.S.; Eldridge, S.M.; et al. RoB 2: A revised tool for assessing risk of bias in randomised trials. *BMJ* **2019**, *366*, l4898. [CrossRef]
32. Page, M.J.; Moher, D.; Bossuyt, P.M.; Boutron, I.; Hoffmann, T.C.; Mulrow, C.D.; Shamseer, L.; Tetzlaff, J.M.; Akl, E.A.; Brennan, S.E.; et al. PRISMA 2020 explanation and elaboration: Updated guidance and exemplars for reporting systematic reviews. *BMJ* **2021**, *372*, n160. [CrossRef]
33. Wyatt, C.C. A 5-year follow-up of older adults residing in long-term care facilities: Utilisation of a comprehensive dental programme. *Gerodontology* **2009**, *26*, 282–290. [CrossRef]
34. Wyatt, C.C.L.; MacEntee, M.I. Caries management for institutionalized elders using fluoride and chlorhexidine mouthrinses. *Community Dent. Oral Epidemiol.* **2004**, *32*, 322–328. [CrossRef]
35. Niessen, L.C. Chlorhexidine varnish, sodium fluoride varnish, and silver diamine fluoride solution can prevent the development of new root caries in elders living in senior homes in Hong Kong. *J. Evid. Based Dent. Pract.* **2012**, *12*, 95–96. [CrossRef]
36. López, R.M.; Uribe, M.R.; Rodríguez, B.O.; Casasempere, I.V. Comparison between amine fluoride and chlorhexidine with institutionalized elders: A pilot study. *Gerodontology* **2013**, *30*, 112–118. [CrossRef]
37. Yi Mohammadi, J.J.; Franks, K.; Hines, S. Effectiveness of professional oral health care intervention on the oral health of residents with dementia in residential aged care facilities: A systematic review protocol. *JBI Database System. Rev. Implement. Rep.* **2015**, *13*, 110–122. [CrossRef]
38. Nct. Effectiveness on SDF Solution and PVP-I Combined NaF Varnish in Preventing Root Caries in Elders. 2018. Available online: https://clinicaltrials.gov/show/NCT03654820 (accessed on 10 September 2021).
39. Mojon, P.; Rentsch, A.; Budtz-Jørgensen, E.; Baehni, P.C. Effects of an oral health program on selected clinical parameters and salivary bacteria in a long-term care facility. *Eur. J. Oral Sci.* **1998**, *106*, 827–834. [CrossRef]
40. Ritter, A.V. The Efficacy of Fluoride on Root Caries Progression May Be Dose-dependent. *J. Evid. Based Dent. Pract.* **2013**, *13*, 177–179. [CrossRef]

41. Marchesan, J.T.; Byrd, K.M.; Moss, K.; Preisser, J.S.; Morelli, T.; Zandona, A.F.; Jiao, Y.; Beck, J. Flossing Is Associated with Improved Oral Health in Older Adults. *J. Dent. Res.* **2020**, *99*, 1047–1053. [CrossRef]
42. Barbe, A.G.; Küpeli, L.S.; Hamacher, S.; Noack, M.J. Impact of regular professional toothbrushing on oral health, related quality of life, and nutritional and cognitive status in nursing home residents. *Int. J. Dent. Hyg.* **2020**, *18*, 238–250. [CrossRef]
43. MacEntee, M.I.; Silver, J.G.; Gibson, G.; Weiss, R. Oral health in a long-term care institution equipped with a dental service. *Community Dent. Oral Epidemiol.* **1985**, *13*, 260–263. [CrossRef]
44. Pearson, A.; Chalmers, J. Oral hygiene care for adults with dementia in residential aged care facilities. *JBI Libr. Syst. Rev.* **2004**, *2*, 1–89. [CrossRef]
45. Al-Nasser, L.; Lamster, I.B. Prevention and management of periodontal diseases and dental caries in the older adults. *Periodontol 2000* **2020**, *84*, 69–83. [CrossRef]
46. Patel, R.; Khan, I.; Pennington, M.; Pitts, N.B.; Robertson, C.; Gallagher, J.E. Protocol for A randomised feasibility trial comparing fluoride interventions to prevent dental decay in older people in care homes (FInCH trial). *BMC Oral Health* **2021**, *21*, 1–12. [CrossRef] [PubMed]
47. ISRCTN. A Randomised Controlled Trial to Evaluate the Cost Effectiveness of Prescribing High Concentration Fluoride Toothpaste to Prevent Tooth Decay in Older Adults. 2017. Available online: http://www.who.int/trialsearch/Trial2.aspx?TrialID=ISRCTN11992428 (accessed on 10 September 2021).
48. Raghoonandan, P.; Cobban, S.J.; Compton, S.M. A scoping review of the use of fluoride varnish in elderly people living in long term care facilities. *Can. J. Dent. Hyg.* **2011**, *45*, 217–222.
49. Wikstrom, M.; Kareem, K.L.; Almstahl, A.; Palmgren, E.; Lingstrom, P.; Wardh, I. Effect of 12-month weekly professional oral hygiene care on the composition of the oral flora in dentate, dependent elderly residents: A prospective study. *Gerodontology* **2017**, *34*, 240–248. [CrossRef] [PubMed]
50. Jabir, E.; McGrade, C.; Quinn, G.; McGarry, J.; Nic Iomhair, A.; Kelly, N.; Srinivasan, M.; Watson, S.; McKenna, G.J. Evaluating the effectiveness of fluoride varnish in preventing caries amongst Long-Term Care Facility Residents. *Gerodontology* **2021**, *39*, 250–256. [CrossRef]
51. Ekstrand, K.; Martignon, S.; Holm-Pedersen, P. Development and evaluation of two root caries controlling programmes for home-based frail people older than 75 years. *Gerodontology* **2008**, *25*, 67–75. [CrossRef]
52. Barbe, A.G.; Kottmann, H.E.; Derman, S.H.M.; Noack, M.J. Efficacy of regular professional brushing by a dental nurse for 3 months in nursing home residents—A randomized, controlled clinical trial. *Int. J. Dent. Hyg.* **2019**, *17*, 327–335. [CrossRef]
53. Brailsford, S.R.; Fiske, J.; Gilbert, S.; Clark, D.; Beighton, D. The effects of the combination of chlorhexidine/thymol- and fluoride-containing varnishes on the severity of root caries lesions in frail institutionalised elderly people. *J. Dent.* **2002**, *30*, 319–324. [CrossRef]
54. Girestam Croonquist, C.; Dalum, J.; Skott, P.; Sjögren, P.; Wårdh, I.; Morén, E. Effects of Domiciliary Professional Oral Care for Care-Dependent Elderly in Nursing Homes—Oral Hygiene, Gingival Bleeding, Root Caries and Nursing Staff's Oral Health Knowledge and Attitudes. *Clin. Interv. Aging* **2020**, *15*, 1305–1315. [CrossRef]
55. Tan, H.P.; Lo, E.C.; Dyson, J.E.; Luo, Y.; Corbet, E.F. A randomized trial on root caries prevention in elders. *J. Dent. Res.* **2010**, *89*, 1086–1090. [CrossRef]
56. Seifo, N.; Robertson, M.; MacLean, J.; Blain, K.; Grosse, S.; Milne, R.; Seeballuck, C.; Innes, N. The use of silver diamine fluoride (SDF) in dental practice. *Br. Dent. J.* **2020**, *228*, 75–81. [CrossRef]
57. Burgess, J.O.; Vaghela, P.M. Silver Diamine Fluoride: A Successful Anticarious Solution with Limits. *Adv. Dent. Res.* **2018**, *29*, 131–134. [CrossRef]
58. Edman, K.; Wårdh, I. Oral health care beliefs among care personnel working with older people—Follow-up of oral care education provided by dental hygienists. *Int. J. Dent. Hyg.* **2022**, *20*, 241–248. [CrossRef]
59. Weening-Verbree, L.F.; Schuller, D.A.A.; Cheung, S.L.; Zuidema, P.; Schans, P.; Hobbelen, D. Barriers and facilitators of oral health care experienced by nursing home staff. *Geriatr. Nurs.* **2021**, *42*, 799–805. [CrossRef]
60. Doshi, M.; Lee, L.; Keddie, M. Effective mouth care for older people living in nursing homes. *Nurs. Older People* **2021**, *33*, 18–23. [CrossRef]
61. Simons, D.; Baker, P.; Jones, B.; Kidd, E.A.; Beighton, D. An evaluation of an oral health training programme for carers of the elderly in residential homes. *Br. Dent. J.* **2000**, *188*, 206–210. [CrossRef]
62. Kiyak, H.A.; Reichmuth, M. Barriers to and enablers of older adults' use of dental services. *J. Dent. Educ.* **2005**, *69*, 975–986. [CrossRef]
63. Lamont, T.; Schwendicke, F.; Innes, N. Why we need a core outcome set for trials of interventions for prevention and management of caries. *Evid.-Based Dent.* **2015**, *16*, 66–68. [CrossRef]

Disclaimer/Publisher's Note: The statements, opinions and data contained in all publications are solely those of the individual author(s) and contributor(s) and not of MDPI and/or the editor(s). MDPI and/or the editor(s) disclaim responsibility for any injury to people or property resulting from any ideas, methods, instructions or products referred to in the content.

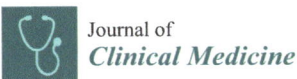 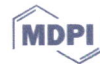

Article

Association between Oral Hygiene Information Sources and Daily Dental and Denture Care Practices in Urban Community-Dwelling Older Adults

Kalliopi Konstantopoulou and Anastassia E. Kossioni *

Department of Prosthodontics, School of Dentistry, National and Kapodistrian University of Athens, 11527 Athens, Greece
* Correspondence: akossion@dent.uoa.gr; Tel.: +30-210-746-1212

Abstract: The purpose of this cross-sectional study was to explore the sources of daily oral hygiene information among urban community-dwelling older adults in Athens, Greece and associate them with their dental and denture care habits. One hundred and fifty-four older adults (aged 71.7 ± 9.2 years) participated in the study, and their dental status, denture use, daily oral care habits according to current gerodontology recommendations, and oral care information sources were investigated. Daily oral hygiene practices were poor, and a small number of individuals recalled having received oral hygiene advice from a dentist. Only 41.7% of the 139 dentate participants performed toothbrushing with fluoride-based toothpaste at least twice a day, and 35.9% completed regular interdental cleaning. Among 54 denture wearers, 68.5% removed their denture(s) at night, and 54% cleaned them at least twice a day. Oral hygiene information sources included dentists (for approximately half of the participants), media, friends/relatives, non-dental health care providers and dental technicians. Dentate participants who had received oral hygiene information from dentists had a greater probability of brushing their teeth with fluoride toothpaste at least twice a day ($p = 0.049$, OR = 2.15) and performing regular interdental cleaning ($p < 0.001$, OR = 29.26). Denture wearers who had received instructions about denture hygiene from dentists were more likely to use a brush and mild soap ($p = 0.016$, OR = 14.67) and remove their denture(s) at night ($p = 0.003$, OR = 8.75). Dentists should improve their oral health prevention and promotion strategies for their older patients.

Keywords: oral hygiene; dentures; information sources; dental devices; home care; geriatric dentistry; aged; independent living

Citation: Konstantopoulou, K.; Kossioni, A.E. Association between Oral Hygiene Information Sources and Daily Dental and Denture Care Practices in Urban Community-Dwelling Older Adults. *J. Clin. Med.* 2023, 12, 2881. https://doi.org/10.3390/jcm12082881

Academic Editor: Andrea Sardella

Received: 10 February 2023
Revised: 30 March 2023
Accepted: 12 April 2023
Published: 14 April 2023

Copyright: © 2023 by the authors. Licensee MDPI, Basel, Switzerland. This article is an open access article distributed under the terms and conditions of the Creative Commons Attribution (CC BY) license (https://creativecommons.org/licenses/by/4.0/).

1. Introduction

Oral health is a fundamental right of all people enabling them to enjoy a high quality of life [1]. It is an integral part of general health and a crucial element of healthy ageing [2]. Oral diseases should be addressed among other non-communicable diseases as a global public health priority [1,3], and countries should promote universal health coverage for oral health by 2030 [4]. Moreover, there is a growing interest in the association between oral and general health and the identification of oral health indicators with high prognostic or diagnostic value for general health deterioration [5,6].

One of the main causes of oral conditions, such as dental caries and periodontal disease, as well as systematic infection, is plaque accumulation due to poor oral hygiene. Periodontal disease and poor oral hygiene in teeth and dentures have been associated with aspiration pneumonia in hospitalised patients and nursing home residents [7,8]. Further, denture wearing during sleep has been associated with a 2.3-fold higher risk of the incidence of aspiration pneumonia in community-dwelling older people [9]. To reduce the number of respiratory pathogens, meticulous dental and denture hygiene and removal of dentures at night are among the recommended measures to prevent aspiration pneumonia in frail older adults [7,10]. According to the Japanese Society of Gerodontology, poor oral hygiene is one of the signs of oral hypofunction that may lead to oral frailty [11].

Three European expert reports by dentists, physicians and dental hygienists working with older people described the necessary measures to promote oral health in older people [12–14]. Among these measures are brushing the teeth at least twice a day with a toothbrush and fluoride toothpaste, cleaning the interdental spaces at least once a day, brushing the dentures at least twice a day with a nonabrasive denture cleanser or liquid soap combined with chemical cleansing agents, and removing the dentures during sleep.

However, although the above daily practices are easy to perform by older individuals (and their carers) and can prevent many oral and general conditions, neglected oral hygiene and poor daily oral care practices are common among older adults [3,8,15–20].

Several structural, intermediate and proximal determinants affect oral health in older adults, including poor general health, frailty, care dependency, poor oral health literacy, negative or wrong beliefs and attitudes towards oral health, lack of interest in oral health, limited professional advice, inadequate oral health policies and commercial activities/information which may manipulate their behaviour [3,4,13,19,21–23].

Dental patients are exposed to various sources of oral health information, including dental professionals, other healthcare workers, relatives, friends, or the media [24,25]. Young and middle-aged people in Iran received oral health information mainly from dentists and television/radio [24]. A study among Brazilian denture wearers with a mean age of 62 years has shown that 77.5% had not received any instructions on denture cleansing and 77.1% on oral care, while an association was recorded between the lack of instructions regarding oral care and the presence of denture stomatitis [26].

Poor professional support from dentists and other healthcare providers, including inadequate, inefficient or ineffective instructions on daily oral hygiene, may lead to poor daily oral care practices and various oral and systemic conditions. However, data on the sources of oral hygiene instructions among community-dwelling older people and their association with performing the recommended oral hygiene practices are scarce. Therefore, the purpose of this study was to explore the sources of daily oral hygiene and care information among urban community-dwelling older adults and associate them with their dental and denture care habits.

2. Materials and Methods

2.1. Study Design

The study had a cross-sectional design. Study participants were community-dwelling older adults who visited the dental school of the National and Kapodistrian University of Athens, Greece, for examination/treatment. The participants' recruitment was conducted according to the following inclusion criteria: (a) being over 60 years of age, (b) being free of cognitive or sensory problems that may affect the ability to communicate with the investigators, (c) being able to speak and understand the Greek language, and (d) offering informed consent to participate. The interviews took place at the first treatment session before any discussion or demonstration of oral hygiene practices by students and faculty.

The research instruments consisted of structured oral interviews and oral clinical examinations. Oral interviews included the recording of participants' sociodemographic characteristics, dental visitations habits, oral and denture hygiene habits, and sources of information about daily oral hygiene. Specific questions investigated the application of currently recommended oral hygiene practices for older adults, including toothbrushing at least twice a day with fluoride toothpaste, interdental brushing at least once a day, denture cleansing at least twice a day with a brush and mild soap, regular use of denture cleansing tablets and removing dentures at night. Dentate/edentulism status and the presence of removable prostheses were also recorded. The sample size was determined using the G*Power 3.1.9.4 software (www.gpower.hhu.de), which pointed at 50 participants [Chi-square test, effect size = 0.4, power of $1 - \beta$ (beta error) = 0.80, α (alpha error) = 0.05, df (degrees of freedom) = 1].

2.2. Statistical Analysis

Data analysis was performed anonymously. Statistical analyses included descriptive statistics and univariate analyses (Chi-square test and Fischer's Exact test). Independent variables with statistically significant or marginally significant ($p < 0.10$) association with the recommended oral and denture hygiene practices were further included in logistic regression analyses. The dependent variables were toothbrushing at least twice a day, using regular interdental cleaning, and removal of dentures at night. The level of statistical significance was set at $p \leq 0.05$. The analysis was performed using statistical software (IBM Corp. Released 2019. IBM SPSS Statistics for Windows, Version 26.0. Armonk, NY, USA: IBM Corp.).

3. Results

3.1. Daily Oral Hygiene Habits and Sources of Oral Care Information

A total of 154 community-dwelling older people (55 males and 99 females) with a mean age of 71.7 ± 9.2 years participated in this study. Participants' sociodemographic characteristics are shown in Table 1. The majority belonged to the age group 60–74 years. Of the total sample, 64% were married, 27.9% were widowed, and 38.4% had attended six or fewer years of formal education. A total of 42.9% reported that they had visited the dentist within the last 12 months. Clinical examination revealed complete edentulism in 9.7% of the participants. The dental hygiene habits and sources of daily dental care information for the dentate older adults ($n = 139$) are reported in Table 2. Forty-two per cent of the respondents cleaned their teeth at least twice a day, as recommended, and 1.4% never. The most frequent method of daily dental hygiene was a manual toothbrush and fluoride toothpaste (92.1%), while interdental cleaning was performed by only 35.9% of the participants.

Table 1. Sociodemographic characteristics and dental visitation habits of study participants.

	n	%
Sociodemographic Characteristics		
Gender		
Male	55	35.7%
Female	99	64.3%
Total	154	100.0%
Age (years)		
<75	92	59.7%
≥75	62	40.3%
Education (years)		
≤6 years	59	38.4%
7–12 years	56	36.4%
>12 years	36	23.4%

Table 2. Dental hygiene habits and sources of daily dental hygiene information among dentate older individuals ($n = 139$).

	n	%
Dental hygiene habits		
Toothbrushing frequency		
≥Twice a day	58	41.7%
Once a day	58	41.7%
<Once a day	21	15.1%
Never	2	1.5%
Toothbrushing means		
Toothbrush and fluoride toothpaste	128	92.1%
Electric toothbrush and fluoride toothpaste	4	2.9%
Toothbrush and water	5	3.6%
No teeth cleaning	2	1.4%

Table 2. *Cont.*

	n	%
Interdental cleaning		
Interdental cleaning on a regular basis	50	35.9%
Interdental brushes	30	21.6%
Dental floss	13	9.3%
Both interdental brushes and dental floss	7	5.0%
Information source for toothbrushing		
Dentist	69	49.6%
Pharmacist	8	5.8%
Relatives/friends	7	5%
Magazines/TV/internet	5	3.6%
Dental technician	1	0.7%
None/cannot remember	49	35.3%
Information source for interdental cleaning		
Dentist	48	34.5%
Pharmacist	3	2.2%
Relatives/friends	1	0.7%
Magazines/TV/internet	3	2.2%
Formal education (School/University, etc.)	1	0.7%
None/cannot remember	82	59.0%

Only 29 (20.9%) of the dentate participants performed the recommended combination of toothbrushing at least twice a day and daily interdental cleaning. The most frequent source of oral hygiene information for toothbrushing and interdental cleaning was the dentist (49.6% and 34.5%, respectively). Other information sources included pharmacists, relatives and friends, magazines, TV, radio or internet, formal education and dental technicians. However, 35.3% and 59.0% reported that they had never obtained or did not remember to have received any information about toothbrushing or interdental cleaning, respectively.

Fifty-four participants (35.1%) used complete or partial removable dentures. Details on denture wearing, denture hygiene habits and related sources of information are presented in Table 3. The age of dentures was 11.6 ± 10.4 years (range 1–50 years). Only 29 (53.7%) of denture wearers cleaned them at least twice a day, as recommended. Mechanical brushing with toothpaste was the most frequent denture hygiene means (55.4%), and only 16.1% used a (tooth)brush and mild soap. Few participants reported brushing only with water or soda and lemon, using sodium hypochlorite or using only denture cleansing tablets. Denture cleansing tablets were used by 12 (22.2%) denture wearers, usually in combination with other methods.

Almost 70% of denture wearers removed their denture (s) at night, as strongly suggested, while 31.5% always used them (Table 3). The dentist was the most common source of denture care information (42.6%), followed by relatives and friends, pharmacists, and dental technicians. Moreover, 51.9% of denture wearers mentioned that the dentist advised them to remove their denture (s) at night. Forty-four per cent did not receive or did not remember to have received any information about daily denture hygiene and care.

Nine denture wearers (16.7%) used denture adhesives; of these participants, seven (13%) always used them, and two (3.7%) sometimes used them. The dentist was the main source of information on the use of denture adhesives (13%), followed by TV/magazines/internet (5.5%), relatives/friends (3.7%) and pharmacists (1.8%). Thirty-seven (66.1%) denture wearers did not know how often dentures should be replaced.

Twenty individuals (12.9%) used a mouth rinse on a daily basis, and 34 (22.1%) occasionally. The main source of information about mouth rinses was the dentist (16.2%), followed by media (5.8%), relatives and friends (5.2%), and pharmacists (1.3%).

Table 3. Dentures' use, dentures' hygiene habits and sources of information about daily dentures' care among denture wearers ($n = 54$).

	n	%
Denture use		
Maxillary complete denture	23	42.6%
Mandibular complete denture	18	33.3%
Maxillary partial denture	21	35.2%
Mandibular partial denture	28	50.0%
Denture hygiene frequency		
≥Twice a day	29	53.7%
Once a day	22	40.7%
Not every day	3	5.6%
Denture hygiene means		
Brushing with mild soap	9	16.7%
Brushing with toothpaste	31	57.4%
Brushing only with water	6	11.1%
Brushing with soda and lemon	1	1.9%
Only rinsing with water	4	7.4%
Use of denture cleansing tablets	12	22.2%
Denture cleansing tablets only	1	1.9%
Use of sodium hypochlorite	1	1.9%
Denture use frequency		
During the day	30	55.6%
Always (24 h)	17	31.5%
During meals only	6	11.1%
When going out only	1	1.9%
Denture removal at night	37	68.5%
Information source for denture hygiene		
Dentist	23	42.6%
Pharmacist	1	1.9%
Relatives and friends	3	5.6%
Dental technician	1	1.9%
None/cannot remember	24	44.4%
Information from the dentist for removing dentures at night		
Yes	28	51.9%
No	26	48.1%

3.2. Factors Affecting the Application of the Recommended Daily Dental Hygiene Practices among Dentate Participants

The association between toothbrushing frequency of at least twice a day among dentate older adults and several independent variables is shown in Table 4. Toothbrushing at least twice a day was statistically significantly associated with not being married ($p = 0.046$), having more years of formal education ($p = 0.006$), visiting the dentist within the past 12 months ($p < 0.001$) and having received relevant information from a dentist (0.003).

Multivariate analysis revealed statistically significant effects of education, marital status, last dental visit, and source of information on toothbrushing frequency (Table 5). Older individuals who were married ($β = 0.76$, OR = 2.15), those who had received at least seven years of education ($β = 0.80$, OR = 2.22), those who visited the dentist within the last 12 months ($β = 1.04$, OR = 2.84) and those informed by the dentist about daily oral hygiene ($β = 0.77$, OR = 2.15) were more likely to brush their teeth at least twice a day (Table 5).

Univariate analyses between regular interdental cleaning and various independent variables are presented in Table 6. More years of formal education and being informed by a dentist were statistically significantly associated with regular interdental cleaning ($p = 0.014$ and $p < 0.001$, respectively). Multivariate analysis (Table 7) demonstrated that only the source of information had a significant effect on interdental cleaning. Participants who were informed about interdental cleaning by their dentists were more likely to regularly use interdental brushes and/or dental floss (β = 3.38, OR = 29.26).

Table 4. The association of sociodemographic characteristics, dental visitation habits and source of dental hygiene information with the recommended toothbrushing frequency in dentate participants.

Independent Variable		n (%)	Toothbrushing Frequency n (%)		p-Value
			<2 Twice/Day	≥2 Twice/Day	
Gender	Male	51 (26.7%)	29 (56.9%)	22 (43.1%)	0.797 [a]
	Female	88 (63.3%)	52 (59.1%)	36 (40.9%)	
Age	≤74 years	89 (64%)	52 (58.4%)	37 (41.6%)	0.466 [b]
	75–84 years	44 (31.7%)	27 (61.4%)	17 (38.6%)	
	≥85 years	6 (4.3%)	2 (33.3%)	4 (66.7%)	
Marital status	Married	90 (64.7%)	58 (64.4%)	32 (35.6%)	0.046 [a]
	Other	49 (35.3%)	23 (46.9%)	26 (53.1%)	
Education	≤6 years	52 (37.4%)	38 (73.1%)	14 (26.9%)	0.006 [a]
	>6 years	87 (62.6%)	43 (49.4%)	44 (50.6%)	
Last dental visit	≤12 months	63 (45.3%)	26 (41.3%)	37 (58.7%)	<0.001 [a]
	>12 months	76 (54.7%)	55 (72.4%)	21 (27.6%)	
Source of oral health information	Dentist	73 (52.5%)	34 (46.6%)	39 (53.4%)	0.003 [a]
	Other	66 (47.5%)	47 (71.2%)	19 (28.8%)	

[a] Chi-square test, [b] Fischer's Exact test.

Table 5. Multivariate analysis between toothbrushing frequency at least twice a day and independent variables.

Predictor Variables	β	SE	p-Value [a]	Odds Ratio
Marital status	0.76	0.40	0.050	2.15
Education	0.80	0.41	0.050	2.22
Last dental visit	1.04	0.39	0.007	2.84
Source of oral health information	0.77	0.39	0.049	2.15

[a] Binary Logistic Regression.

Table 6. The association of sociodemographic characteristics, dental visitation habits and source of daily dental hygiene information with regular interdental cleaning in dentate participants.

Independent Variable		n (%)	Interdental Cleaning on a Regular Basis n (%)		p-Value
			No	Yes	
Gender	Male	51 (26.7%)	36 (70.6%)	15 (29.4%)	0.220 [a]
	Female	88 (63.3%)	53 (60.2%)	35 (39.8%)	
Age	≤74 years	89 (64%)	54 (62.7%)	35 (39.3%)	0.485 [b]
	75–84 years	44 (31.7%)	30 (68.2%)	14 (31.8%)	
	≥85 years	6 (4.3%)	5 (83.3%)	1 (16.7%)	
Marital status	Married	90 (64.7%)	56 (62.2%)	34 (37.8%)	0.548 [a]
	Other	49 (35.3%)	33 (67.3%)	16 (32.7%)	
Education	≤6 years	52 (37.4%)	40 (82.7%)	12 (17.3%)	0.014 [a]
	>6 years	87 (62.6%)	49 (56.3%)	38 (43.7%)	
Last dental visit	≤12 months	63 (45.3%)	38 (60.3%)	25 (39.7%)	0.406 [a]
	>12 months	76 (54.7%)	51 (67.1%)	25 (32.9%)	
Source of oral health information	Dentist	73 (52.5%)	9 (18.8%)	39 (81.2%)	<0.001 [a]
	Other	66 (47.5%)	80 (87.9%)	11 (12.1%)	

[a] Chi-square test, [b] Fischer's Exact test.

Table 7. Multivariate analysis between interdental cleaning and independent variables.

Predictor Variable	β	SE	p-Value [a]	Odds Ratio
Education	0.52	0.51	0.327	1.67
Source of oral health information	3.38	0.49	<0.001	29.26

[a] Binary Logistic Regression.

The factors affecting the combination of tooth brushing at least twice a day and regular interdental cleaning are presented in Table 8 and include more years of formal education, a dental visit within the past 12 months, and having received relevant instructions from a dentist ($p = 0.012$, $p = 0.042$ and $p < 0.001$, respectively). The multivariate analysis showed that older adults who had obtained oral hygiene information directly from the dentist had a statistically significantly higher probability of brushing their teeth at least twice per day and performing regular interdental cleaning (β = 2.40, OR = 11.03) (Table 9).

Table 8. The association of sociodemographic characteristics, dental visitation habits and source of daily dental hygiene information with toothbrushing frequency at least twice a day and interdental cleaning at least once a day.

Independent Variable		n (%)	Toothbrushing Frequency ≥ Twice a Day and Interdental Cleaning on a Regular Basis n (%)		p-Value
			No	Yes	
Gender	Male	51 (26.7%)	41 (80.4%)	10 (19.6%)	0.782 [a]
	Female	88 (63.3%)	69 (78.4%)	19 (21.6%)	
Age	≤74 years	89 (64%)	71 (79.8%)	18 (20.2%)	0.915 [b]
	75–84 years	44 (31.7%)	34 (77.3%)	10 (22.7%)	
	≥85 years	6 (4.3%)	5 (83.3%)	1 (16.7%)	
Marital status	Married	90 (64.7%)	73 (81.1%)	17 (18.9%)	0.438 [a]
	Other	(35.3%)	37 (75.5%)	12 (24.5%)	
Education	≤6 years	52 (37.4%)	47 (90.4%)	5 (9.6%)	0.012 [a]
	>6 years	87 (62.6%)	63 (72.4%)	24 (27.6%)	
Last dental visit	≤12 months	63 (45.3%)	45 (71.4%)	18 (28.6%)	0.042 [a]
	>12 months	76 (54.7%)	65 (85.5%)	111 (14.5%)	
Source of oral health information for teeth brushing and interdental cleaning	Dentist	73 (52.5%)	23 (18.8%)	22 (81.2%)	<0.001 [a]
	Other	66 (47.5%)	87 (51.1%)	7 (48.9%)	

[a] Chi-square test, [b] Fischer's Exact test.

Table 9. Multivariate analysis between toothbrushing frequency at least twice a day combined with interdental cleaning and independent variables.

Predictor Variables	β	SE	p-Value [a]	Odds Ratio
Education	0.60	0.60	0.314	1.82
Last dental visit	0.86	0.50	0.087	2.37
Source of oral health information	2.40	0.52	<0.001	11.03

[a] Binary Logistic Regression.

3.3. Factors Affecting the Application of the Recommended Daily Denture Hygiene and Care Practices

The frequency of denture hygiene was not statistically significantly associated with any of the independent parameters investigated. Source of information about denture hygiene (by a dentist) and last dental visit within the past 12 months were significantly

(p = 0.001) and marginally significantly (p = 0.066) associated with denture cleaning using mechanical brushing and mild soap, while gender, age, marital status, and education did not have any significant effect. In the multivariate analysis, only the source of information remained significant (p = 0.016). Participants who had received instructions about denture hygiene from the dentist were more likely to use a brush and soap (β = 2.69, OR = 14.67).

Furthermore, direct information from the dentist led to an increased prevalence of denture removal at night (p = 0.001) (Table 10). Logistic regression has shown that those informed by the dentist about the appropriate frequency of denture use had a higher probability of removing their denture (s) at night (β = 2.17, OR = 8.75, p = 0.003) (Table 11).

Table 10. The association of sociodemographic characteristics, dental visitation habits and information from the dentist with denture removal at night.

Independent Variable		n (%)	Denture Removal at Night n (%)		p-Value
			Yes	No	
Gender	Male	17 (31.5%)	11 (64.7%)	6 (35.3%)	0.683 [a]
	Female	37 (68.5%)	26 (70.3%)	11 (29.7%)	
Age	≤74 years	23 (42.6%)	14 (60.9%)	9 (39.1%)	0.668 [b]
	75–84 years	23 (42.6%)	17 (73.9%)	6 (26.1%)	
	≥85 years	8 (14.8%)	6 (75.0%)	2 (25.5%)	
Marital status	Married	31 (57.4%)	20 (64.5%)	11 (35.5%)	0.462 [a]
	Other	23 (42.6%)	17 (73.9%)	6 (26.1%)	
Education	≤6 years	29 (53.7%)	22 (77.4%)	7 (22.6%)	0.211 [a]
	>6 years	25 (46.3%)	15 (60%)	10 (40%)	
Last dental visit	≤12 months	22 (39.3%)	13 (59.1%)	9 (40.9%)	0.216 [a]
	>12 months	32 (60.7%)	24 (75.0%)	8 (25.0%)	
Information from the dentist for removing dentures at night	Yes	28 (51.9%)	25 (89.3%)	3 (10.7%)	0.001 [a]
	No	26 (48.1%)	12 (46.2%)	14 (53.8%)	

[a] Chi-square test, [b] Fischer's Exact test.

Table 11. The association between denture removal at night and information from the dentist.

Predictor Variable	β	SE	p-Value [a]	Odds Ratio
Information from the dentist for removing dentures at night	2.17	0.73	0.003	8.75

[a] Binary Logistic Regression.

4. Discussion

Under the limitations of the present study, the participants had received daily oral hygiene and care information from various sources, including dentists, media (television, magazines and the internet), formal education, relatives, friends, and other care providers, such as pharmacists and dental technicians. The oral care information obtained from dentists was associated with better adherence to the currently recommended daily oral care practices for both teeth and dentures for older adults. However, many participants reported that they had not received any kind of oral hygiene information. Moreover, for many participants, the reported dental and denture daily care habits were poor.

Almost half of the dentate participants reported that they had obtained toothbrushing instructions from their dentist but only 34.5% on interdental cleaning. Many studies have shown that the dentist is the main source of oral health information to her/his patients. As in the present study, a younger and middle-aged sample in Iran indicated that the most common oral health information source was the dentist (52.6%), followed by TV/radio, books/newspapers, family/friends and the internet, and only 1% had not obtained any relevant information [24]. Partially dentate adults in Brazil obtained information about oral hygiene mainly from their dentist or undergraduate dental students (62.2%), 5.5% from the media, and 0.8% from relatives [25]. Dental advice led to a higher possibility of having adequate oral health literacy among younger and middle-aged Brazilian immigrants in Canada [27].

Forty-three per cent of the participants reported that their dentist had educated them on denture cleaning, and 51.9% on removing the dentures at night. Lower percentages were reported by middle-aged and older individuals in Brazil (22.5%) [26] and Iran (39.6%) [28] but were higher in Turkey (90%) [29].

The findings in the present study revealed that many participants did not perform the recommended daily oral and denture hygiene practices [12–14]. A positive finding was the combination of a toothbrush and fluoride toothpaste (95%). Similar findings in adult and older populations have been reported in other countries [30,31]. The use of fluoride toothpaste has expanded in the past decades, particularly in developed countries. It is a major contributor to decay control and has been included in the list of essential medicines by WHO [4]. Electric toothbrushes were used by a very small number of participants (3%). Although electric toothbrushes seem to be equally or even more effective in dental plaque removal compared to conventional ones, further studies are needed to examine their applicability and affordability in older individuals [32].

Regarding toothbrushing frequency, 42% of the participants brushed their teeth at least twice a day compared to 31% in a previous study among older adults in the same geographical area [33], which is considered significant progress. However, there is large variability in relevant findings among countries [30,31,34,35].

Only 36% per cent of the participants regularly cleaned the interdental areas with dental floss and/or interdental brushes. Although there is a large variation in the frequency of interdental cleaning between studies, rates are significantly lower compared to toothbrushing [30,31]. It should be noted that only 21% of the study participants combined toothbrushing with fluoride toothpaste at least twice a day and regular interdental cleaning, and these habits have been associated with related instructions from their dentist.

Many participants (35%) used mouth rinses daily or occasionally, but only 16.2% after dental advice, as it is highly recommended to control potential side effects. Other information sources such as the media, relatives and friends and other healthcare workers played an important role in promoting this habit. A systematic review of randomised clinical trials demonstrated the wide use of mouth rinses, especially those which contain chlorhexidine, fluorides and essential oils, in the older population [36]. These findings clearly indicate that more emphasis is needed on educating non-dental healthcare providers and the public about the proper use of various mouth rinses.

Mechanical brushing with toothpaste was the most common denture hygiene practice (55.4%) despite the existing recommendations to avoid toothpaste. Previous studies among denture wearers in American, Asian and European countries also reported mechanical brushing alone (36.5–100%) or with toothpaste (29.2–88.9%) as the most prevalent denture cleaning method [26,28,34,37–43]. However, only 54% of the study participants cleaned their dentures at least twice a day, and only 22.2% used denture cleansing tablets as recommended [12–14].

Less than 70% of denture wearers removed their dentures at night, and the main contributor to this practice was previous dental advice. However, few denture wearers across the globe (23.6–58.5%) remove their dentures at night [26,28,37–41,44,45], although proper hygiene and nocturnal removal of dentures can reduce the incidence of aspiration pneumonia, a leading cause of death from infection among frail older persons [9,46–48].

Although the dentist was the main source of information about the use of denture adhesives, the media, relatives and friends also played a significant role. Denture adhesives support the quality of life of denture wearers [49], but their use should be based on professional advice [50].

Women reported better daily oral hygiene practices compared to men but not to a statistically significant level. Several previous studies in adult and older populations have associated female gender with higher level of oral health literacy and better toothbrushing and denture hygiene habits [24,41,51,52]. Participants with more than six years of education were twice as likely to brush their teeth at least twice a day. Lower educational level has been frequently reported as a significant predictor of poorer oral health literacy among middle-aged and older people [26,30,51,53–57]. Last dental visit was another independent predictor for increased toothbrushing frequency. However, only 45.3% of the dentate participants had visited the dentist in the past 12 months, and this percentage decreased to 39.3% in denture wearers.

Many participants did not recall having received detailed information about dental and denture care practices from any source. This score was 35.3% for toothbrushing, 59% for interdental cleaning, and 44.4% for daily denture hygiene. Patients tend to forget oral health instructions provided by their dentists [58], and this may explain both a large number of those with poor reported oral hygiene practices as well as those who reported that they had not received any information from any source. Almost one-third of a Brazilian sample of adults up to 64 years old also reported that they did not have any access to oral health information [59].

Older individuals face various degrees of declines in intrinsic capacities, such as cognitive and visual impairment, hearing loss and limited mobility [60], which may limit access to the dentist, their understanding of the provided instructions and the actual daily hygiene practices. The type of information from the dentist may have a significant effect on the level of denture cleaning [29]. Those who had obtained both written and verbal advice had the highest level of denture cleaning, followed by those who were informed only verbally or only in written [29]. It seems that the use of multiple oral health information sources may improve oral hygiene practices. Moreover, easy-to-read oral health education material enriched oral health literacy among older adults [61]. Access to digital technology may help even those with limited access to dental offices, as web-based oral health promotion programmes for older adults have been shown to improve oral health knowledge, attitudes and self-efficacy [62]. However, this requires digital literacy promotion programmes for older people.

Dental practitioners should improve their communication skills with older adults [63] and provide comprehensive oral health information adapted to individual levels of capacity. Moreover, non-dental care providers who play an important role in oral hygiene counselling of older adults and their carers should receive appropriate oral health education and training [18]. Finally, effective policies are needed to improve the oral health literacy of the public for self-care and care of others [18].

Study Limitations

Study participants belonged to a functionally independent urban dental school sample, restricting the generalisation of the findings to functionally dependent older population groups and those living in rural areas. Also, there is a high possibility of recall bias as patients may have forgotten their dentist providing information about dental and denture hygiene. In addition, the reported oral hygiene practices, dental visitation habits and sources of oral health information may not correspond completely to reality since some participants may have adapted their answers to satisfy the investigators (Hawthorne effect). Finally, the clinical examination included only the number of natural teeth and the presence of the dentures without investigating other oral health indicators.

5. Conclusions

Under the limitations of the present study, the application of currently recommended daily oral hygiene practices was associated with previous relevant instructions from a dentist. However, only a small number of individuals recalled having received oral health prevention and promotion advice from a dentist. Appropriate policies should be developed and implemented to improve oral health knowledge and practices among older adults taking into consideration their specific characteristics and the heterogeneity of ageing.

Dental practitioners should improve communication with their older patients with an emphasis on effective, detailed and repetitive advice. More effective and tailor-made educational strategies should be developed, including digital technology. Finally, oral health education should be provided to non-dental health care professionals who meet older adults more often than dentists.

Author Contributions: Conceptualization, A.E.K.; methodology, A.E.K.; formal analysis, K.K. and A.E.K.; investigation, K.K. and A.E.K.; resources, A.E.K.; data curation, K.K.; writing—original draft preparation, K.K.; writing—review and editing, A.E.K.; supervision, A.E.K.; project administration, A.E.K. All authors have read and agreed to the published version of the manuscript.

Funding: This research received no external funding.

Institutional Review Board Statement: The study was conducted in accordance with the Declaration of Helsinki and approved by the Ethics and Research Committee of the Dental School of the National and Kapodistrian University of Athens, Greece (#346/2018).

Informed Consent Statement: Informed consent was obtained from the participants.

Data Availability Statement: The data presented in this study are available on request from the corresponding author. The data are not publicly available due to ethical restrictions.

Acknowledgments: We would like to deeply thank Dimokritos Papalexopoulos for his contribution to the data curation.

Conflicts of Interest: The authors declare no conflict of interest.

References

1. World Health Organization. Draft Global Strategy on Oral Health. 2021. Available online: https://cdn.who.int/media/docs/default-source/searo/india/health-topic-pdf/noncommunicable-diseases/draft-discussion-paper--annex-3-(global-strategy-on-oral-health)-.pdf?sfvrsn=aa03ca5b_3&download=true (accessed on 30 January 2023).
2. World Health Organization. Health in Older Age. In Book World Report on Ageing and Health; WHO Press, World Health Organization: Geneva, Switzerland, 2015; pp. 43–85. ISBN 978-92-4-069481-1.
3. Peres, M.A.; Macpherson, L.M.; Weyant, R.J.; Daly, B.; Venturelli, R.; Mathur, M.R.; Listl, S.; Celeste, R.K.; Guarnizo-Herreño, C.C.; Kearns, C.; et al. Oral diseases: A global public health challenge. *Lancet* **2019**, *394*, 249–260. [CrossRef] [PubMed]
4. World Health Organization. Global Oral Health Status Report: Towards Universal Health Coverage for Oral Health by 2030. World Health Organization. 2022. Available online: https://www.who.int/publications/i/item/9789240061484 (accessed on 30 January 2023).
5. Romandini, M.; Baima, G.; Antonoglou, G.; Bueno, J.; Figuero, E.; Sanz, M. Periodontitis, Edentulism, and Risk of Mortality: A Systematic Review with Meta-analyses. *J. Dent. Res.* **2020**, *100*, 37–49. [CrossRef] [PubMed]
6. Liu, F.; Song, S.; Ye, X.; Huang, S.; He, J.; Wang, G.; Hu, X. Oral health-related multiple outcomes of holistic health in elderly individuals: An umbrella review of systematic reviews and meta-analyses. *Front. Public Health* **2022**, *10*, 1104. [CrossRef] [PubMed]
7. Scannapieco, F.A. Poor Oral Health in the Etiology and Prevention of Aspiration Pneumonia. *Dent. Clin. N. Am.* **2021**, *65*, 307–321. [CrossRef]
8. Ástvaldsdóttir, Á.; Boström, A.-M.; Davidson, T.; Gabre, P.; Gahnberg, L.; Englund, G.S.; Skott, P.; Ståhlnacke, K.; Tranaeus, S.; Wilhelmsson, H.; et al. Oral health and dental care of older persons—A systematic map of systematic reviews. *Gerodontology* **2018**, *35*, 290–304. [CrossRef]
9. Iinuma, T.; Arai, Y.; Abe, Y.; Takayama, M.; Fukumoto, M.; Fukui, Y.; Iwase, T.; Takebayashi, T.; Hirose, N.; Gionhaku, N.; et al. Denture Wearing during Sleep Doubles the Risk of Pneumonia in the Very Elderly. *J. Dent. Res.* **2014**, *94*, 28S–36S. [CrossRef]
10. van der Maarel-Wierink, C.D.; Vanobbergen, J.N.; Bronkhorst, E.M.; Schols, J.M.G.A.; de Baat, C. Oral health care and aspiration pneumonia in frail older people: A systematic literature review. *Gerodontology* **2012**, *30*, 3–9. [CrossRef]
11. Minakuchi, S.; Tsuga, K.; Ikebe, K.; Ueda, T.; Tamura, F.; Nagao, K.; Furuya, J.; Matsuo, K.; Yamamoto, K.; Kanazawa, M.; et al. Oral hypofunction in the older population: Position paper of the Japanese Society of Gerodontology in 2016. *Gerodontology* **2018**, *35*, 317–324. [CrossRef]
12. Kossioni, A.E.; Hajto-Bryk, J.; Janssens, B.; Maggi, S.; Marchini, L.; McKenna, G.; Müller, F.; Petrovic, M.; Roller-Wirnsberger, R.E.; Schimmel, M.; et al. Practical Guidelines for Physicians in Promoting Oral Health in Frail Older Adults. *J. Am. Med. Dir. Assoc.* **2018**, *19*, 1039–1046. [CrossRef]
13. Charadram, N.; Maniewicz, S.; Maggi, S.; Petrovic, M.; Kossioni, A.; Srinivasan, M.; Schimmel, M.; Mojon, P.; Müller, F.; Soiza, R.L.; et al. Development of a European consensus from dentists, dental hygienists and physicians on a standard for oral health care in care-dependent older people: An e-Delphi study. *Gerodontology* **2020**, *38*, 41–56. [CrossRef]

14. Krausch-Hofmann, S.; Palmers, E.; Declerck, D.; Duyck, J. Development of practice guidelines for daily oral care in care-dependent older adults to complement the InterRAI suite of instruments using a modified Delphi approach. *Int. J. Older People Nurs.* **2020**, *16*, e12351. [CrossRef] [PubMed]
15. Petersen, P.E.; Kandelman, D.; Arpin, S.; Ogawa, H. Global oral health of older people—Call for public health action. *Community Dent Health* **2010**, *27*, 257–267. [PubMed]
16. Thomson, W.M. Epidemiology of oral health conditions in older people. *Gerodontology* **2014**, *31*, 9–16. [CrossRef]
17. Ornstein, K.A.; DeCherrie, L.; Gluzman, R.; Ba, E.S.S.; Kansal, J.; Shah, T.; Katz, R.; Soriano, T.A. Significant Unmet Oral Health Needs of Homebound Elderly Adults. *J. Am. Geriatr. Soc.* **2014**, *63*, 151–157. [CrossRef]
18. Kossioni, A.E.; Hajto-Bryk, J.; Maggi, S.; McKenna, G.; Petrovic, M.; Roller-Wirnsberger, R.E.; Schimmel, M.; Tamulaitienė, M.; Vanobbergen, J.; Müller, F. An Expert Opinion from the European College of Gerodontology and the European Geriatric Medicine Society: European Policy Recommendations on Oral Health in Older Adults. *J. Am. Geriatr. Soc.* **2017**, *66*, 609–613. [CrossRef]
19. Watt, R.G.; Daly, B.; Allison, P.; Macpherson, L.M.D.; Venturelli, R.; Listl, S.; Weyant, R.J.; Mathur, M.R.; Guarnizo-Herreño, C.C.; Celeste, R.K.; et al. Ending the neglect of global oral health: Time for radical action. *Lancet* **2019**, *394*, 261–272. [CrossRef]
20. GBD 2017 Oral Disorders Collaborators; Bernabe, E.; Marcenes, W.; Hernandez, C.R.; Bailey, J.; Abreu, L.G.; Alipour, V.; Amini, S.; Arabloo, J.; Arefi, Z.; et al. Global, Regional, and National Levels and Trends in Burden of Oral Conditions from 1990 to 2017: A Systematic Analysis for the Global Burden of Disease 2017 Study. *J. Dent. Res.* **2020**, *99*, 362–373. [CrossRef] [PubMed]
21. Strayer, M.S. Perceived barriers to oral health care among the homebound. *Spéc. Care Dent.* **1995**, *15*, 113–118. [CrossRef] [PubMed]
22. Kossioni, E.A. Current Status and Trends in Oral Health in Communitydwelling Older Adults: A Global Perspective. *Oral Health Prev Dent* **2013**, *11*, 331–340. [CrossRef]
23. Janssens, B.; Kossioni, A. Oral health promotion in primary and institutional care. In *Geodontology Essentials for Healthcare Professionals, Practical Issues in Geriatrics*, 1st ed.; Kossioni, A., Maggi, S., Eds.; Springer Nature Switzerland AG: Cham, Switzerland, 2020; pp. 131–174. ISBN 978-3-030-41468-9. [CrossRef]
24. Sistani, M.N. Oral health literacy and information sources among adults in Tehran, Iran. *Community Dent. Health* **2013**, *5*, 178–182. [CrossRef]
25. Ribeiro, D.G.; Jorge, J.H.; Varjão, F.M.; Pavarina, A.C.; Garcia, P.P.N.S. Evaluation of partially dentate patients' knowledge about caries and periodontal disease. *Gerodontology* **2011**, *29*, e253–e258. [CrossRef] [PubMed]
26. Marchini, L.; Tamashiro, E.; Nascimento, D.F.F.; Cunha, V.P.P. Self-reported denture hygiene of a sample of edentulous attendees at a University dental clinic and the relationship to the condition of the oral tissues. *Gerodontology* **2004**, *21*, 226–228. [CrossRef]
27. Calvasina, P.; Lawrence, H.P.; Hoffman-Goetz, L.; Norman, C.D. Brazilian immigrants' oral health literacy and participation in oral health care in Canada. *BMC Oral Health* **2016**, *16*, 18. [CrossRef] [PubMed]
28. Torabi Parizi, M.; Taheri, S.h.; Amini, P.; Karimi Afshar, M.; Karimi Afshar, M. Evaluation of denture hygiene among removable denture wearers referred to clinics of Kerman, Iran. *J. Oral Health Oral Epidemiol.* **2013**, *2*, 44–48.
29. Cankaya, Z.T.; Yurdakos, A.; Kalabay, P.G. The association between denture care and oral hygiene habits, oral hygiene knowledge and periodontal status of geriatric patients wearing removable partial dentures. *Eur. Oral Res.* **2020**, *54*, 9–15. [CrossRef] [PubMed]
30. Olusile, A.O.; Adeniyi, A.A.; Orebanjo, O. Self-rated oral health status, oral health service utilization, and oral hygiene practices among adult Nigerians. *BMC Oral Health* **2014**, *14*, 140. [CrossRef]
31. Norderyd, O.; Kochi, G.; Papias, A.; Köhler, A.A.; Helkimo, A.N.; Brahm, C.-O.; Lindmark, U.; Lindfors, N.; Mattsson, A.; Rolander, B.; et al. Oral health of individuals aged 3–80 years in Jönköping, Sweden, during 40 years (1973–2013). I. Review of findings on oral care habits and knowledge of oral health. *Swed. Dent. J.* **2015**, *39*, 57–68.
32. Nobre, C.V.C.; Gomes, A.M.M.; Gomes, A.A.; Nascimento, A.P.C. Assessment of the efficacy of the utilisation of conventional and electric toothbrushes by the older adults. *Gerodontology* **2014**, *37*, 297–302. [CrossRef]
33. Gkavela, G. Survey of the Oral health Status and Oral Care Habits of Independent Community-Dwelling Older Adults and Association with Medical and Socio-Economic Factors. Ph.D. Thesis, Dental School, National and Kapodistrian University of Athens, Athens, Greece, 2019.
34. Skorupka, W.; Żurek, K.; Kokot, T.; Nowakowska-Zajdel, E.; Fatyga, E.; Niedworok, E.; Muc-Wierzgoń, M. Assessment of Oral Hygiene in Adults. *Cent. Eur. J. Public Health* **2012**, *20*, 233–236. [CrossRef]
35. Piyakhunakorn, P.; Sermsuti-Anuwat, N. The Associations between Oral Health Literacy and Oral Health-Related Behaviours among Community-Dwelling Older People in Thailand. *Glob. J. Health Sci.* **2021**, *13*, 1. [CrossRef]
36. Pérez-Nicolás, C.; Pecci-Lloret, M.P.; Guerrero-Gironés, J. Use and efficacy of mouthwashes in elderly patients: A systematic review of randomized clinical trials. *Ann. Anat.-Anat. Anz.* **2023**, *246*, 152026. [CrossRef]
37. Takamiya, A.S.; Monteiro, D.R.; Barão, V.A.R.; Pero, A.C.; Compagnoni, M.A.; Barbosa, D.B. Complete denture hygiene and nocturnal wearing habits among patients attending the Prosthodontic Department in a Dental University in Brazil. *Gerodontology* **2010**, *28*, 91–96. [CrossRef]
38. Chowdhary, R.; Chandraker, N.K. Clinical survey of denture care in denture-wearing edentulous patients of Indian population. *Geriatr. Gerontol. Int.* **2010**, *11*, 191–195. [CrossRef] [PubMed]
39. Bacali, C.; Nastase, V.; Constantiniuc, M.; Lascu, L.; Badea, M.E. Oral Hygiene Habits of Complete Denture Wearers in Central Transylvania, Romania. *Oral Health Prev. Dent.* **2021**, *19*, 107–113. [CrossRef] [PubMed]

40. Cinquanta, L.; Varoni, E.M.; Barbieri, C.; Sardella, A. Patient attitude and habits regarding removable denture home hygiene and correlation with prosthesis cleanliness: A cross-sectional study of elderly Italians. *J. Prosthet. Dent.* **2021**, *125*, 1–7. [CrossRef]
41. Baran, I.; Nalçacı, R. Self-reported denture hygiene habits and oral tissue conditions of complete denture wearers. *Arch. Gerontol. Geriatr.* **2009**, *49*, 237–241. [CrossRef]
42. Barreiro, D.M.; Scheid, P.A.; May, L.; Unfer, B.; Braun, K.O. Evaluation of procedures employed for the maintenance of removable dentures in elderly individuals. *Oral Health Prev. Dent.* **2009**, *7*, 243–249.
43. Wu, J.-H.; Yang, Y.-H.; Wang, C.-H.; Lee, H.-E.; Du, J.-K. Effects of denture maintenance on satisfaction levels of Taiwanese elderly using removable partial dentures: A pilot study. *Gerodontology* **2011**, *29*, e458–e463. [CrossRef] [PubMed]
44. Santos, M.B.F.; Carvalho, R.M.; Guimarães, T.S.S.C.; Santos, J.F.F.; Marchini, L. Longitudinal study of removable partial dentures and hygiene habits. *Braz. Dent. Sci.* **2007**, *10*, 281. [CrossRef]
45. Ercalik-Yalcinkaya, S.; Özcan, M. Association between Oral Mucosal Lesions and Hygiene Habits in a Population of Removable Prosthesis Wearers. *J. Prosthodont.* **2014**, *24*, 271–278. [CrossRef]
46. Sjogren, P.; Nilsson, E.; Forsell, M.; Johansson, O.; Hoogstraate, J.; Sjögren, P. A Systematic Review of the Preventive Effect of Oral Hygiene on Pneumonia and Respiratory Tract Infection in Elderly People in Hospitals and Nursing Homes: Effect Estimates and Methodological Quality of Randomized Controlled Trials. *J. Am. Geriatr. Soc.* **2008**, *56*, 2124–2130. [CrossRef]
47. Müller, F. Oral Hygiene Reduces the Mortality from Aspiration Pneumonia in Frail Elders. *J. Dent. Res.* **2014**, *94*, 14S–16S. [CrossRef] [PubMed]
48. Janssens, J.-P.; Krause, K.-H. Pneumonia in the very old. *Lancet Infect. Dis.* **2004**, *4*, 112–124. [CrossRef]
49. Kossioni, A. Prevalence and Factors Associated with the Use of Denture Adhesives by Older Complete Denture Wearers. *Eur. J. Prosthodont. Restor. Dent.* **2018**, *26*, 197–201. [CrossRef]
50. Bartlett, D.; Carter, N.; Felton, D.; Goffin, G.; Kawai, Y.; Muller, F.; Polyzois, G.; Walls, A. *White Paper on Guidelines for the Use of Denture Adhesives and Their Benefits for Oral and General Health*; Oral Health Foundation: Warwickshire, UK, 2019.
51. Mohammadi, T.M.; Malekmohammadi, M.; Hajizamani, H.R.; Mahani, S.A. Oral health literacy and its determinants among adults in Southeast Iran. *Eur. J. Dent.* **2018**, *12*, 439–442. [CrossRef] [PubMed]
52. Sfeatcu, R.; Balgiu, B.A.; Mihai, C.; Petre, A.; Pantea, M.; Tribus, L. Gender Differences in Oral Health: Self-Reported Attitudes, Values, Behaviours and Literacy among Romanian Adults. *J. Pers. Med.* **2022**, *12*, 1603. [CrossRef] [PubMed]
53. Sermsuti-Anuwat, N.; Piyakhunakorn, P. Association Between Oral Health Literacy and Number of Remaining Teeth Among the Thai Elderly: A Cross-Sectional Study. *Clin. Cosmet. Investig. Dent.* **2021**, *13*, 113–119. [CrossRef]
54. Márquez-Arrico, C.F.; Almerich-Silla, J.-M.; Montiel-Company, J.-M. Oral health knowledge in relation to educational level in an adult population in Spain. *J. Clin. Exp. Dent.* **2019**, *11*, e1143–e1150. [CrossRef]
55. Baskaradoss, J.K. Relationship between oral health literacy and oral health status. *BMC Oral Health* **2018**, *18*, 172. [CrossRef]
56. McQuistan, M.R.; Qasim, A.; Shao, C.; Straub-Morarend, C.L.; Macek, M.D. Oral health knowledge among elderly patients. *J. Am. Dent. Assoc.* **2015**, *146*, 17–26. [CrossRef]
57. Wanichsaithong, P.; Goodwin, M.; Pretty, I.A. Development and pilot study of an oral health literacy tool for older adults. *J. Investig. Clin. Dent.* **2019**, *10*, e12465. [CrossRef] [PubMed]
58. Asimakopoulou, K.; Daly, B.; Dunne, S.; Packer, M.; Millar, B.; Misra, S. Dentist–patient communication: What do patients and dentists remember following a consultation? Implications for patient compliance. *Patient Prefer. Adherence* **2013**, *7*, 543–549. [CrossRef] [PubMed]
59. Batista, M.J.; Lawrence, H.P.; Sousa, M.D.L.R.D. Oral health literacy and oral health outcomes in an adult population in Brazil. *BMC Public Health* **2017**, *18*, 1–9. [CrossRef] [PubMed]
60. Integrated care for older people (ICOPE). *Guidance for Person-Centred Assessment and Pathways in Primary Care*; World Health Organization: Geneva, Switzerland, 2019.
61. Sun, K.-T.; Shieh, T.-M.; Hsia, S.-M.; Ningrum, V.; Lin, X.-Y.; Shih, Y.-H. Easy to Read Health Education Material Improves Oral Health Literacy of Older Adults in Rural Community-Based Care Centers: A Quasi-Experimental Study. *Healthcare* **2021**, *9*, 1465. [CrossRef]
62. Mariño, R.J.; Marwaha, P.; Barrow, S.-Y. Web-based oral health promotion program for older adults: Development and preliminary evaluation. *Int. J. Med. Inform.* **2016**, *91*, e9–e15. [CrossRef]
63. Åstrøm, A.N.; Özkaya, F.; Nasir, E.; Tsakos, G. The dentist-patient relationship and oral health–related quality of life among older adults: A cohort study. *Gerodontology* **2022**, *11*, 12663. [CrossRef]

Disclaimer/Publisher's Note: The statements, opinions and data contained in all publications are solely those of the individual author(s) and contributor(s) and not of MDPI and/or the editor(s). MDPI and/or the editor(s) disclaim responsibility for any injury to people or property resulting from any ideas, methods, instructions or products referred to in the content.

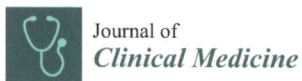 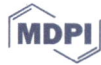

Review

Oral Health Factors Related to Rapid Oral Health Deterioration among Older Adults: A Narrative Review

Jhanvi P. Desai and Rohit U. Nair *

Department of Preventive and Community Dentistry, The University of Iowa College of Dentistry and Dental Clinics, Iowa City, IA 52242, USA
* Correspondence: rohit-nair@uiowa.edu

Abstract: Older adults who face systemic health issues and lack adequate social support are at risk for oral health deterioration. How rapidly such changes take place depends on the severity of their medical condition and their ability to access oral health services in a timely manner. The management of dental caries and periodontal disease in this cohort is made complex by the interaction of local and host factors such as the presence of dry mouth, involvement of root surfaces, and altered wound healing. in addition to enhanced maintenance needs to avoid recurrence or progression. Tooth replacement can be beneficial in restoring oral function, allowing patients to enjoy a healthy and nutritious diet but requires careful consideration to avoid further damage to remaining dental units. Establishing a dental home for the older adult can facilitate routine surveillance, disease prevention, and patient/caregiver education to achieve oral health goals commensurate with overall health. This narrative review details oral health factors that are related to rapid oral health deterioration among older adults.

Keywords: oral hygiene; root caries; tooth loss; xerostomia; dependent oral care; ill-fitting partial dentures; dental care utilization

Citation: Desai, J.P.; Nair, R.U. Oral Health Factors Related to Rapid Oral Health Deterioration among Older Adults: A Narrative Review. *J. Clin. Med.* **2023**, *12*, 3202. https://doi.org/10.3390/jcm12093202

Academic Editor: Marco Tatullo

Received: 20 January 2023
Revised: 11 April 2023
Accepted: 24 April 2023
Published: 29 April 2023

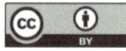

Copyright: © 2023 by the authors. Licensee MDPI, Basel, Switzerland. This article is an open access article distributed under the terms and conditions of the Creative Commons Attribution (CC BY) license (https://creativecommons.org/licenses/by/4.0/).

1. Introduction

Older adults constitute a unique and diverse demographic group in countries and societies around the world. Medical advances, financial and social support, and improvements in living conditions have all contributed to increased longevity, with global life expectancy increasing to nearly 73 years as of 2019 and that in OECD countries exceeding 79 years around the same time [1]. The evolution of medical and dental specialties that focus on patient-centered care for the older adult highlight the complexity of care needs that might be seen in this patient population [2].

The concept of rapid oral health deterioration (ROHD) provides a critical thinking framework for dental practitioners to systematically analyze the risk of older adult patients to experience progressive oral health decline that may be precipitated by a combination of systemic health events and oral health factors [3]. By leading the provider through an expert's clinical decision-making style and weighing the relative impact of general health conditions, social support, and oral conditions (Figure 1), the ROHD model allows for risk stratification and facilitates broad guidance for treatment approaches while reconciling providers' biases relating to patient care [4]. Increasingly, we see this and other similar models being successfully adopted in dental school curricula in response to the growing need for oral health services for older adults and other patients with special needs [5–8]. This review paper will focus on oral health factors related to ROHD among older adults as proposed by Marchini and colleagues, namely, oral hygiene, periodontal conditions, number of teeth/restorations, prosthetic status, presence of oral lesions, and utilization of dental services (Figure 2) [3].

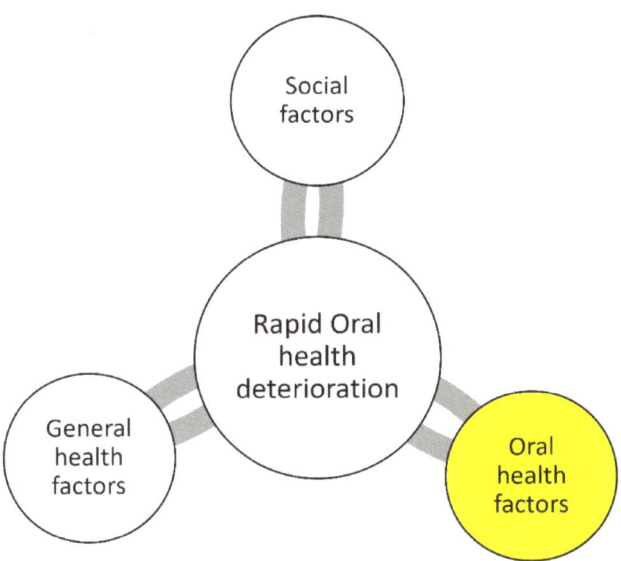

Figure 1. Factors contributing to rapid oral health deterioration. Adapted from Marchini et al [3].

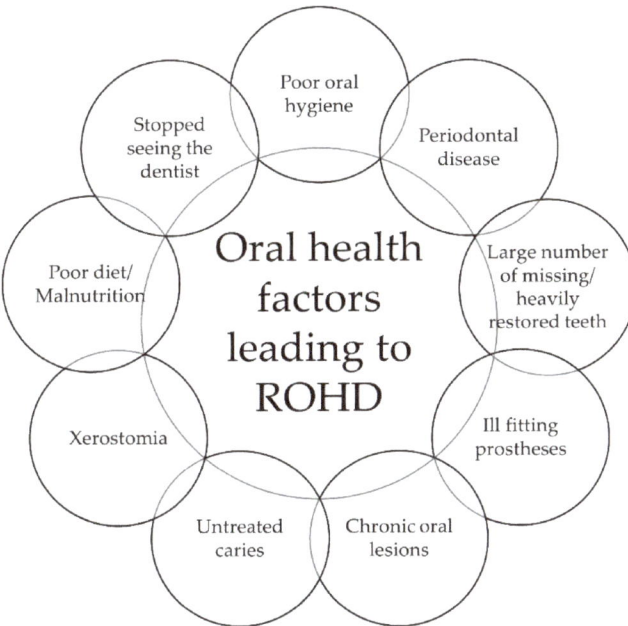

Figure 2. Oral health factors leading to rapid oral health deterioration. Adapted from Marchini et al [3].

2. Methods

Although there is general agreement over the fact that older adults experience oral health decline due to oral, systemic, and social factors, such changes are not documented in the literature exclusively using the term "rapid oral health deterioration". To find information for this narrative review, we conducted a literature search within the PubMed database using search terms relating to each of the nine oral health risk factors originally proposed by Marchini et al. [3] in combination with terms that represent the older adult population. The search was limited to peer-reviewed publications that were indexed as articles or reviews. Terms used included "Dental Caries" [Mesh], "Dental Devices, Home Care" [Mesh], "Mouth Diseases" [Mesh], "No-Show Patients" [Mesh], "Oral Hygiene" [Mesh], "Periodontal Diseases" [Mesh], "Root Caries" [Mesh], "Toothbrushing" [Mesh] AND "Aged" [Mesh], "Aged, 80 and over" [Mesh], "Dental Care for Aged" [Mesh], "Frail Elderly" [Mesh], ROHD [tw], and rapid oral health deterioration [tw]. Abstracts of publications that resulted from this search were reviewed and shortlisted for inclusion based on the scope of this narrative review.

3. Discussion

3.1. Oral Health Factors related to ROHD among Older Adults

3.1.1. Oral Hygiene

The likelihood of older adults maintaining a healthy, functional dentition throughout their lifespan depends on their ability to perform or receive daily oral hygiene care and to periodically access professional maintenance services [9]. This assumes particular significance for patients who have extensively restored dentitions or long-standing periodontal disease and those who are dependent for care. Oral health risk factors resulting from poor oral hygiene may predispose individuals to developing certain systemic health conditions, for example, diabetes mellitus or cardiovascular disease. Older adults can progress through the stages of rapid oral health deterioration after experiencing a major health event that diminishes their functional ability, requires new living arrangements/additional caregiver support, or disrupts normal oral physiology such as salivary flow. Although a causal relationship is difficult to establish, periodontal disease is a known risk factor for developing aspiration pneumonia, especially in institutionalized older adults with dysphagia. Regular oral hygiene maintenance can reduce the incidence of respiratory complications in this cohort [10].

Oral hygiene has been associated with cognitive conditions such as Alzheimer's disease (AD) that affect the patient's ability to perform activities of daily living [11]. The chronic inflammatory potential of periodontal disease may be somewhat associated with the risk of developing such progressive neurocognitive disorders, and poor oral health has been frequently cited as a modifiable risk factor for developing dementia [12–16]. Although much can be achieved through preventive approaches, the task of ensuring routine oral hygiene maintenance in older adults with cognitive disorders poses additional challenges. A team approach that involves the patient, caregivers, dental professionals, and occupational therapists may be beneficial when trying to restore oral self-care routines in such patients but might need to be modified based on the severity of their cognitive condition [17,18].

In the case of frail and/or dependent older adults, providing oral hygiene training to nursing assistants at long-term care facilities has been shown to improve residents' oral health status [19]. Caregivers' own attitudes toward dependent individuals' oral health have been linked to their own oral health behaviors [20]. Poor or worsening manual dexterity can be the result of experiencing stroke, progressive musculoskeletal conditions like rheumatoid or osteo arthritis, neurological conditions like Parkinson's disease, chronic pain such as that from fibromyalgia, etc. This can hinder older adults' ability to independently perform daily oral hygiene and may necessitate the use of suitable oral hygiene aids [21]. It has been suggested that this cohort's caries risk increases as they become functionally dependent toward the end of life [22]. Oral hygiene aids with physical modifications, such as adaptive toothbrush handles, triple-headed toothbrushes, Collis-curve brushes, floss holders/single-use floss picks, interdental brushes of varying sizes, water flossers, and electric toothbrushes, all facilitate better plaque removal in these individuals. Chemotherapeutic aids such as 1.1% sodium fluoride dentifrices (5000 ppm) and 0.12% chlorhexidine gluconate mouth rinse are known to be effective in providing additional protection against caries progression and periodontal disease. Since these are prescription-based agents, the patient and caregiver should be advised on the appropriate use of these products by the provider. Moreover, the dental provider will need to actively monitor for any side effects associated with these products [23,24].

A well-established oral hygiene routine that consists of brushing with a fluoridated toothpaste and flossing, either independently or with assistance from a caregiver, can deter the immediate impact of systemic health events on oral health until the patient's primary dental care provider can assess their new needs and modify existing approaches to care [25].

3.1.2. Periodontal Disease

Periodontal disease is one of the direct consequences of poor oral hygiene. A survey of US adults aged 65 years and over found that more than 60% of this group experienced some form of periodontal disease of varying severity [26]. While this may be the result of years of unmet oral hygiene needs, it poses a special risk for oral health decline in this population. Guarding the aging dentition from periodontal disease is particularly challenging considering the impact that aging has on wound-healing mechanisms, bone physiology, the oral microbiome, xerostomia, and the ability to ensure plaque control [27].

From an oral health standpoint, in the absence of adequate hygiene maintenance, local and systemic factors result in progressive deterioration of the supporting dental tissues causing gingival recession, bone loss, and increased tooth mobility. The functional impact of these changes is seen in older adults' ability to chew food adequately and a tendency to choose softer foods that are easier to masticate but which may be rich in fermentable carbohydrates. The nutritional value of these food choices aside, there is an increased risk for root caries in the periodontally compromised dentition especially if accompanied by dry mouth [28].

Untreated periodontal disease can lead to tooth loss. Although it is possible to function on a reduced dentition, the presence of well-distributed, opposing dental units offers patients a better chance of sustaining a favorable oral health-related quality of life. The ability to function with a removable partial prosthesis also depends on the health of abutment teeth. Periodontal disease around strategic teeth can result in tooth mobility or gradual shifting under traumatic occlusal forces. Long-term changes in tooth position due to periodontal disease may render removable prostheses unusable, further affecting older adults' quality of life. The presence of a removable prosthesis has also been shown to negatively impact the periodontal condition of abutment teeth, resulting in greater gingival recession, clinical attachment loss, caries, and fractures as compared to non-abutment teeth. A degree of manual dexterity is required to independently place and remove mechanically retained prostheses, to clean dentures, and to perform oral/peri-implant hygiene procedures. It is necessary to factor in patient's ability to maintain oral hygiene, their adherence to a recall schedule, and the need for repairs and other maintenance procedures for the prosthesis when determining the periodontal prognosis of the abutment teeth [29].

From a systemic health perspective, active management of periodontal disease by performing periodic in-office scaling, root planning, and maintenance procedures can improve glycemic control, at least in the short-term, by minimizing a source of chronic inflammation [30,31]. A consensus report by the International Diabetes Federation and the European Federation of Periodontology confirms the safety and efficacy of periodontal therapy in diabetic patients and attests to modest improvements in HbA1C values up to 3 months after therapy [32]. Chaffee et al. studied the association between chronic periodontal disease and obesity and confirmed a positive relation between the two although it is difficult to infer if either condition poses a risk for the other [33].

3.1.3. Presence of Untreated Dental Caries

Risk factors such as high sugar consumption, reduced salivary flow, reduced oral clearance due to lack of oral hygiene maintenance and/or xerostomia, reduced salivary buffering capacity, use of removable of prosthesis, and lack of fluoride exposure all contribute to both coronal and root caries development in older adults [34]. In fact, higher coronal caries experience in older adults is considered a risk predictor for root caries [35]. The combination of these risk factors can accelerate oral health deterioration.

Data from the National Health and Nutritional Examination Survey (NHANES) 2011–2016 highlighted the wide prevalence of dental caries among older adults; 96% of this cohort had experienced dental caries, and nearly one in every six individuals had untreated dental caries [36]. A sugar-rich diet allows demineralization of teeth to outpace remineralization resulting in caries. Thus, a carbohydrate-rich diet which may be softer in consistency and easier to prepare, may be preferred by patients with functional disability that results in challenges in mastication. However, this translates into more sugar intake which can magnify the risk of caries. In addition, other risk factors associated with this disease in older adults include belonging to disadvantaged sociodemographic groups, presence of systemic diseases, and lack of general and preventive oral health behaviors [37,38].

Adults over 65 years of age also experience the highest burden of untreated root caries among all age groups [39]. Root caries has a multifactorial etiology and is subject to some unique dental anatomical, histological, and microbiological features. Some habits, especially the use of tobacco in older adults, has been reported to have a positive correlation with root caries. Oral hygiene practices such as daily toothbrushing and interdental cleaning are linked with a lower incidence of root caries. Fundamentally, root caries develops on teeth that have had clinical attachment loss, a mechanism that is different from that related to other smooth surface caries. The presence of periodontal disease with biofilm formation and retention, as well as a lack of routine in-office cleaning, has a positive correlation to root caries experience [40]. Active root caries lesions require prompt intervention owing to their potential for rapid extension and involvement of nearby pulpal and periodontal tissues. The incidence of root caries can be reduced by modifying patients' dietary habits, promoting self-care, and utilizing preventive services. Even without tooth loss, the presence of untreated caries increases the risk of experiencing pain and swelling and has the potential to affect an older individual's quality of life.

3.1.4. Restorative Status

Oral health-related quality of life is positively impacted by the retention of healthy natural teeth [41]. Depending on the extent of tooth loss, older adults may be rehabilitated with conventional or implant-supported complete/partial dentures, tooth or implant-supported fixed dental prostheses, or single-unit restorations. Complete denture prostheses are a comprehensive solution that minimize the disease burden resulting from poorly maintained dental hard tissues. These are, however, limited by the quality and stability of the foundational tissues they are designed to function on. Chronic changes in the supporting tissues because of residual ridge resorption makes it necessary for extensive removable denture prostheses to be periodically maintained with occlusal adjustments, relines, etc. The loss of retention encountered with removable prostheses can be overcome, to some extent, using tooth overdenture abutments with pre-machined attachments. This approach, however, requires careful maintenance to avoid developing recurrent caries/periodontal disease in the abutment teeth and subsequent prosthetic failure.

For the edentulous patient, implant supported overdentures offer a reliable way to improve retention and stability by placing multiple fixtures and compatible retentive elements along the span of the prosthesis [42]. These too can fail if not adequately maintained. Implant therapy itself may not be a feasible option for frail older adults due to the complexity of procedures involved, associated comorbidity, and increased need for peri-implant and prosthetic maintenance. Careful case selection, cleansable prosthetic design, personal and professional care regimens, and patient education will be critical to ensuring that middle-aged individuals who now have implant-supported restorations are not at risk of developing peri-implant disease or prosthetic failure as they approach old age and frailty themselves. Boven et al. report that although implant-supported dentures vastly improved patient comfort, improved patient satisfaction did not always improve their general or health-related quality of life, suggesting that there are other factors at play [43].

The shortened dental arch concept can be an effective treatment approach for the partially dentate patient who is unable to receive fixed prostheses and is maladaptive to removable prostheses [44]. Studies have shown that dental arches comprising the anterior and premolar regions meet the requirements of a functional dentition [45]. Research on occlusal stability, masticatory efficiency, and temporomandibular joint function support the design and maintenance of shortened arches in patients receiving fixed prostheses, providing an alternative to distal extension RPDs with which patients tend to be non-compliant. Moynihan et al. systematically reviewed the impact of wearing dentures on dietary intake but could not discern a clear association between the two. Nevertheless, the presence of stable, retentive tooth replacements can improve the overall experience of eating and restore esthetics where desired [46].

3.1.5. Functional Dentition and Nutritional Status

Although there has been a significant global decline in the prevalence and incidence of severe tooth loss, older adults continue to be the most likely group to experience such adverse oral health events [47]. While this might be the outcome of accumulated oral health needs across their lifespan, the consequences of tooth loss have a significant impact on older adults' quality of life at a time when they may not be able to adapt to rehabilitative procedures owing to other systemic/functional limitations. The presence and severity of tooth loss have also been associated with mortality resulting from metabolic, digestive, and cardiovascular disease [48,49].

The relationship between nutrition and oral health is bidirectional and dynamic in nature. A balanced diet helps preserve oral health while a functioning oral cavity enables the gastrointestinal system to assimilate dietary elements resulting in benefits to one's overall health. While oral health, diet, and nutrition are closely linked, food choices vary widely among people due to personal preferences, cultural influences, access to food resources, and several other factors [50].

Marcenes et al. studied the relationship between dental status, food selection, nutrition, and body mass index (BMI) in a national sample of adults aged 65 years and over living in Great Britain. They found that older adults with a functional dentition comprising 21 or more teeth were likely to have a healthier diet that was rich in fruits and vegetables and have a favorable BMI [51]. While it is intuitive to link the number of remaining functional dental units with older adults' risk of developing malnutrition, the multifactorial nature of the latter condition must be emphasized. Bakker et al. found in a cross-sectional observational study of 1325 community-dwelling adults aged 75 years and over that although malnourished older adults reported problems with speech and mastication, there was no significant association between malnutrition and oral health problems, including edentulism. However, respondents' health-related quality of life (HRQoL) was associated with malnutrition, suggesting that a combination of oral, systemic, and social factors was likely at play [52].

Gil-Montoya et al., in a cross-sectional study of 2860 adults in Spain aged 65 years and older, validated the use of the oral health-related quality of life (OHRQoL) assessment to identify older adults who are at risk of malnutrition due to oral problems [53]. In addition to the number of remaining teeth, other factors, such as presence of xerostomia, poor appetite or trouble swallowing, also play an important role in shaping older adult's likelihood of facing nutritional problems [54,55].

Impaired dental status among older adults is linked to chewing difficulty, dysphagia, and oral pain due to chronic inflammation and persistent infections, all of which lead to dietary limitations. Masticatory efficiency is affected by tooth loss, number of functional occluding teeth, and presence of a prosthesis. With limited masticatory efficiency, older adults may be at risk of making poor dietary choices. Softer foods often tend to be high in sugars and fats and low in protein and fiber. This in turn affects systemic health by increasing risk of coronary artery disease, diabetes, gastrointestinal issues, etc. [56]. In a nationwide survey of 4820 adults aged 50 years and over who had at least 18 teeth or who wore dentures, Sahyoun et al. found that self-perceived ill-fitting of dentures negatively impacted this cohort's inclusion of vegetables and other essential nutrients in their diet, resulting in significantly lower serum levels of vitamins C and E, beta carotene, folic acid, etc., in comparison to dentate peers [57].

In a study conducted by Maitre et al. in France, 23% of older adults in the study sample were picky eaters with food selectivity being highest among nursing home residents. The findings of this study reiterated that greater food selectivity correlates with an increase of malnutrition risk and is parallel to the effect of eating difficulties on malnutrition [58]. Sheiham et al. in Great Britain showed that older adults who had less than 21 natural teeth were on an average 3 or more times likely to be obese while individuals with fewer than 11 teeth were significantly more likely to be underweight [59].

Older adults face a higher risk for dehydration due to reduced muscle mass, decline in kidney function, disability, and reduced thirst [60]. This, in combination with factors including antisialagogue drugs, radiation therapy, or comorbidities such as Sjogren's syndrome, can predispose older adults to xerostomia. Having a poor dentition may result in body image issues, decreasing social interactions, and being at risk of psychosocial disorders. Conditions such as loneliness and depression may cause affected individuals to resort to non-nutritional binging on comfort food, resulting in a vicious cycle that further compromises oral and general health [61].

3.1.6. Conditions Affecting Oral Soft Tissues

Candidiasis is a very common mycotic infection of the oral cavity [62]. Although it can be seen across the lifespan, there are several risk factors that predispose older adults developing oral candidiasis in [63]. These include long-term antibiotic therapy, poor oral/denture hygiene, dry mouth, chronic immunosuppressive conditions, and diabetes mellitus, among others, all of which are commonly encountered in this cohort. Buranarom et al., in a cross-sectional study of 53 independent adults aged 65 years and over, reported that patients with hyposalivation were nearly four times more likely to have oral Candida colonization [64]. A similar trend was noted in a cohort study by Deng et al., where more than half the number of subjects who received irradiation to the oral cavity developed oral candidiasis compared to only about 12% of the nonirradiated group. Xerostomia, mouth and throat soreness, and dysphagia were significantly higher in the former group, underscoring a complex situation that favors the progression of such infections in the medically compromised host [65]. Effective management of oral Candida infections can also have a beneficial effect on salivary flow. Ohga et al. reported significantly higher whole salivary flow rates following antifungal therapy with miconazole gel to eliminate oral Candida spp. in a group of 52 mostly older adult patients. This was accompanied by improvement in self-reported xerostomia and oral pain scores [66].

Denture stomatitis is an inflammatory, erythematous condition of denture-bearing oral mucosal tissues. As with candidiasis, it too has a complex etiology and could be the result of denture materials, poorly fitting dentures, inadequate denture hygiene, continuous wearing of removable dentures, poor denture plaque control, or bacterial and fungal contamination of denture surfaces [67]. All these factors facilitate the growth of opportunistic pathogens such as Candida albicans on affected tissues. The combination of mucosal infections and prosthetic malfunction makes this a significant quality of life issue for older denture wearers, especially when declining systemic health impacts their ability to receive oral health services.

Angular cheilitis is an inflammatory condition affecting the commissures of the mouth. It can result from a deficiency of essential nutrients including iron and vitamin B12, drooling, and denture-related issues, among other reasons. In denture wearers, the lack of adequate vertical dimension at occlusion can result in inversion of the angles of the mouth causing maceration and erythema. Chronic overloading of maxillary anterior denture-bearing tissues leads to the replacement of alveolar bone with fibrous tissues resulting in a "flabby ridge" that compromises denture stability [68]. Chronic irritation can result in the fibrous growths in vestibular areas adjacent to denture borders, causing discomfort and necessitating surgical removal prior to remaking or repairing prostheses. Unresolved mechanical tissue trauma, as with chemical irritants such as tobacco and alcohol, can result in precancerous leukoplakic and erythroplakic changes and subsequently increase the risk for oral squamous cell carcinoma [69]. In an analytical cross-sectional study of 821 participants aged 60–100 years in Brazil, Saintrain et al. showed that injuries to the oral cavity were significantly associated with age, retirement status, level of education, and the presence of dentures [70]. Furthermore, teeth with lost restorations, fractured teeth, or those with erosive or attritional wear can cause traumatic ulcers on the tongue/cheek mucosa if left unaddressed.

Older adults may need additional surveillance of soft tissue injuries to prevent progression and to monitor suspected malignant lesions to ensure timely referral for management. Older adults are particularly vulnerable to head and neck cancers with close to half of all new cases diagnosed in the United States between 1973 and 2008 occurring in patients aged 65 years and over [71]. This number is likely to rise as the global aging population increases and more sophisticated diagnostic tools become available. Considering the impact that multimodality therapy–surgery, radiation, chemotherapy–can have on oral soft tissues, supportive care such as the management of mucositis, xerostomia, and dysphagia is critical to the patient's quality of life [72]. As discussed earlier, all of these are also directly related to their risk for developing secondary oral complications such as dental caries and periodontal disease.

3.1.7. Xerostomia

Xerostomia is the subjective perception of oral dryness that may or may not be accompanied by an actual decline in salivary flow. Ship and colleagues estimated at least 30% of older adults experience dry mouth, with this number being as high as 72% among institutionalized older adults. In the same study, the prevalence of xerostomia was 100% in older adults with Sjogren's syndrome and those who had experienced cancer-related head and neck radiation [34,35]. Salivary gland hypofunction can lead to xerostomia; however, both are not necessarily correlated. It is important to note that both xerostomia and salivary hypofunction cause decrease in oral health-related quality of life, and the perception of dry mouth may not only be a result of salivary quantity but changes in the salivary composition as well.

Older adults are more likely to be prescribed multiple medications, as they may be managing concomitant systemic conditions. Xerostomia associated with polypharmacy is common in patients who use of five or more medications which most often have antisialagogic effects. Classes of drugs like anticholinergics, antidepressants, antipsychotics, diuretics, anxiolytics, antihistamines, antihypertensives, and analgesic drugs are frequently implicated in causing dry mouth in older adults. Since older adults are more likely to take multiple prescription medications as compared to the rest of the population, they are also most vulnerable to the side effects of these drugs and their impact on oral disease experience [73]. History of radiation to the head and neck, diseases of salivary glands, diabetes, alcoholic cirrhosis, and autoimmune disorders such as lupus and Sjogren's syndrome are some biological factors leading to dry mouth. Certain social and psychological factors, such as depression, stress, and anxiety, are also recognized as etiologic factors [74].

Reduced salivary flow allows micro-organisms to aggregate and adhere better in the oral environment, which causes the biofilm to stagnate longer, leading to loss of tooth structure, gingivitis, periodontal disease, dental caries, and halitosis. Since immunological functions of saliva are altered due to age as well as salivary hypofunction, older adults face a higher risk for opportunistic infections such as candidiasis because of hyposalivation. Candida species often harbor in the fissures of the tongue, leading to symptoms of burning tongue [75]. Studies highlight dry mouth as a local contributory factor in debilitating oral conditions such as burning mouth syndrome, which is characterized by the presence of a burning sensation of the oral mucosa in the absence of clinically apparent mucosal alterations. This disorder is often a challenge to diagnose and negatively impacts the patient's oral health-related quality of life [76]. In edentulous patients, reduced quality and quantity of saliva can negatively impact denture retention and cause discomfort while chewing due to insufficient lubrication between the denture base and supporting tissues. Depending on the severity of the condition, older adults who experience xerostomia may alter food choices, preferring items with higher moisture content to be able to comfortably masticate food and experience a variety of flavors and textures [77].

3.1.8. Utilization of Dental Services

As the global older adult population grows and continues to retain teeth for longer, their oral health needs are projected to increase as well [78]. However, a disparity exists when it comes to the utilization of dental services by older adults. There are many factors that affect older patients' ability to see a dentist or establish a dental home. As per the Health Policy Institute's 2019 Annual Dental Industry report, the utilization of dental services among older adults was influenced by dental insurance, household income, perceived affordability, and overall health outcomes. Older adults on public dental insurance programs utilized dental care the least, and race and/or ethnicity-related disparities in dental service utilization were apparent [79–82].

According to the CDC, there is a higher prevalence of untreated caries, edentulism, and periodontal disease among older adults from minority groups [83]. There is some association between poor oral health, self-perceptions of oral health, and affordability among older adults coming from disadvantaged ethnic minorities. This is a barrier to oral care by itself since such patients may not seek out oral care unless they are facing a dental emergency [84]. Occupational status and education among older adults were also found to be important predictors of the utilization of dental services [85]. Rural-dwelling older adults as well as those living in long-term care facilities typically were reported to have fewer visits to the dentist, making location of residence a predictor in understanding dental use by this group. Residents of long-term care facilities were found to face a combination of other barriers, such as poor functional status, difficulty in making visits to dental providers, and the unavailability of dentists who provide dental care within the nursing home settings [86].

From a functional standpoint, poor systemic health and multiple comorbidities are predictors of low dental service uptake among older adults. A study by Kuthy et al. suggested that individuals who had frequent medical visits and spent more resources on medications/medical visits tended to use dental services less. This can be correlated to the shift in focus from oral health to chronic conditions that impair activities of daily living [87]. One psychosocial predictor of using dental services among older adults is a social support network. Older adults who experience social isolation due to loss of a spouse, close friends, or relocation to a new community tend to utilize dental services less. This could be due to a lack of interpersonal ties and social connectedness resulting in lapsed oral health behaviors including seeing a dentist on a regular basis [88].

Lastly, dental providers' attitude can be both an enabler and barrier to the use of dental services among older adults. Dentists' beliefs, stereotypes, and skill levels with older patients can encourage or discourage use of dental services among this population. This is also compounded by shortage of skilled geriatric oral health care professionals making it harder for patients to access those providers with expertise in the geriatric dentistry [89].

4. Summary

Oral health and systemic health are closely related. When viewed through the lens of the rapid oral health deterioration conceptual framework, it becomes possible to identify specific risk factors that increase older adults' likelihood of experiencing a sharp decline in their oral health following a significant health event (Table 1). Good oral hygiene, performed independently or with help from a caregiver, offers protection from dental caries and periodontal disease. Retaining healthy teeth and replacing missing teeth strategically can facilitate speech, function, and esthetics while improving older adults' quality of life.

General health conditions or therapies to manage these can alter normal oral physiology and render older adults susceptible to unwanted side effects such as xerostomia. A combination of these and other social factors plays a role in their ability to choose and consume a nutritious diet. Oral soft tissue lesions require prompt management not only to ensure comfortable functioning with removable prostheses but also to minimize the risk of developing cancer from long-standing irritation. It is essential that older adults have a dental home in addition to a medical home to ensure that they are receiving timely preventive oral care and have access to the expertise needed to arrest rapid oral health deterioration.

Table 1. Interrelated nature of oral factors contributing to rapid oral health deterioration.

Oral Health Factors Leading to ROHD	Contributing Factors	Effects on Oral Health
Poor oral hygiene	Major health event, frailty, decreased manual dexterity, dependence on daily oral care, cognitive decline	Plaque retention, gingival inflammation, risk for periodontal disease, increased caries risk, halitosis
Periodontal disease	Inadequate oral hygiene maintenance, systemic risk factors or chronic inflammatory conditions, metabolic factors such as obesity, diabetes mellitus	Occlusal instability, tooth movement, tooth mobility, tooth loss, halitosis
Number of remaining teeth/restorations	Untreated dental caries, untreated periodontal disease, access to dental services	Multisurface restorations needing maintenance, interrupted dental arches, reduced masticatory ability, psychological impact of tooth loss
Sequelae of wearing fixed or removable dental prostheses	Condition of denture-bearing tissues, patient perception, ill-fitting dentures, worn-out artificial teeth, difficulty with placing and removing dentures, poor denture hygiene	Maladaptation to dentures, failure of abutment teeth, denture stomatitis, reduced masticatory ability, oral candidiasis
Presence of oral lesions	Poor denture hygiene, denture irritation, loss of occlusal vertical dimension, continuous denture usage, head and neck cancer, radiotherapy to this region	Candidiasis, traumatic ulcers, angular cheilitis, flabby tissue, dry mouth, burning mouth syndrome, radiation mucositis, decreased OHRQoL
Untreated dental caries	Poor oral hygiene maintenance, untreated periodontal disease, high sugar exposure, dry mouth, presence of prostheses, low access to dental care	Pain, reversible or irreversible pulpitis, increased risk for tooth fracture, tooth loss
Xerostomia	Polypharmacy, xerogenic medications, head and neck radiotherapy, salivary gland diseases, diabetes, autoimmune disorders such as Sjogren's syndrome or lupus	Dental caries, difficulty wearing dentures, decreased OHRQoL
Dietary choices	Loss of functional occluding units, dietary choices which have high sugar, insufficient calorie intake, availability of caregiver support	Increased caries risk, obesity, nutritional deficiencies related to proteins, vitamins, and minerals; dehydration; increased risk for malnutrition; frailty
Inability to utilize dental services	Caregiver availability, financial limitations, transportation barriers, institutionalization, poor systemic health, dental workforce issues	Discontinued dental visits, lack of surveillance of progressive oral conditions

Author Contributions: J.P.D. and R.U.N.; resources, J.P.D. and R.U.N.; data curation, J.P.D. and R.U.N.; writing—original draft preparation, J.P.D. and R.U.N.; writing—review and editing, J.P.D. and R.U.N. All authors have read and agreed to the published version of the manuscript.

Funding: This research received no external funding.

Institutional Review Board Statement: Not applicable.

Informed Consent Statement: Not applicable.

Data Availability Statement: Not applicable.

Acknowledgments: The authors sincerely thank Christopher A. Childs MLS, Clinical Education Librarian at Hardin Library for the Health Sciences, University of Iowa, for sharing his expertise and guiding our early literature search efforts.

Conflicts of Interest: The authors declare no conflict of interest.

References

1. Roser, M.; Ortiz-Ospina, E.; Ritchie, H. Life Expectancy. 2013. Available online: https://ourworldindata.org/life-expectancy (accessed on 20 March 2023).
2. Brummel-Smith, K.; Butler, D.; Frieder, M.; Gibbs, N.; Henry, M.; Koons, E.; Loggers, E.; Porock, D.; Reuben, D.B. Person-centered care: A definition and essential elements. *J. Am. Geriatr. Soc.* **2016**, *64*, 15–18.
3. Marchini, L.; Hartshorn, J.E.; Cowen, H.; Dawson, D.V.; Johnsen, D.C. A Teaching Tool for Establishing Risk of Oral Health Deterioration in Elderly Patients: Development, Implementation, and Evaluation at a U.S. Dental School. *J. Dent. Educ.* **2017**, *81*, 1283–1290. [CrossRef] [PubMed]
4. Marshall, T.A.; Marchini, L.; Cowen, H.; Hartshorn, J.E.; Holloway, J.A.; Straub-Morarend, C.L.; Gratton, D.; Solow, C.M.; Colangelo, N.; Johnsen, D.C. Critical Thinking Theory to Practice: Using the Expert's Thought Process as Guide for Learning and Assessment. *J. Dent. Educ.* **2017**, *81*, 978–985. [CrossRef] [PubMed]
5. Slack-Smith, L.; Hearn, L.; Wilson, D.; Wright, F. Geriatric dentistry, teaching and future directions. *Aust. Dent. J.* **2015**, *60*, 125–130. [CrossRef] [PubMed]
6. Ettinger, R.L.; Goettsche, Z.S.; Qian, F. Predoctoral Teaching of Geriatric Dentistry in U.S. Dental Schools. *J. Dent. Educ.* **2017**, *81*, 921–928. [CrossRef]
7. Craig, T.; Johnsen, D.C.; Dds, J.E.H.; Cowen, H.; Ashida, S.; Thompson, L.; Msc, C.P.; Xie, X.J.; Marchini, L. Teaching rapid oral health deterioration risk assessment: A 5-year report. *J. Dent. Educ.* **2020**, *84*, 1159–1165. [CrossRef]
8. Craig, T.W.; Comnick, C.L.; Leary, K.S.; Hartshorn, J.E.; Johnsen, D.C.; Marchini, L. A tool for incorporating interprofessional perspectives into dental students decision-making: A 2-year follow-up on this learning outcome. *Clin. Exp. Dent. Res.* **2022**, *8*, 1295–1301. [CrossRef]
9. Coll, P.P.; Lindsay, A.; Meng, J.; Gopalakrishna, A.; Raghavendra, S.; Bysani, P.; O'Brien, D. The Prevention of Infections in Older Adults: Oral Health. *J. Am. Geriatr. Soc.* **2019**, *68*, 411–416. [CrossRef]
10. Pace, C.C.; McCullough, G.H. The Association Between Oral Microorgansims and Aspiration Pneumonia in the Institutionalized Elderly: Review and Recommendations. *Dysphagia* **2010**, *25*, 307–322. [CrossRef]
11. Chalmers, J.M. Behavior management and communication strategies for dental professionals when caring for patients with dementia. *Spéc. Care Dent.* **2000**, *20*, 147–154. [CrossRef] [PubMed]
12. Noble, J.M.; Scarmeas, N.; Papapanou, P.N. Poor Oral Health as a Chronic, Potentially Modifiable Dementia Risk Factor: Review of the Literature. *Curr. Neurol. Neurosci. Rep.* **2013**, *13*, 384. [CrossRef] [PubMed]
13. Harding, A.; Robinson, S.; Crean, S.; Singhrao, S.K. Can Better Management of Periodontal Disease Delay the Onset and Progression of Alzheimer's Disease? *J. Alzheimer's Dis.* **2017**, *58*, 337–348. [CrossRef]
14. Delwel, S.; Binnekade, T.T.; Perez, R.S.G.M.; Hertogh, C.M.P.M.; Scherder, E.J.A.; Lobbezoo, F. Oral hygiene and oral health in older people with dementia: A comprehensive review with focus on oral soft tissues. *Clin. Oral Investig.* **2017**, *22*, 93–108. [CrossRef] [PubMed]
15. Jablonski, R.A.; Kolanowski, A.M.; Azuero, A.; Winstead, V.; Jones-Townsend, C.; Geisinger, M.L. Randomised clinical trial: Efficacy of strategies to provide oral hygiene activities to nursing home residents with dementia who resist mouth care. *Gerodontology* **2018**, *35*, 365–375. [CrossRef] [PubMed]
16. Jungbauer, G.; Stähli, A.; Zhu, X.; Alberi, L.A.; Sculean, A.; Eick, S. Periodontal microorganisms and Alzheimer disease—A causative relationship? *Periodontology 2000* **2022**, *89*, 59–82. [CrossRef] [PubMed]
17. Marchini, L.; Ettinger, R.; Caprio, T.; Jucan, A. Oral health care for patients with Alzheimer's disease: An update. *Spéc. Care Dent.* **2019**, *39*, 262–273. [CrossRef]
18. Uchimura, M.; Tsutsumi, T.; Kikutani, T.; Inaba, S.; Saitou, N. Restoration of the habit of routine tooth brushing teeth in patients with severe dementia. *Nippon. Ronen Igakkai Zasshi. Jpn. J. Geriatr.* **2001**, *38*, 366–371. [CrossRef] [PubMed]
19. Hartshorn, J.E.; Cowen, H.J.; Comnick, C.L. Cluster randomized control trial of nursing home residents' oral hygiene following the Mouth Care Matters education program for certified nursing assistants. *Spéc. Care Dent.* **2021**, *41*, 372–380. [CrossRef] [PubMed]
20. Vanagas, G.; Milašauskienė, Ž.; Grabauskas, V.; Mickevičienė, A. Associations between parental skills and their attitudes toward importance to develop good oral hygiene skills in their children. *Medicina* **2009**, *45*, 718–723. [CrossRef] [PubMed]
21. Milleman, K.; Milleman, J.; Bosma, M.L.; McGuire, J.A.; Sunkara, A.; DelSasso, A.; York, T.; Cecil, A.M. Role of Manual Dexterity on Mechanical and Chemotherapeutic Oral Hygiene Regimens. *J. Dent. Hyg.* **2022**, *96*, 35–45. [PubMed]
22. Chen, X.; Clark, J.J.; Preisser, J.S.; Naorungroj, S.; Shuman, S.K. Dental Caries in Older Adults in the Last Year of Life. *J. Am. Geriatr. Soc.* **2013**, *61*, 1345–1350. [CrossRef] [PubMed]
23. James, P.; Worthington, H.V.; Parnell, C.; Harding, M.; Lamont, T.; Cheung, A.; Whelton, H.; Riley, P. Chlorhexidine mouthrinse as an adjunctive treatment for gingival health. *Cochrane Database Syst. Rev.* **2017**, *2021*, CD008676. [CrossRef]
24. Robinson, P.; Deacon, S.; Deery, C.; Heanue, M.; Walmsley, D.; Worthington, H.; Glenny, A.-M.; Shaw, B.C. Manual versus powered toothbrushing for oral health. *Cochrane Database Syst. Rev.* **2005**, CD002281. [CrossRef]
25. Marchesan, J.; Byrd, K.; Moss, K.; Preisser, J.; Morelli, T.; Zandona, A.; Jiao, Y.; Beck, J. Flossing Is Associated with Improved Oral Health in Older Adults. *J. Dent. Res.* **2020**, *99*, 1047–1053. [CrossRef] [PubMed]

26. Eke, P.I.; Wei, L.; Borgnakke, W.S.; Thornton-Evans, G.; Zhang, X.; Lu, H.; McGuire, L.C.; Genco, R.J. Periodontitis prevalence in adults ≥ 65 years of age, in the USA. *Periodontol. 2000* **2016**, *72*, 76–95. [CrossRef]
27. Curtis, D.A.; Lin, G.; Rajendran, Y.; Gessese, T.; Suryadevara, J.; Kapila, Y.L. Treatment planning considerations in the older adult with periodontal disease. *Periodontol. 2000* **2021**, *87*, 157–165. [CrossRef]
28. López, R.; Smith, P.C.; Göstemeyer, G.; Schwendicke, F. Ageing, dental caries and periodontal diseases. *J. Clin. Periodontol.* **2017**, *44*, S145–S152. [CrossRef]
29. Carreiro, A.; Dias, K.D.C.; Lopes, A.L.C.; Resende, C.M.B.M.; Martins, A.R.L.D.A. Periodontal Conditions of Abutments and Non-Abutments in Removable Partial Dentures over 7 Years of Use. *J. Prosthodont.* **2016**, *26*, 644–649. [CrossRef] [PubMed]
30. Preshaw, P.M.; Alba, A.L.; Herrera, D.; Jepsen, S.; Konstantinidis, A.; Makrilakis, K.; Taylor, R. Periodontitis and diabetes: A two-way relationship. *Diabetologia* **2012**, *55*, 21–31. [CrossRef]
31. Kocher, T.; König, J.; Borgnakke, W.; Pink, C.; Meisel, P. Periodontal complications of hyperglycemia/diabetes mellitus: Epidemiologic complexity and clinical challenge. *Periodontol. 2000* **2018**, *78*, 59–97. [CrossRef]
32. Sanz, M.; Ceriello, A.; Buysschaert, M.; Chapple, I.; Demmer, R.T.; Graziani, F.; Herrera, D.; Jepsen, S.; Lione, L.; Madianos, P.; et al. Scientific evidence on the links between periodontal diseases and diabetes: Consensus report and guidelines of the joint workshop on periodontal diseases and diabetes by the International Diabetes Federation and the European Federation of Periodontology. *J. Clin. Periodontol.* **2017**, *45*, 138–149. [CrossRef] [PubMed]
33. Chaffee, B.W.; Weston, S.J. Association Between Chronic Periodontal Disease and Obesity: A Systematic Review and Meta-Analysis. *J. Periodontol.* **2010**, *81*, 1708–1724. [CrossRef] [PubMed]
34. Turner, M.D.; Ship, J.A. Dry Mouth and Its Effects on the Oral Health of Elderly People. *J. Am. Dent. Assoc.* **2007**, *138*, S15–S20. [CrossRef] [PubMed]
35. Liu, B.; Dion, M.R.; Jurasic, M.M.; Gibson, G.; Jones, J.A. Xerostomia and salivary hypofunction in vulnerable elders: Prevalence and etiology. *Oral Surg. Oral Med. Oral Pathol. Oral Radiol.* **2012**, *114*, 52–60. [CrossRef] [PubMed]
36. Zhang, J.; Leung, K.C.; Sardana, D.; Wong, M.C.; Lo, E.C. Risk predictors of dental root caries: A systematic review. *J. Dent.* **2019**, *89*, 103166. [CrossRef] [PubMed]
37. Tonetti, M.S.; Bottenberg, P.; Conrads, G.; Eickholz, P.; Heasman, P.; Huysmans, M.C.; Lopez, R.; Madianos, P.; Müller, F.; Needleman, I.; et al. Dental caries and periodontal diseases in the ageing population: Call to action to protect and enhance oral health and well-being as an essential component of healthy ageing—Consensus report of group 4 of the joint EFP/ORCA workshop on the boundaries between caries and periodontal diseases. *J. Clin. Periodontol.* **2017**, *44* (Suppl. S18), S135–S144. [CrossRef] [PubMed]
38. De Mata, C.; McKenna, G.; Burke, F.M. Caries and the older patient. *Dent. Update* **2011**, *38*, 376–378. [CrossRef] [PubMed]
39. Hayes, M.; Da Mata, C.; Cole, M.; McKenna, G.; Burke, F.; Allen, P.F. Risk indicators associated with root caries in independently living older adults. *J. Dent.* **2016**, *51*, 8–14. [CrossRef]
40. Gavriilidou, N.N.; Belibasakis, G.N. Root caries: The intersection between periodontal disease and dental caries in the course of ageing. *Br. Dent. J.* **2019**, *227*, 1063–1067. [CrossRef]
41. Tan, H.; Peres, K.; Peres, M. Retention of Teeth and Oral Health–Related Quality of Life. *J. Dent. Res.* **2016**, *95*, 1350–1357. [CrossRef]
42. Turkyilmaz, I.; Company, A.M.; McGlumphy, E.A. Should edentulous patients be constrained to removable complete dentures? The use of dental implants to improve the quality of life for edentulous patients. *Gerodontology* **2010**, *27*, 3–10. [CrossRef] [PubMed]
43. Boven, G.C.; Raghoebar, G.M.; Vissink, A.; Meijer, H.J.A. Improving masticatory performance, bite force, nutritional state and patient's satisfaction with implant overdentures: A systematic review of the literature. *J. Oral Rehabil.* **2014**, *42*, 220–233. [CrossRef]
44. Armellini, D.; von Fraunhofer, J.A. The shortened dental arch: A review of the literature. *J. Prosthet. Dent.* **2004**, *92*, 531–535. [CrossRef] [PubMed]
45. Aukes, J.N.S.C.; Käyser, A.F.; Felling, A.J.A. The subjective experience of mastication in subjects with shortened dental arches. *J. Oral Rehabil.* **1988**, *15*, 321–324. [CrossRef] [PubMed]
46. Moynihan, P.; Varghese, R. Impact of Wearing Dentures on Dietary Intake, Nutritional Status, and Eating: A Systematic Review. *JDR Clin. Transl. Res.* **2021**, *7*, 334–351. [CrossRef] [PubMed]
47. Kassebaum, N.J.; Bernabé, E.; Dahiya, M.; Bhandari, B.; Murray, C.J.L.; Marcenes, W. Global Burden of Severe Tooth Loss: A Systematic Review and Meta-Analysis. *J. Dent. Res.* **2014**, *93* (Suppl. S7), 20S–28S. [CrossRef] [PubMed]
48. Li, Q.; Chalmers, J.; Czernichow, S.; Neal, B.; Taylor, B.A.; Zoungas, S.; Poulter, N.; Woodward, M.; Patel, A.; De Galan, B.; et al. Oral disease and subsequent cardiovascular disease in people with type 2 diabetes: A prospective cohort study based on the Action in Diabetes and Vascular Disease: Preterax and Diamicron Modified-Release Controlled Evaluation (ADVANCE) trial. *Diabetologia* **2010**, *53*, 2320–2327. [CrossRef]
49. Kim, S.Y.; Lee, C.H.; Yoo, D.M.; Kwon, M.J.; Kim, J.H.; Kim, J.-H.; Byun, S.-H.; Park, B.; Lee, H.-J.; Choi, H.G. Is the Number of Missing Teeth Associated with Mortality? A Longitudinal Study Using a National Health Screening Cohort. *Front. Med.* **2022**, *9*, 1749. [CrossRef]
50. Walls, A.W.G.; Steele, J.G.; Sheiham, A.; Marcenes, W.; Moynihan, P.J. Oral Health and Nutrition in Older People. *J. Public Heal. Dent.* **2000**, *60*, 304–307. [CrossRef]

51. Marcenes, W.; Steele, J.G.; Sheiham, A.; Walls, A.W.G. The relationship between dental status, food selection, nutrient intake, nutritional status, and body mass index in older people. *Cad. Saude Publica* **2003**, *19*, 809–815. [CrossRef]
52. Bakker, M.H.; Vissink, A.; Spoorenberg, S.L.; Jager-Wittenaar, H.; Wynia, K.; Visser, A. Are Edentulousness, Oral Health Problems and Poor Health-Related Quality of Life Associated with Malnutrition in Community-Dwelling Elderly (Aged 75 Years and Over)? A Cross-Sectional Study. *Nutrients* **2018**, *10*, 1965. [CrossRef] [PubMed]
53. Gil-Montoya, J.A.; Subirá, C.; Ramón, J.M.; González-Moles, M.A. Oral Health-Related Quality of Life and Nutritional Status. *J. Public Heal. Dent.* **2008**, *68*, 88–93. [CrossRef] [PubMed]
54. Salmi, A.; Komulainen, K.; Nihtilä, A.; Tiihonen, M.; Nykänen, I.; Hartikainen, S.; Suominen, A.L. Eating problems among old home care clients. *Clin. Exp. Dent. Res.* **2022**, *8*, 959–968. [CrossRef]
55. Leung, D.Y.; Leung, A.Y.; Chi, I. Factors associated with chewing problems and oral dryness among older Chinese people in Hong Kong. *Gerodontology* **2014**, *33*, 106–115. [CrossRef]
56. Kazemi, S.; Savabi, G.; Khazaei, S.; Savabi, O.; Esmaillzadeh, A.; Keshteli, A.H.; Adibi, P. Association between food intake and oral health in elderly: SEPAHAN systematic review no. 8. *Dent. Res. J.* **2011**, *8* (Suppl. S1), S15–S20.
57. Sahyoun, N.R.; Krall, E. Low dietary quality among older adults with self-perceived ill-fitting dentures. *J. Am. Diet. Assoc.* **2003**, *103*, 1494–1499. [CrossRef]
58. Maitre, I.; Van Wymelbeke, V.; Amand, M.; Vigneau, E.; Issanchou, S.; Sulmont-Rossé, C. Food pickiness in the elderly: Relationship with dependency and malnutrition. *Food Qual. Preference* **2014**, *32*, 145–151. [CrossRef]
59. Sheiham, A.; Steele, J.G.; Marcenes, W.; Finch, S.; Walls, A.W.G. The relationship between oral health status and body mass index among older people: A national survey of older people in Great Britain. *Brit. Dent. J.* **2002**, *192*, 703–706. [CrossRef]
60. Hooper, L.; Bunn, D.; Jimoh, F.O.; Fairweather-Tait, S.J. Water-loss dehydration and aging. *Mech. Ageing Dev.* **2014**, *136–137*, 50–58. [CrossRef]
61. Gerontological Society of America. Interprofessional Solutions for Improving Oral Health in Older Adults: Addressing Access Barriers, Creating Oral Health Champions. July 2017. Available online: https://www.geron.org/images/gsa/documents/gsa2017oralhealthwhitepaper.pdf (accessed on 29 November 2022).
62. Dreizen, S. Oral candidiasis. *Am. J. Med.* **1984**, *77*, 28–33.
63. Rossie, K.; Guggenheimer, J. Oral candidiasis: Clinical manifestations, diagnosis, and treatment. *Pr. Periodontics Aesthetic Dent. PPAD* **1997**, *9*, 635–641.
64. Buranarom, N.; Komin, O.; Matangkasombut, O. Hyposalivation, oral health, and Candida colonization in independent dentate elders. *PLoS ONE* **2020**, *15*, e0242832. [CrossRef] [PubMed]
65. Deng, Z.; Kiyuna, A.; Hasegawa, M.; Nakasone, I.; Hosokawa, A.; Suzuki, M. Oral candidiasis in patients receiving radiation therapy for head and neck cancer. *Otolaryngol. Neck Surg.* **2010**, *143*, 242–247. [CrossRef] [PubMed]
66. Ohga, N.; Yamazaki, Y.; Sato, J.; Asaka, T.; Morimoto, M.; Hata, H.; Satoh, C.; Kitagawa, Y. Elimination of oral candidiasis may increase stimulated whole salivary flow rate. *Arch. Oral Biol.* **2016**, *71*, 129–133. [CrossRef]
67. Gendreau, L.; Loewy, Z.G. Epidemiology and Etiology of Denture Stomatitis. *J. Prosthodont.* **2011**, *20*, 251–260. [CrossRef]
68. Budtz-Jorgensen, E. Oral mucosal lesions associated with the wearing of removable dentures. *J. Oral Pathol. Med.* **1981**, *10*, 65–80. [CrossRef] [PubMed]
69. Randall, D.A.; Wilson Westmark, N.L.; Neville, B.W. Common Oral Lesions. *Am. Fam. Physician* **2022**, *105*, 369–376. [PubMed]
70. Saintrain, M.V.D.L.; Bandeira, A.B.V.; Pequeno, L.L.; Bizerril, D.O.; Marques, P.L.P.; Viana, F.A.C. Oral health of older people: Tracking soft tissue injuries for the prevention of oral cancer. *Rev. Esc. Enferm. USP* **2018**, *52*. [CrossRef] [PubMed]
71. National Cancer Institute. Surveillance, Epidemiology, and End Results Program. Available online: http://www.seer.cancer.gov (accessed on 27 November 2022).
72. VanderWalde, N.A.; Fleming, M.; Weiss, J.; Chera, B.S. Treatment of Older Patients with Head and Neck Cancer: A Review. *Oncology* **2013**, *18*, 568–578. [CrossRef]
73. Singh, M.L.; Papas, A. Oral Implications of Polypharmacy in the Elderly. *Dent. Clin. N. Am.* **2014**, *58*, 783–796. [CrossRef] [PubMed]
74. Wiener, R.C.; Wu, B.; Crout, R.; Wiener, M.; Plassman, B.; Kao, E.; McNeil, D. Hyposalivation and Xerostomia in Dentate Older Adults. *J. Am. Dent. Assoc.* **2010**, *141*, 279–284. [CrossRef]
75. Bergdahl, M.; Bergdahl, J. Burning mouth syndrome: Prevalence and associated factors. *J. Oral Pathol. Med.* **2007**, *28*, 350–354. [CrossRef] [PubMed]
76. Sun, A.; Wu, K.-M.; Wang, Y.-P.; Lin, H.-P.; Chen, H.-M.; Chiang, C.-P. Burning mouth syndrome: A review and update. *J. Oral Pathol. Med.* **2013**, *42*, 649–655. [CrossRef]
77. Quandt, S.A.; Savoca, M.R.; Leng, X.; Chen, H.; Bell, R.A.; Gilbert, G.H.; Anderson, A.M.; Kohrman, T.; Arcury, T.A. Dry Mouth and Dietary Quality in Older Adults in North Carolina. *J. Am. Geriatr. Soc.* **2011**, *59*, 439–445. [CrossRef]
78. Calabrese, J.M.; Rawal, K. Demographics and Oral Health Care Utilization for Older Adults. *Dent. Clin. North Am.* **2021**, *65*, 241–255. [CrossRef] [PubMed]
79. Hovland, E.J. The Surgeon General's report on oral health. *LDA J.* **2000**, *59*, 13–14.
80. Vujicic, M.; Buchmueller, T.; Klein, R. Dental Care Presents the Highest Level of Financial Barriers, Compared to Other Types of Health Care Services. *Heal. Aff.* **2016**, *35*, 2176–2182. [CrossRef]

81. Scannapieco, F.A.; Amin, S.; Salme, M.; Tezal, M. Factors associated with utilization of dental services in a long-term care facility: A descriptive cross-sectional study. *Spéc. Care Dent.* **2016**, *37*, 78–84. [CrossRef] [PubMed]
82. Center for Medicare Advocacy Dental/Oral Health. Available online: https://www.medicareadvocacy.org/medicare-info/dental-coverage-under-medicare/ (accessed on 1 January 2023).
83. Centers for Disease Control and Prevention. Oral Health Surveillance Report: Trends in Dental Caries and Sealants, Tooth Retention, and Edentulism, United States, 1999–2004 to 2011–2016. Atlanta, GA: Centers for Disease Control and Prevention, U.S. Department of Health, and Human Services. 2019. Available online: https://www.cdc.gov/oralhealth/publications/OHSR-2019-index.html (accessed on 15 December 2022).
84. Ahluwalia, K.P.; Sadowsky, D. Oral disease burden and dental services utilization by Latino and African-American seniors in Northern Manhattan. *J. Community Health* **2003**, *28*, 267–280. [CrossRef]
85. Roberts-Thomson, K.; Brennan, D.S.; Spencer, A.J. Social inequality in the use and comprehensiveness of dental services. *Aust. J. Public Health* **2010**, *19*, 80–85. [CrossRef] [PubMed]
86. Kiyak, H.A.; Reichmuth, M. Barriers to and Enablers of Older Adults' Use of Dental Services. *J. Dent. Educ.* **2005**, *69*, 975–986. [CrossRef] [PubMed]
87. Kuthy, R.A.; Strayer, M.S.; Caswell, R.J. Determinants of dental user groups among an elderly, low-income population. *Health Serv. Res.* **1996**, *30*, 809–825.
88. Avlund, K.; Holm-Pedersen, P.; Morse, U.E.; Viitanen, M.; Winblad, B. Social relations as determinants of oral health among persons over the age of 80 years. *Community Dent. Oral Epidemiol.* **2003**, *31*, 454–462. [CrossRef] [PubMed]
89. Dolan, T.A.; Atchison, K.; Huynh, T.N. Access to Dental Care Among Older Adults in the United States. *J. Dent. Educ.* **2005**, *69*, 961–974. [CrossRef] [PubMed]

Disclaimer/Publisher's Note: The statements, opinions and data contained in all publications are solely those of the individual author(s) and contributor(s) and not of MDPI and/or the editor(s). MDPI and/or the editor(s) disclaim responsibility for any injury to people or property resulting from any ideas, methods, instructions or products referred to in the content.

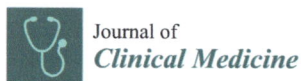 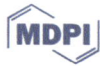

Review

Assessment and Improvement of Masticatory Performance in Frail Older People: A Narrative Review

Martin Schimmel [1,2,*], Noemi Anliker [1], Gabriela Panca Sabatini [1,3], Marcella Silva De Paula [1,4], Adrian Roman Weber [1] and Pedro Molinero-Mourelle [1]

1. Department of Reconstructive Dentistry and Gerodontology, School of Dental Medicine, University of Bern, 3010 Bern, Switzerland
2. Division of Gerodontology and Removable Prosthodontics, University Clinics of Dental Medicine, University of Geneva, 1211 Geneva, Switzerland
3. Department of Prosthodontics, University of São Paulo (USP), São Paulo 05508-900, Brazil
4. Department of Prevention and Oral Rehabilitation, Universidade Federal de Goiás, Goiania 74690-900, Brazil
* Correspondence: martin.schimmel@unibe.ch

Abstract: According to the World Health Organization (WHO), the estimated number of older adults is around 962 million and is projected to increase to 2.1 billion by 2050. The oral frailty concept is associated with gradual oral function loss in relation to aging. There is a need to emphasize the improvement of oral function based on an evaluation of masticatory performance in patients with various oral conditions or systemic diseases and especially in the frail elderly. The present narrative review presents an overview of the current state of the assessment and improvement of masticatory performance in frail older people. To fully encompass oral frailty, oro-facial hypofunction, or oro-facial fitness, dental Patient Reported Outcomes (dPROs) should be included; nevertheless, there are limited evidence-based rehabilitation approaches. The concept of oral frailty, oro-facial hypofunction, or oro-facial fitness should involve dental Patient Reported Outcomes (dPROs), and in this sense, there are only a few evidence-based rehabilitation procedures to improve oro-facial hypofunction besides prosthodontics. It must be considered that reduced neuroplastic capacity in old individuals might preclude a positive outcome of these strategies that might need to be accompanied by functional training and nutritional counseling.

Keywords: geriatrics; frail elderly; frailty; oral health; tooth loss; dental care for age

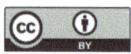

1. Introduction

According to the World Health Organization (WHO), as of 2020, the number of older adults (defined as people aged 60 years and older) worldwide is estimated to be around 962 million. This number is projected to increase to 2.1 billion by 2050, which represents a significant demographic shift toward an aging population [1].

This shift is related to an increased life expectancy and a reduced birth rate, as observed primarily in the Western world, but the same effect is present in developing countries. Nowadays, the so-called baby boomer generation has arrived at medical and dental practices, and this trend will be progressing during the next ten to twenty years [2]. Due to the current social aspects, especially in industrialized countries, these individuals have high expectations in relation to their oral health and orofacial function. If teeth need replacement, many of them expect stable, functional, esthetic and predictable tooth replacements. In this sense, this group of patients is little inclined to make compromises regarding their social life and food choice and often demonstrate a high willingness to invest in "high technology" treatment and prostheses [3].

Aging is a continuous process, and during this period, individuals will be subjected to progressive degenerative changes in their state of mental, cognitive, and general health [4]. In the last period of life, during old age, individuals might become frail or finally dependent on care. Laslett [5] introduced the term third age, which compromises a phase of retirement with social integration, high levels of activity and often very active baby boomers. Later, the term "fourth age" was introduced, which is characterized by a unique excess of women over men, higher levels of comorbidity and institutionalization, and greater consumption of medical and care services [6]. In a specific description, "third age" exemplifies positive characteristics, and "fourth age" dysfunction and death on biological, functional, or quality of life characteristics [7].

Considering this current epidemiological trend, aging is related to frailty, which is defined as "a state of vulnerability to poor resolution of homeostasis following a stress and is a consequence of a cumulative decline in multiple physiological systems over a lifespan". Often, individuals will expect a gradual decline of the physiological health reserve; nevertheless, the frailty state includes multiple interrelated physiological system disorders that will decline in a more accelerated way with the consequent initiation of the failure of homeostatic mechanisms [8].

With respect to the frailty state, it is important to remark that complex aging mechanisms are involved in this state, which will promote a continuous cumulative decline in the physiological systems that will weaken the homeostasis of these individuals, making them more vulnerable to the consequent changes in the state of health [9]. For dental medicine, oral frailty is a relatively new concept that can be associated with gradual oral function loss in relation to aging [10]. This state is characterized by the presence of whole limitations and deficiencies that produce a rapid deterioration in daily oral functions, such as tooth loss, poor oral hygiene, the existence of insufficient dental prostheses and/or difficulty chewing associated with age-related swallowing changes [8].

Tooth loss plays a significant role in the oral health and quality of life of frail older people since this condition triggers a deterioration of all masticatory and swallowing functions [11]. In the Western world, this condition has been decreasing in the last 20 years due to the improvements in oral health prevention and care, especially for edentulism [12]. Nevertheless, it is still highly prevalent in frail and dependent older adults. Edentulism increases exponentially with age; it is often associated with multimorbidity and is highly dependent on socio-economics factors [13]. In addition to tooth loss, oral health challenges in the old population include dental caries, periodontal disease, dry mouth, oral precancer/cancer, denture-related conditions, masticatory impairment, dysphagia and aspiration pneumonia [14,15]. The consequent oral and dental care of this patient should be: ensuring access to dental care for the elderly, establishing an infection- and pain-free oral cavity, long-term prevention of oral infections, fostering oral health-related quality of life factors (such as keeping 20 teeth or more and avoidance of removable dental prostheses), the maintenance or improving masticatory function and ensuring acceptable oral aesthetic appearance and the maintenance of patient autonomy [16]. The needs for care within the frail aged population are undergoing rapid changes as the baby boomer generation reaches retirement age. Traditional top-down healthcare decision-making that relies on passive acceptance of offered treatments is no longer sufficient. Normative and expressed needs may diverge, and patients are increasingly participating in research to inform best practices. Thus, there is a growing need for more collaborative, partnership-based decision-making with the patient to ensure that care aligns with their needs and preferences [17].

Considering the previous statements, there is a need to emphasize the improvement of oral function based on an evaluation of masticatory performance in patients with various oral conditions or systemic diseases and especially in the frail elderly. The aim of the present narrative review is to present a concise but comprehensive overview of the current state of the assessment and improvement of masticatory performance in frail older people.

2. A Conceptual Model of Oro-Facial Health with an Emphasis on Function

Historically, trends in dental medicine have often led to an artificial separation in dental education, research, patient care and public health policy from general medicine and its disciplines [18]. This obvious limitation is now changing and evolving, and therefore current educational trends will allow current and future clinicians to consider the orofacial system in a broader context of health and function. In relation to these changes, in the last decade, both in undergraduate and postgraduate dental education and in daily clinical practice, the domains of quality of life and patient-centered values have gained importance with an emphasis on oro-facial function [19].

In 2014, the Meikirch model was developed with a new dynamic definition of the health concept [20]. The definition was not only based on static immunological systems state but health results throughout the life course when individuals' potentials—and social and environmental determinants—suffice to respond satisfactorily to the demands of life. During life, the biologically given potential decreases as a result of the general, irreversible process of aging. Parallel to this decline and compensating for the possible negative implications on the orofacial functional capacity, the personally acquired potential increases, ensuring the state of health [21]. Most oro-facial conditions, such as periodontitis, tooth loss, impaired oral food processing or hyposalivation, are chronic and hence require attention for prolonged periods of time. Conditions of the orofacial system might be the origin or even can modify general diseases such as aspiration pneumonia, or general conditions such as cancer and the treatment thereof might manifest themselves in the oral cavity and hamper oro-facial function [15,22]. Nowadays, a common view is that health care should provide a cure, whereas providing long-term care and maintaining the quality of life (QoL) to an acceptable standard, from a person's point of view, has gained little attention so far [17,23,24].

The oral health-related quality of life (OHRQoL) is a concept that is based on the idea of patient-based medicine and is a useful tool that clinicians and researchers can use to understand or assess the oral state, dental treatment or a related condition [25,26]. OHRQoL includes biological, social, and psychological aspects and is gaining importance in the context of oro-facial frailty and oro-facial hypofunction. It should be considered that oral function, oro-facial pain, oro-facial appearance and psychosocial impact are related to the reasons why patients seek help from dental and medical professionals [27,28].

As part of the conceptual health, to achieve favorable treatment outcomes, researchers and clinicians measure the different states that are involved in dental medicine, such as the biological status, the clinical status and the patient functional status (chewing function, oral diadochokinesis) [29]. Based on this state, specific dental Patient-Reported Outcomes (dPROs) have been developed to measure the influence of oral health on aspects of daily living, patient satisfaction with dental care, oral health and treatment outcome and patients' self-perception of oral health, dental treatment or esthetics [29]. This state can be measured by means of questionnaires (instruments) or by a qualitative approach that is oriented to reflect the multidimensional model of OHRQoL. These methodologies have been widely investigated and validated and currently are one of the most used and useful tools for assessing oral health status. Among others, the most used in gerodontology are a denture satisfaction index (DSI); visual analog scales (VAS), an oral health impact profile (OHIP) and the Geriatric Oral Health Assessment Index (GOHAI) [30–33].

The use of these questionnaires can give a baseline assessment and, therefore, valuable information and diagnosis to develop a proper treatment plan to improve the masticatory ability, especially in such patients that are dependent or impaired [34]. Considering the conceptual model of oro-facial health and considering the limitations of frail ancient populations, some physiological requirements are in relation to oral function. It should be noted that oral function not only includes eating, swallowing or speaking ability as physical aspects but also has psychosocial and environmental aspects.

The condition of being fit in terms of oro-facial health, commonly referred to as the vitality of the oro-facial system, involves the lack of effective management of physical and mental ailments, pain, and negative environmental or social aspects. This enables individuals to meet the demands of everyday life while also facilitating natural oro-facial functions such as sensation, taste, touch, bite, mastication, deglutition, articulation, yawning, singing, kissing and different countenances. Comorbid diseases such as frailty may negatively affect the oro-facial functional capacity and may result in dysfunction and disease. It was described that an association between the presence of poor oral health status is associated with polypharmacy and multimorbidity, and therefore, orofacial fitness will be affected [35]. Although the interest in this topic has been growing, there is still a lack of widespread, validated, easy-to-use instruments that help to distinguish between states of orofacial fitness as opposed to orofacial hypofunction [24].

3. Factors Influencing Mastication

Mastication is one of the most important physiological functions since it is interrelated with eating and swallowing depends on it [36]. It is well documented how the aging process is related to a deterioration of the masticatory function involving the decrease of occlusal forces and the motor function of the tongue and peri-oral muscles [37]. The main consequence of functional progressive aging will be an impairment of the masticatory efficiency, food bolus formation and swallowing, and therefore digestion and nutrient absorption will be compromised, leading to insufficient nutrition [37,38]. As with any other body function, masticatory function is a multifactorial process that involves orofacial structures and function, individuals' physiological aspects, the environment and general health [24].

Masticatory function depends not only on tooth- and prosthesis-related factors. Edentulous adults have usually already reached an advanced age and thus frequently exhibit age-related comorbidities [39].

Increasing evidence also suggests that not only impaired cognitive function leads to oral dysfunction but indeed, masticatory difficulties could be a causal contributor to the onset of neurodegenerative diseases such as dementia [40–45]. The favorable masticatory function could therefore be a protecting factor in terms of increased cerebral blood flow in patients that already suffer from neurodegenerative conditions [46].

With increasing disease, saliva-inhibiting medications are also taken more frequently, which can lead to a variety of problems. The lack of saliva causes poorly retained removable dentures and often pain due to the lack of the mucosa protective effect of saliva. In addition, food cannot be lubricated, which greatly complicates the shaping and oral/esophageal transport of the food bolus. Thus, chewing efficiency is also significantly dependent on saliva quantity and consistency [47].

Also, the influence of the tongue, palate, cheek, and lip on chewing function should not be underestimated. As food particles are crushed between the chewing surfaces, these structures shape the bolus and reposition it between the dentition between masticatory cycles [48,49]. For example, stroke patients whose innervation, strength, and mobility of these structures are impaired also show decreased masticatory efficiency [50]. The decline in muscular coordination ability may be a physiological sign of aging, as it is with handwriting, but its effect on chewing function is poorly documented [51]. In contrast, a decline in chewing ability has been demonstrated in patients with neurodegenerative diseases [52]. In the advanced stage of Alzheimer's dementia, the brain no longer knows how to generate chewing and swallowing movements, and even when food is placed in the patient's mouth, feeding difficulty occurs in older adults with dementia [53,54].

Another aspect related to masticatory function is the age-related atrophy of the large jaw sphincters, which is further accelerated by edentulism [55]. Newton et al. have shown that overdentures supported by natural roots counteract the atrophy of jaw elevators [56]. To date, there is limited evidence, but it appears that implant-supported/retained dentures may also inhibit this atrophy [57]. This underscores the preventive benefits of implant-supported restorations in the edentulous patient.

Although the masticatory function of edentulous patients can be significantly increased by stabilizing, especially the lower denture, this does not automatically have a positive influence on diet or nutritional status [24]. Nutrition of the elderly depends on many factors, such as limited mobility, appetite, budget, depression and long-established habits [58]. Therefore, about up to one-third of the old living at home show malnutrition or undernutrition, and the proportion is likely to be even higher among institutionalized seniors [59,60]. In a Geneva study, it was shown that in a population sample of people over 80, 40% had less than three foods or spoiled foods, and 10% had no food at all in the refrigerator [61].

Chewing as a physiological function includes food-related aspects such as appetite, expectation, smell, taste, texture, temperature, preferences and conditioning. As previously mentioned, the multifactorial of the masticatory function not only involves the oral function but co-factors of oral food processing, such as the vision, the smell, the taste, the rheological properties, individuals' expectations and the cultural/religious context.

4. Assessment of the Masticatory Performance in Frail Older People

It is evident how individual progressive aging will produce a series of changes at the oro-facial level that will be aggravated by tooth loss. Setting aside the classic extraoral physical signs and the intraoral state that characterize the edentulous state, the most critical change is chewing impairment [11,62,63]. If this situation is considered, it is of paramount importance for the clinician to be able to assess this state of mastication.

Numerous methodological procedures have been used to describe the masticatory process, but there is occasional overlap in the terminology used to describe these techniques. It is crucial to standardize these terms to enable comparisons across studies. Care should especially be taken to distinguish between the terms "chewing efficiency/performance" for an objective clinical evaluation of the chewing function and "masticatory ability", which comprises the subjective evaluation by the individual [64].

Therefore, the objective evaluation of the mastication will be based on the individual's chewing efficiency or chewing performance, which may be assessed using well-validated tests. Furthermore, it was previously mentioned within the scope of the current oral health concept that there is a need to also use an evaluation from the individual's point of view to further assess compensation mechanisms. Due to alterations in the orofacial systems, as individuals age and become frail, their chewing behavior tends to change. Peyron et al. have shown that for every year of life, there is an average increase of 0.3 cycles per sequence, which refers to the number of chewing cycles performed before swallowing [65]. Additionally, there is a gradual increase in the mean summed EMG (electromyographic) activity per sequence, which is a measure of the muscle activity involved in chewing. Furthermore, older individuals also tend to exhibit changes in cycle and opening duration at the beginning of the chewing sequence. Specifically, these durations decrease with age, which suggests that there may be alterations in the coordination of chewing movements as individuals get older [65]. Considering these statements, the best way to evaluate mastication will be based on a combination of patient-based and laboratory-based methods [36].

Hence, from a clinical point of view, the sole evaluation of chewing efficiency/performance is not sufficient to comprehend the old and/or frail patients' adaptive or maladaptive behavior in relation to mastication or bolus preparation.

5. Chewing Efficiency

Objective evaluations might comprise the use assessment with "breakable" foodstuff or test food such as nuts or silicone cubes (Optocal), plastic or elastic test foods including chewing gum or wax, or finally, shearable specimens including gummy jelly of various hardness.

The glossary of prosthodontic terms defines chewing or masticatory efficiency as the "degree of effort needed to grind food to a standardized level of comminution" [66] and has been assessed by several methods, as shown in Table 1. One important term is median particle size, which is used to describe the food bolus. When investigating how crumbly foods such as nuts break down during chewing until they form a food bolus consisting of small particles, this bolus can be studied. When analyzing the distribution of particle size using techniques such as optical scanning or sieving, this can be quantified in terms of the median particle size. By chewing the food a specific number of times, the particle size distribution can be used to evaluate masticatory or chewing performance [64]. As an objective test to analyze particle size distribution, the empirical equation of the Rosin-Rammler formula can be used, which is defined by two parameters—the median particle size (D50) and the cumulative distribution of particle sizes in a sample [67]. A further example is the "carrot test"; carrots as test food were applied in research to define a minimum masticatory efficacy of healthy individuals to be classified as such with regard to chewing function. Carrots were also used in geriatric research to screen for deficient masticatory function with a simpler evaluation based on the visual evaluation of chewed carrots. Tests assessing chewing efficiency with these breakable test foods might still be the gold standard of assessing masticatory function due to their long history and widespread application in research; however, they are expensive and laborious to use due to the need for laboratory-based analysis and furthermore, might not be safe in frail elders who might suffer from dysphagia.

Another objective to describe chewing efficiency is shearing tests. Elastic "shearable" foodstuff refers to foods that have a certain level of elasticity. This property is often associated with certain types of meat, such as beef or pork, as well as some plant-based foods, including mushrooms. The amount of deformation that occurs before the food breaks depends on the food's elasticity and other properties, such as its moisture content and texture. Considering these different aspects, researchers at the University of Auvergne developed a model food material that is designed to simulate the mechanical properties of natural foods, such as hardness, elasticity, and texture. It is a standardized, non-nutritive material made from a mixture of synthetic polymers, invented by the University of Auvergne, faculty of dental surgery in France. Likewise, the Glucosensor© test (GC, Lucerne, Switzerland) is a technique that involves crushing a jelly within a 20-s time frame and dissolving it in water to determine the quantity of glucose (mg/dL) released. A specimen is deemed to have inferior masticatory function when the glucose concentration measured is less than 100 mg/dL [37]. This test is widely applied in Japan and was adapted for the diagnoses of oral hypofunction by the Japanese Society of Gerodontology [10].

In terms of texture, a plastic "deformable" foodstuff is a food material that can be easily molded or reshaped without breaking or cracking. In order to facilitate the objective measurement of chewing function, color mixing tests have been developed. Two-color test foods (i.e., wax, chewing gum, colored gelatin) are used [68–71]. The degree of color mixing achieved and the shape of the resulting bolus obtained after a given number of chewing cycles can be used as a measure of chewing efficiency. The two-color mixing test correlates significantly with the "sieve method" and is particularly suitable for subjects with reduced chewing function [72].

Own investigations [70,73] could show that the color mixing degree of a two-color chewing gum can be approximately described by a logarithmic function (log10) with the base "number of chewing cycles". Here, the test subject is offered conventional, commercially available chewing gum in the colors blue and pink as a test food. The chewing gum is placed on the tongue, and the subject is asked to chew it for 20 chewing cycles on his/her preferred chewing side. It is then removed from the oral cavity and pressed in clear plastic film to a thickness of one mm. Both sides of the rolled-out chewing gum are then digitized using a flatbed scanner, and the two resulting images are copied into an image template of a specified size and number of pixels. The software Viewgum© [74] can be used to determine the variance of the color tones; this can be used to determine chewing efficiency. The color variance (Variance of Hue, VOH) shows a strong association with the number of chewing cycles and can be described by a logarithmic to linear curve, depending on the sample material. Hence, samples with a low color mixing degree show a high variance in the color distribution and indicate a poor chewing function [75]. Furthermore, van der Bilt et al. demonstrated that these two-colour mixing-ability tests might be more suitable for assessing chewing function in individuals with impaired mastication [70,75–78].

The group of Kaya et al. observed a correlation between a bolus kneading test based on the analysis of VOH and D50 (chewing efficiency) [76]. Both methods were able to differentiate masticatory performance differences. Nonetheless, the two-color chewing gum mixing ability test can still be considered reliable for assessing masticatory performance and chewing performance, especially in non-clinical settings for individuals with dysphagia or reduced chewing function. A simplified version of this color mixing test is also suitable for use in a dental practice, hospital or nursing home. For this, the bolus taken from the oral cavity is first evaluated visually using a scale and provides quick and simple information about the individual chewing efficiency (Figure 1).

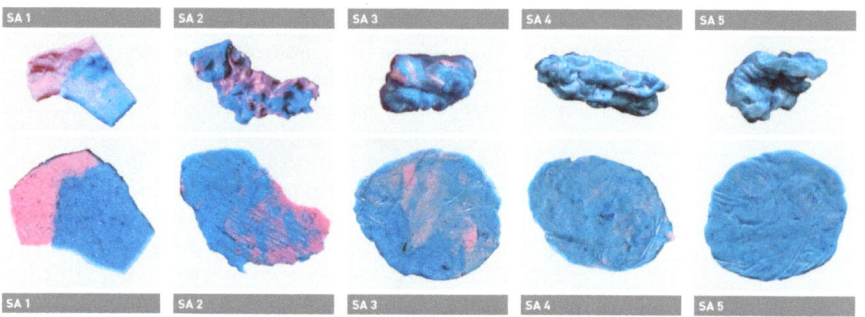

Figure 1. The Subjective Assessment Scale (SA) allows for the quick and simple evaluation of chewing efficiency by judging color mixture and bolus formation [63]. If the patient shows a degree of mixing of SA 1 or SA 2, it can be assumed that she/he has difficulty enjoying normal meals.

If the patient shows a degree of mixing of 1 or 2, it can be assumed that he or she has difficulty enjoying normal meals. For example, if no material at all is available for testing the chewing function when a patient is admitted to the geriatric hospital, simply biting the examiner's finger [79] or chewing a carrot on a trial basis [80] can provide an initial indication of whether the patient can be served pureed or normal meals.

Table 1. Recommended methods of assessment of chewing efficiency/performance, i.e., objective clinical assessment for frail older adults.

Test	Methodology	Functioning
Color mixing-ability test	Two-colored chewing gum	Might contain sugar, older adults might not be familiar with chewing gum, easy to control bolus, easy to evaluate, easy to evaluate (scale) [14,81].
Color mixing-ability test	Two-colored wax	Older adults might not be comfortable with chewing on wax, easy to control bolus, easy to evaluate, easy to evaluate (scale) [82].
Glucosensor © (GC)	Glucose extraction from gum jelly	Needs specialized equipment and specimens [83].
Carrot-test	Carrot slices	Always available, hardness might be difficult to control, easy to evaluate (scale) [80].
Bite force	Force gauge	Force gauges for bite force are often not available. Bite force, however, is a good predictor of chewing function [47].
Occlusal contacts in the four supporting zones (Eichner Classification)	Needs light and a good overview	Easiest way to extrapolate on chewing function. Main predictor of chewing function [8].

6. Chewing Ability

Considering the limitations of solely assessing chewing function with clinical tests, the chewing ability will be assessed with qualitative semi-structured interviews or validated questionnaires, such as the temporomandibular joint disability index (TDI), and the eating Related Quality of Life. However, in a recent study, there were no conclusive significant correlations between the subdomains of chewing ability or the nutritional variables. This could be due to the lack of standardized and validated methods for assessing masticatory ability for various cultural or geographical backgrounds. Although there is no widely accepted questionnaire, some instruments comprise questions that relate to chewing ability and some to specific compensatory mechanisms if chewing is impaired, as shown in Table 2.

Table 2. Examples of methods that relate to chewing ability, i.e., subjective evaluation of chewing.

Index	Methodology
TMJ Disability Index (TDI) [84]	Various items relate to difficulties in chewing certain examples of food items with varying consistencies. Hence, the TDI might be applicable to older adults with various cultural backgrounds.
Open or semi-structured interviews [85]	Individual evaluation of oral health and function, possible compensatory mechanisms, eating habits, and further adaptation processes. i.e., self-reported chewing difficulties, food avoidance,
Eating Related Quality of Life ERQoL [85,86]	Enjoyment of eating and social and emotional issues around eating, eating comfort
Denture satisfaction index [87]	VAS-scale-based instrument with certain items relating to chewing ability

7. Improvement the Masticatory Performance in Frail Older People

When considering different treatment modalities in the rehabilitation of edentulous individuals, Muller et al. [57] described the masticatory performance with two implant overdentures (IOD) in patients depending on their ADL (activities of daily living). The intervention group received two interforaminal short implants ($n = 16$), while the control group ($n = 18$) obtained conventional relines. The results showed that IODs were more stable and resulted in significantly higher denture satisfaction and OHRQoL compared to the control group. The study also showed an improvement in maximum voluntary bite force and masseter muscle thickness in the intervention group, indicating that IODs may benefit edentulous patients who require assistance even late in life [57].

In view of the different numbers and types of reestablishments of masticatory units, McKenna G et al. [88] conducted a randomized controlled trial in 2014, comparing removable dental partial prostheses to shortened dental arches restored with bridgework. Both groups showed significant improvement in masticatory performance ($p < 0.0001$) with no significant difference between the groups ($p = 0.1689$); however, significantly higher OHRQoL and reduced caries incidence in the group with fixed dental prostheses [88].

Several studies have examined various factors related to oral health, medical conditions, and nutrition that may affect masticatory function. In a 10-year longitudinal survey by the group of Sato et al. with the inclusion of 349 older adults, they found that occlusal support did not have a significant impact on masticatory ability. However, the number of food items that could be chewed had significantly decreased in subjects who remained in Zone A (subjects' largest number of eatable items), suggesting that other factors beyond occlusal support (number of occluding pairs) may play a role in masticatory ability in very old individuals [62]. Adherence to a familiar Mediterranean diet in a sample of older Greek adults was discussed by the group of Bousiou et al. [89]. They detected that lower masticatory performance, higher BMI, smoking, and a larger number of drugs per day negatively affected adherence to the Mediterranean diet in older adults. Nevertheless, increased masticatory performance was an independent predictor of better adherence to the Mediterranean diet [89].

Based on the findings of animal and human experimental studies investigating the interplay of mastication, nutrition, cognition, and activities of daily living. Weijenberg et al. (2011) suggested a causal relationship between mastication and cognition [51]. Even though the healthy brain has an amazing capacity to adapt to changes and create new neural pathways, which is called neuroplasticity, when it comes to prosthodontic rehabilitation and the loss of periodontal receptors and neural pathways, the adaptive capacities of older patients may be limited. Additionally, there are currently no reliable predictors for the success of treatment in these cases. This highlights the importance of carefully considering the potential impact of invasive treatment concepts on the functional and cognitive abilities of aged patients.

A valuable alternative could be the alteration of the preexisting dental prosthesis to optimize masticatory function and simultaneously limit the adaption process needed [90,91]. A different option for complete dentures and IODs involves creating a duplicate prosthesis. This approach allows for the preservation of various aspects of the existing prosthesis, such as vertical dimension and aesthetics, while also fabricating a new prosthesis that offers improved hygiene [92].

The number and time of clinical visits during the fabrication of a new prosthesis should be limited and adjusted to patients' medical conditions and, furthermore, be as atraumatic as possible. Different treatment modalities were proposed to limit the number of dental visits, i.e., the acquisition of the definitive impression and jaw relation in one session [93,94]. Nevertheless, it is crucial to evaluate each patient's unique needs and ensure that the post-treatment care is designed to be easily manageable, with a focus on facilitation, especially in terms of the deconstructability and maintenance of denture and oral hygiene [3].

In terms of medical conditions, amyotrophic lateral sclerosis (ALS) is a progressive neurodegenerative disease that affects motor neurons. As the disease progresses, it leads to muscle weakness and atrophy, which can affect the ability to speak, swallow and breathe. Schimmel et al. [95] conducted a matched case-control study to investigate the oral function of ALS patients. The study involved 26 ALS patients and 26 matched controls, and the results showed that ALS patients had significantly lower chewing performance, lip force, tongue force, saliva weight, and fat-free mass index compared to controls. ALS patients also had a higher EAT-10 score. In addition, low chewing performance in ALS patients was found to be correlated with low bite and tongue force. Chewing performance, fat-free mass index, and saliva weight were identified as the most important discriminant parameters between the two groups [95].

In a longitudinal study with stroke patients, the group by Schimmel et al. evaluated chewing performance, lip and bite force, and masseter muscle thickness compared to controls over a 2-year period. Results showed impaired chewing efficiency and lower lip forces in stroke patients with no significant improvement over time. Bite forces were not different between sides, but hand-grip strength was significantly impaired and did not improve. Impaired chewing efficiency and reduced lip force are quantifiable symptoms in stroke patients that may require oro-facial rehabilitation [63].

The Japanese Society of Gerodontology proposes diagnostic criteria and management strategies to reduce the risk of oral dysfunction among older people, defining it as a presentation of seven oral signs or symptoms and recommending more evidence from clinical studies to clarify their diagnostic criteria and management strategies. Clinical signs include poor oral hygiene (total number of microorganisms [CFU/mL is 106.5 or more]), oral dryness (moisture checker < 27.0), reduced occlusal force (<200 N), decreased tongue-lip motor function (the number of any counts of pa/ta/or/ka/ produced per second is less than 6), decreased tongue pressure (maximum tongue pressure is less than 30 kPa), decreased masticatory function (the glucose concentration obtained by chewing gelatin gummies is less than 100 mg/dL) and deterioration of swallowing function (the total score of EAT-10 is 3 or higher) [10].

Schimmel et al. propose a conceptual model of oro-facial health that emphasizes the relationship between oro-facial function and an individual's ability to lead an independent life until death. According to this model, a well-functioning oro-facial system is characterized by the absence of positive coping of physical and mental disease, pain and negative environmental and social factors. Conversely, oral hypofunction occurs due to physiological aging, comorbid medical conditions, and a lack of reliable assessment tools to distinguish between states of optimal oro-facial fitness and hypofunction [24].

8. Conclusions

- To fully encompass oral frailty, oro-facial hypofunction, or oro-facial fitness, dental patient reported outcomes (dPROs) should be included.
- Currently, there are few evidence-based rehabilitation approaches apart from prosthodontics to ameliorate oro-facial hypofunction.
- Older adults may have decreased neuroplasticity, which may hinder the effectiveness of such interventions, thus necessitating functional training and nutritional counseling to complement these strategies.
- The concept of oral frailty, oro-facial hypofunction or oro-facial fitness should involve dental patient reported outcomes (dPROs).
- Reduced neuro-plastic capacity in old individuals might preclude a positive outcome of these strategies that might need to be accompanied by functional training and nutritional counseling.

Author Contributions: Conceptualization, M.S. and P.M.-M.; methodology, M.S.; validation, M.S.; formal analysis, M.S., N.A., G.P.S. and P.M.-M.; investigation, M.S., N.A., G.P.S. and P.M.-M.; resources, M.S.; data curation, M.S., N.A., G.P.S., A.R.W. and P.M.-M.; writing—original draft preparation, N.A., G.P.S., P.M.-M., A.R.W., M.S.D.P. and M.S.; writing—review and editing, N.A., G.P.S., M.S.D.P., A.R.W., P.M.-M. and M.S.; visualization, M.S.; supervision, M.S. and P.M.-M.; project administration, M.S. All authors have read and agreed to the published version of the manuscript.

Funding: This research received no external funding.

Institutional Review Board Statement: Not applicable.

Informed Consent Statement: Not applicable.

Data Availability Statement: The data that support the findings of this study are available from the corresponding author upon reasonable request.

Conflicts of Interest: The authors declare no conflict of interest.

References

1. World Health Organization. Available online: https://www.who.int/news-room/fact-sheets/detail/ageing-and-health (accessed on 22 April 2023).
2. Neue Zürcher Zeitung. Available online: https://www.nzz.ch/die_babyboomer_kommen_ins_rentenalter-ld.492953?reduced=true (accessed on 22 April 2023).
3. Schimmel, M.; Müller, F.; Suter, V.; Buser, D. Implants for Elderly Patients. *Periodontology 2000* **2017**, *73*, 228–240. [CrossRef] [PubMed]
4. Müller, F.; Srinivasan, M.; Krause, K.H.; Schimmel, M. Periodontitis and Peri-Implantitis in Elderly People Experiencing Institutional and Hospital Confinement. *Periodontology 2000* **2022**, *90*, 138–145. [CrossRef] [PubMed]
5. Laslett, P. The Emergence of the Third Age. *Ageing Soc.* **2008**, *7*, 133–160. [CrossRef]
6. Suzman, R.M.; Willis, D.P.; Manton, K.G. (Eds.) *Social Gerontology: The Oldest Old*; Oxford University Press: New York, NY, USA, 1992.
7. Gilleard, C.; Higgs, P. The Fourth Age and the Concept of a "Social Imaginary": A Theoretical Excursus. *J. Aging Stud.* **2013**, *27*, 368–376. [CrossRef] [PubMed]
8. Dibello, V.; Zupo, R.; Sardone, R.; Lozupone, M.; Castellana, F.; Dibello, A.; Daniele, A.; De Pergola, G.; Bortone, I.; Lampignano, L.; et al. Oral Frailty and Its Determinants in Older Age: A Systematic Review. *Lancet Health Longev.* **2021**, *2*, e507–e520. [CrossRef]

9. Strandberg, T.E.; Nieminen, T. *Future Perspectives on the Role of Frailty in Cardiovascular Diseases*; Springer: Berlin/Heidelberg, Germany, 2020; Volume 1216, ISBN 9783030333294.
10. Minakuchi, S.; Tsuga, K.; Ikebe, K.; Ueda, T.; Tamura, F.; Nagao, K.; Furuya, J.; Matsuo, K.; Yamamoto, K.; Kanazawa, M.; et al. Oral Hypofunction in the Older Population: Position Paper of the Japanese Society of Gerodontology in 2016. *Gerodontology* **2018**, *35*, 317–324. [CrossRef]
11. Kosaka, T.; Kida, M.; Kikui, M.; Hashimoto, S.; Fujii, K.; Yamamoto, M.; Nokubi, T.; Maeda, Y.; Hasegawa, Y.; Kokubo, Y.; et al. Factors Influencing the Changes in Masticatory Performance: The Suita Study. *JDR Clin. Transl. Res.* **2018**, *3*, 405–412. [CrossRef]
12. Schneider, C.; Zemp, E.; Zitzmann, N.U. Oral Health Improvements in Switzerland over 20 Years. *Eur. J. Oral Sci.* **2017**, *125*, 55–62. [CrossRef]
13. Slade, G.D.; Akinkugbe, A.A.; Sanders, A.E. Projections of U.S. Edentulism Prevalence Following 5 Decades of Decline. *J. Dent. Res.* **2014**, *93*, 959–965. [CrossRef]
14. Bousiou, A.; Konstantopoulou, K.; Polychronopoulou, A.; Halazonetis, D.J.; Schimmel, M.; Kossioni, A.E. Sociomedical and Oral Factors Affecting Masticatory Performance in an Older Population. *Clin. Oral Investig.* **2022**, *26*, 3477–3486. [CrossRef]
15. Müller, F. Oral Hygiene Reduces the Mortality from Aspiration Pneumonia in Frail Elders. *J. Dent. Res.* **2015**, *94*, 14S–16S. [CrossRef] [PubMed]
16. Schimmel, M. Preventive Strategies in Geriatric Dental Medicine. *Oral Health Prev. Dent.* **2016**, *14*, 291–292. [CrossRef] [PubMed]
17. Brocklehurst, P.R.; McKenna, G.; Schimmel, M.; Kossioni, A.; Jerković-Ćosić, K.; Hayes, M.; da Mata, C.; Müller, F. How Do We Incorporate Patient Views into the Design of Healthcare Services for Older People: A Discussion Paper. *BMC Oral Health* **2018**, *18*, 61. [CrossRef]
18. Ship, J.A. Oral Health in the Elderly—What's Missing? *Oral Surg. Oral Med. Oral Pathol. Oral Radiol. Endodontol.* **2004**, *98*, 625–626. [CrossRef] [PubMed]
19. Kossioni, A.; McKenna, G.; Müller, F.; Schimmel, M.; Vanobbergen, J. Higher Education in Gerodontology in European Universities. *BMC Oral Health* **2017**, *17*, 71. [CrossRef]
20. Bircher, J.; Kuruvilla, S. Defining Health by Addressing Individual, Social, and Environmental Determinants: New Opportunities for Health Care and Public Health. *J. Public Health Policy* **2014**, *35*, 363–386. [CrossRef]
21. Bircher, J.; Hahn, E.G. Will the Meikirch Model, a New Framework for Health, Induce a Paradigm Shift in Healthcare? *Cureus* **2017**, *9*, e1081. [CrossRef]
22. Szczesniak, M.M.; Maclean, J.; Zhang, T.; Graham, P.H.; Cook, I.J. Persistent Dysphagia after Head and Neck Radiotherapy: A Common and under-Reported Complication with Significant Effect on Non-Cancer-Related Mortality. *Clin. Oncol.* **2014**, *26*, 697–703. [CrossRef]
23. Chebib, N.; Abou-Ayash, S.; Maniewicz, S.; Srinivasan, M.; Hill, H.; McKenna, G.; Holmes, E.; Schimmel, M.; Brocklehurst, P.; Müller, F. Exploring Older Swiss People's Preferred Dental Services for When They Become Dependent. *Swiss Dent. J.* **2020**, *130*, 876–884.
24. Schimmel, M.; Aarab, G.; Baad-Hansen, L.; Lobbezoo, F.; Svensson, P. A Conceptual Model of Oro-Facial Health with an Emphasis on Function. *J. Oral Rehabil.* **2021**, *48*, 1283–1294. [CrossRef]
25. Reissmann, D.R. Dental Patient-Reported Outcome Measures Are Essential for Evidence-Based Prosthetic Dentistry. *J. Evid. Based. Dent. Pract.* **2019**, *19*, 1–6. [CrossRef] [PubMed]
26. Reissmann, D.R. Methodological Considerations When Measuring Oral Health–Related Quality of Life. *J. Oral Rehabil.* **2021**, *48*, 233–245. [CrossRef] [PubMed]
27. John, M.T.; Rener-Sitar, K.; Baba, K.; Čelebić, A.; Larsson, P.; Szabo, G.; Norton, W.E.; Reissmann, D.R.; Rashighi, M.; Harris, J.E. Patterns of Impaired Oral Health-Related Quality of Life Dimensions. *Physiol. Behav.* **2017**, *43*, 519–527. [CrossRef]
28. John, M.T.; Sekulić, S.; Bekes, K.; Al-Harthy, M.H.; Michelotti, A.; Reissmann, D.R.; Nikolovska, J.; Sanivarapu, S.; Lawal, F.B.; List, T.; et al. Why Patients Visit Dentists—A Study in All World Health Organization Regions. *J. Evid. Based. Dent. Pract.* **2020**, *20*, 101459. [CrossRef] [PubMed]
29. Bader, J.D.; Shugars, D.A.; White, B.A.; Rindal, D.B. Evaluation of Audit-Based Performance Measures for Dental Care Plans. *J. Public Health Dent.* **1999**, *59*, 150–157. [CrossRef]
30. Yeung, A.W.K.; Wong, N.S.M. The Historical Roots of Visual Analog Scale in Psychology as Revealed by Reference Publication Year Spectroscopy. *Front. Hum. Neurosci.* **2019**, *13*, 86. [CrossRef]
31. Slade, G.; Spencer, A. Development and Evaluation of the Oral Health Impact Profile. *Community Dent. Health* **1994**, *11*, 3–11. [PubMed]
32. Hassel, A.J.; Rolko, C.; Koke, U.; Leisen, J.; Rammelsberg, P. A German Version of the GOHAI. *Community Dent. Oral Epidemiol.* **2008**, *36*, 34–42. [CrossRef]
33. Allyson Ross, D.; Ware, J.E. *Development of a Dental Satisfaction Questionnaire*; The Rand Corporation: Santa Monica, CA, USA, 1982; pp. 298–309.
34. Elgestad Stjernfeldt, P.; Faxén-Irving, G.; Wårdh, I. Masticatory Ability in Older Individuals: A Qualitative Interview Study. *Gerodontology* **2021**, *38*, 199–208. [CrossRef]

35. Anliker, N.; Molinero-Mourelle, P.; Weijers, M.; Bukvic, H.; Bornstein, M.M.; Schimmel, M. Dental Status and Its Correlation with Polypharmacy and Multimorbidity in a Swiss Nursing Home Population: A Cross-Sectional Study. *Clin. Oral Investig.* **2023**, in press. [CrossRef]
36. Woda, A.; Hennequin, M.; Peyron, M.A. Mastication in Humans: Finding a Rationale. *J. Oral Rehabil.* **2011**, *38*, 781–784. [CrossRef] [PubMed]
37. Imamura, Y.; Chebib, N.; Ohta, M.; Mojon, P.; Schulte-Eickhoff, R.M.; Schimmel, M.; Graf, C.; Sato, Y.; Müller, F. Masticatory Performance in Oral Function Assessment: Alternative Methods. *J. Oral Rehabil.* **2023**, *50*, 383–391. [CrossRef] [PubMed]
38. Chen, J.E.L. *Fundamentals of Eating and Sensory Perception*; Wiley: Hoboken, NJ, USA, 2012; ISBN 9781444330120.
39. Micheelis, W.; Schiffner, U.; Hoffmann, T.; Reis, U.; Schroeder, E. *Vierte Deutsche Mundgesundheitsstudie (DMS IV): Neue Ergebnisse Zu Oralen Erkrankungsprävalenzen, Risikogruppen Und Zum Zahnärztlichen Versorgungsgrad in Deutschland 2005*; Institut der Deutschen Zahnärzte: Köln, Germany, 2007; Volume 101, ISBN 3934280943.
40. Da, D.; Ge, S.; Zhang, H.; Zeng, X. Association between Occlusal Support and Cognitive Impairment in Older Chinese Adults: A Community-Based Study. *Front. Aging Neurosci.* **2023**, *15*, 1146335. [CrossRef] [PubMed]
41. Ahmed, S.E.; Mohan, J.; Parithimar, K.; Kandasamy, S.; Raju, R.; Champakesan, B. Influence of Dental Prostheses on Cognitive Functioning in Elderly Population: A Systematic Review. *J. Pharm. Bioallied Sci.* **2021**, *13* (Suppl. S1), S788–S794. [CrossRef]
42. Nakamura, T.; Zou, K.; Shibuya, Y.; Michikawa, M. Oral Dysfunctions and Cognitive Impairment/Dementia. *J. Neurosci. Res.* **2021**, *99*, 518–528. [CrossRef]
43. Ki, S.; Yun, J.; Kim, J.; Lee, Y. Association between Dental Implants and Cognitive Function in Community-Dwelling Older Adults in Korea. *J. Prev. Med. Public Health* **2019**, *52*, 333–343. [CrossRef]
44. Klotz, A.L.; Hassel, A.J.; Schröder, J.; Rammelsberg, P.; Zenthöfer, A. Oral Health-Related Quality of Life and Prosthetic Status of Nursing Home Residents with or without Dementia. *Clin. Interv. Aging* **2017**, *12*, 659–665. [CrossRef]
45. Kamiya, K.; Narita, N.; Iwaki, S. Improved Prefrontal Activity and Chewing Performance as Function of Wearing Denture in Partially Edentulous Elderly Individuals: Functional near-Infrared Spectroscopy Study. *PLoS ONE* **2016**, *11*, e0158070. [CrossRef]
46. Chuhuaicura, P.; Dias, F.J.; Arias, A.; Lezcano, M.F.; Fuentes, R. Mastication as a Protective Factor of the Cognitive Decline in Adults: A Qualitative Systematic Review. *Int. Dent. J.* **2019**, *69*, 334–340. [CrossRef]
47. Ikebe, K.; Matsuda, K.; Morii, K.; Furuya-Yoshinaka, M.; Nokubi, T.; Renner, R.P. Association of Masticatory Performance with Age, Posterior Occlusal Contacts, Occlusal Force, and Salivary Flow in Older Adults. *Int. J. Prosthodont.* **2006**, *19*, 475–481.
48. Kikutani, T.; Tamura, F.; Nishiwaki, K.; Kodama, M.; Suda, M.; Fukui, Y.; Takahashi, N.; Yoshida, M.; Akagawa, Y.; Kimura, M. Oral Motor Function and Masticatory Performance in the Community-Dwelling Elderly. *Odontology* **2009**, *97*, 38–42. [CrossRef] [PubMed]
49. Mazari, A.; Heath, M.R.; Prinz, J.F. Contribution of the Cheeks to the Intraoral Manipulation of Food. *Dysphagia* **2007**, *22*, 117–121. [CrossRef] [PubMed]
50. Schimmel, M.; Leemann, B.; Christou, P.; Kiliaridis, S.; Herrmann, F.R.; Müller, F. Quantitative Assessment of Facial Muscle Impairment in Patients with Hemispheric Stroke. *J. Oral Rehabil.* **2011**, *38*, 800–809. [CrossRef] [PubMed]
51. Weijenberg, R.A.F.; Scherder, E.J.A.; Lobbezoo, F. Mastication for the Mind-The Relationship between Mastication and Cognition in Ageing and Dementia. *Neurosci. Biobehav. Rev.* **2011**, *35*, 483–497. [CrossRef] [PubMed]
52. Miura, H.; Yamasaki, K.; Kariyasu, M.; Miura, K.; Sumi, Y. Relationship between Cognitive Function and Mastication in Elderly Females. *J. Oral Rehabil.* **2003**, *30*, 808–811. [CrossRef]
53. Chang, C.C.; Roberts, B.L. Feeding Difficulty in Older Adults with Dementia. *J. Clin. Nurs.* **2008**, *17*, 2266–2274. [CrossRef]
54. Ikeda, M.; Brown, J.; Holland, A.J.; Fukuhara, R.; Hodges, J.R. Changes in Appetite, Food Preference, and Eating Habits in Frontotemporal Dementia and Alzheimer's Disease. *J. Neurol. Neurosurg. Psychiatry* **2002**, *73*, 371–376. [CrossRef]
55. Newton, J.P.; Yemm, R.; Abel, R.W.; Menhinick, S. Changes in Human Jaw Muscles with Age and Dental State. *Gerodontology* **1993**, *10*, 16–22. [CrossRef]
56. Newton, J.P.; McManus, F.C.; Menhenick, S. Jaw Muscles in Older Overdenture Patients. *Gerodontology* **2004**, *21*, 37–42. [CrossRef]
57. Müller, F.; Duvernay, E.; Loup, A.; Vazquez, L.; Herrmann, F.R.; Schimmel, M. Implant-Supported Mandibular Overdentures in Very Old Adults: A Randomized Controlled Trial. *J. Dent. Res.* **2013**, *92*, 446–450. [CrossRef]
58. Müller, F.; Nitschke, I. Mundgesundheit, Zahnstatus Und Ernährung Im Alter. *Z. Gerontol. Geriatr.* **2005**, *38*, 334–341. [CrossRef] [PubMed]
59. Dormenval, V.; Budtz-Jørgensen, E.; Mojon, P.; Bruyère, A.; Rapin, C.H. Nutrition, General Health Status and Oral Health Status in Hospitalised Elders. *Gerodontology* **1995**, *12*, 73–80. [CrossRef] [PubMed]
60. Nordström, G. The Impact of Socio- Medical Factors and Oral Status on Dietary Intake in the Eighth Decade of Life. *Aging Clin. Exp. Res.* **1990**, *2*, 371–385. [CrossRef] [PubMed]
61. Boumendjel, N.; Herrmann, F.; Girod, V.; Sieber, C.; Rapin, C. Refrigerator Content and Hospital Admission in Old People for Personal Use Only. Not to Be Reproduced without Permission of The Lancet. *Lancet* **2000**, *356*, 2000. [CrossRef] [PubMed]
62. Sato, N.; Ono, T.; Kon, H.; Sakurai, N.; Kohno, S.; Yoshihara, A.; Miyazaki, H. Ten-Year Longitudinal Study on the State of Dentition and Subjective Masticatory Ability in Community-Dwelling Elderly People. *J. Prosthodont. Res.* **2016**, *60*, 177–184. [CrossRef]
63. Schimmel, M.; Leemann, B.; Schnider, A.; Herrmann, F.R.; Kiliaridis, S.; Müller, F. Changes in Oro-Facial Function and Hand-Grip Strength during a 2-Year Observation Period after Stroke. *Clin. Oral Investig.* **2013**, *17*, 867–876. [CrossRef]

64. Gonçalves, T.M.S.V.; Schimmel, M.; van der Bilt, A.; Chen, J.; van der Glas, H.W.; Kohyama, K.; Hennequin, M.; Peyron, M.A.; Woda, A.; Leles, C.R.; et al. Consensus on the Terminologies and Methodologies for Masticatory Assessment. *J. Oral Rehabil.* **2021**, *48*, 745–761. [CrossRef]
65. Peyron, M.A.; Blanc, O.; Lund, J.P.; Woda, A. Influence of Age on Adaptability of Human Mastication. *J. Neurophysiol.* **2004**, *92*, 773–779. [CrossRef]
66. Manly, R.S.; Braley, L.C. Masticatory Performance and Efficiency. *J. Dent. Res.* **1950**, *29*, 448–462. [CrossRef]
67. Rosin, P.; Rammler, E. The Rosin-Rammler Particle Size Distribution. *J. Inst. Fuel* **1933**, *5*, 275–277.
68. Liedberg, B.; Öwall, B. Masticatory Ability in Experimentally Induced Xerostomia. *Dysphagia* **1991**, *6*, 211–213. [CrossRef] [PubMed]
69. Prinz, J.F. Quantitative Evaluation of the Effect of Bolus Size and Number of Chewing Strokes on the Intra-Oral Mixing of a Two-Colour Chewing Gum. *J. Oral Rehabil.* **1999**, *26*, 243–247. [CrossRef] [PubMed]
70. Schimmel, M.; Christou, P.; Herrmann, F.; Müller, F. A Two-Colour Chewing Gum Test for Masticatory Efficiency: Development of Different Assessment Methods. *J. Oral Rehabil.* **2007**, *34*, 671–678. [CrossRef] [PubMed]
71. Speksnijder, C.M.; Abbink, J.H.; Van Der Glas, H.W.; Janssen, N.G.; Van Der Bilt, A. Mixing Ability Test Compared with a Comminution Test in Persons with Normal and Compromised Masticatory Performance. *Eur. J. Oral Sci.* **2009**, *117*, 580–586. [CrossRef] [PubMed]
72. Van Der Bilt, A.; Mojet, J.; Tekamp, F.A.; Abbink, J.H. Comparing Masticatory Performance and Mixing Ability. *J. Oral Rehabil.* **2010**, *37*, 79–84. [CrossRef] [PubMed]
73. Schimmel, M.; Leemann, B.; Christou, P.; Kiliaridis, S.; Schnider, A.; Herrmann, F.R.; Müller, F. Oral Health-Related Quality of Life in Hospitalised Stroke Patients. *Gerodontology* **2011**, *28*, 3–11. [CrossRef]
74. Viewgum. Available online: www.dhal.com (accessed on 23 April 2023).
75. Halazonetis, D.J.; Schimmel, M.; Antonarakis, G.S.; Christou, P. Novel Software for Quantitative Evaluation and Graphical Representation of Masticatory Efficiency. *J. Oral Rehabil.* **2013**, *40*, 329–335. [CrossRef]
76. Kaya, M.S.; Güçlü, B.; Schimmel, M.; Akyüz, S. Two-Colour Chewing Gum Mixing Ability Test for Evaluating Masticatory Performance in Children with Mixed Dentition: Validity and Reliability Study. *J. Oral Rehabil.* **2017**, *44*, 827–834. [CrossRef]
77. Schimmel, M.; Katsoulis, J.; Genton, L.; Müller, F.; Bern, C.; Kosaka, T.; Kida, M.; Kikui, M.; Hashimoto, S.; Fujii, K.; et al. Masticatory Function and Nutrition in Old Age. *JDR Clin. Transl. Res.* **2018**, *3*, 449–454.
78. Buser, R.; Ziltener, V.; Samietz, S.; Fontolliet, M.; Nef, T.; Schimmel, M. Validation of a Purpose-Built Chewing Gum and Smartphone Application to Evaluate Chewing Efficiency. *J. Oral Rehabil.* **2018**, *45*, 845–853. [CrossRef]
79. Heath, M.R. The Effect of Maximum Biting Force and Bone Loss upon Masticatory Function and Dietary Selection of the Elderly. *Int. Dent. J.* **1982**, *32*, 345–356. [PubMed]
80. Wöstmann, B.; Brinkert, B.; Melchheier, A.; Zenginel, M.R.P. Chewing Efficiency Screening Test for Non-Dental-Professionals. *J. Dent. Res.* **2011**, *90*, 1598.
81. Schimmel, M.; Rachais, E.; Al-Haj Husain, N.; Müller, F.; Srinivasan, M.; Abou-Ayash, S. Assessing Masticatory Performance with a Colour-Mixing Ability Test Using Smartphone Camera Images. *J. Oral Rehabil.* **2022**, *49*, 961–969. [CrossRef] [PubMed]
82. Liedberg, B.; Öwall, B. Oral Bolus Kneading and Shaping Measured with Chewing Gum. *Dysphagia* **1995**, *10*, 101–106. [CrossRef]
83. Takeshima, T.; Fujita, Y.; Maki, K. Factors Associated with Masticatory Performance and Swallowing Threshold According to Dental Formula Development. *Arch. Oral Biol.* **2019**, *99*, 51–57. [CrossRef]
84. TMJ Disability Index. Available online: http://www.nppt.com/files/forms/tmj-03-2016.pdf (accessed on 23 April 2023).
85. Moynihan, P.; Chu, M.; Moores, C.; Ibrahim, A. Eating-Related Quality of Life in People Who Wear Complete Dentures. *Proc. Nutr. Soc.* **2023**, *82*, 2023. [CrossRef]
86. Moynihan, P.; Varghese, R. Impact of Wearing Dentures on Dietary Intake, Nutritional Status, and Eating: A Systematic Review. *JDR Clin. Transl. Res.* **2022**, *7*, 334–351. [CrossRef]
87. de Souza, R.F.; Ribeiro, A.B.; Oates, T.W.; Feine, J.S. The McGill Denture Satisfaction Questionnaire Revisited: Exploratory Factor Analysis of a Binational Sample. *Gerodontology* **2020**, *37*, 233–243. [CrossRef]
88. McKenna, G.; Allen, P.F.; O'Mahony, D.; Flynn, A.; Cronin, M.; Damata, C.; Woods, N. Comparison of Functionally Orientated Tooth Replacement and Removable Partial Dentures on the Nutritional Status of Partially Dentate Older Patients: A Randomised Controlled Clinical Trial. *J. Dent.* **2014**, *42*, 653–659. [CrossRef]
89. Bousiou, A.; Konstantopoulou, K.; Martimianaki, G.; Peppa, E.; Trichopoulou, A.; Polychronopoulou, A.; Halazonetis, D.J.; Schimmel, M.; Kossioni, A.E. Oral Factors and Adherence to Mediterranean Diet in an Older Greek Population. *Aging Clin. Exp. Res.* **2021**, *33*, 3237–3244. [CrossRef]
90. Heckmann, S.M.; Heußinger, S.; Linke, J.J.; Graef, F.; Pröschel, P. Improvement and Long-Term Stability of Neuromuscular Adaptation in Implant-Supported Overdentures. *Clin. Oral Implants Res.* **2009**, *20*, 1200–1205. [CrossRef] [PubMed]
91. Lin, C.S. Functional Adaptation of Oromotor Functions and Aging: A Focused Review of the Evidence From Brain Neuroimaging Research. *Front. Aging Neurosci.* **2020**, *11*, 354. [CrossRef] [PubMed]
92. Lindquist, T.J.; Ettinger, R.L. Patient Management and Decision Making in Complete Denture Fabrication Using a Duplicate Denture Procedure: A Clinical Report. *J. Prosthet. Dent.* **1999**, *82*, 499–503. [CrossRef] [PubMed]
93. Daher, T.; Dermendjian, S.; Morgano, S.M. Obtaining Maxillomandibular Records and Definitive Impressions in a Single Visit for a Completely Edentulous Patient with a History of Combination Syndrome. *J. Prosthet. Dent.* **2008**, *99*, 489–491. [CrossRef] [PubMed]

94. Utz, K.H.; Müller, F.; Kettner, N.; Reppert, G.; Koeck, B. Functional Impression and Jaw Registration: A Single Session Procedure for the Construction of Complete Dentures. *J. Oral Rehabil.* **2004**, *31*, 554–561. [CrossRef]
95. Schimmel, M.; Leuchter, I.; Héritier Barras, A.C.; Leles, C.R.; Abou-Ayash, S.; Viatte, V.; Esteve, F.; Janssens, J.P.; Mueller, F.; Genton, L. Oral Function in Amyotrophic Lateral Sclerosis Patients: A Matched Case–Control Study. *Clin. Nutr.* **2021**, *40*, 4904–4911. [CrossRef]

Disclaimer/Publisher's Note: The statements, opinions and data contained in all publications are solely those of the individual author(s) and contributor(s) and not of MDPI and/or the editor(s). MDPI and/or the editor(s) disclaim responsibility for any injury to people or property resulting from any ideas, methods, instructions or products referred to in the content.

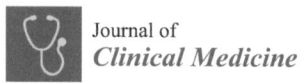

Journal of Clinical Medicine

Article

An Overview of Systemic Health Factors Related to Rapid Oral Health Deterioration among Older People

Gert-Jan van der Putten [1,2,*] and Cees de Baat [3]

1. Orpea Dagelijks Leven, 7327 AA Apeldoorn, The Netherlands
2. Department of Dentistry, Radboud University Nijmegen Medical Centre, 6525 GA Nijmegen, The Netherlands
3. Fresh Unieke Mondzorg, 2411 NT Bodegraven, The Netherlands
* Correspondence: gert-janvanderputten@radboudumc.nl

Abstract: The oral health of older individuals can be negatively impacted by various systemic health factors, leading to rapid oral health deterioration. This paper aims to present an overview of the published evidence on systemic health factors that contribute to rapid oral health deterioration in older individuals, and to explore the implications of these factors for both general healthcare and oral healthcare provision. Older people are at risk of experiencing adverse reactions to medications due to multimorbidity, polypharmacy, and changes in pharmacokinetics and pharmacodynamics. Hyposalivation, a significant side effect of some medications, can be induced by both the type and number of medications used. Frailty, disability, sarcopenia, care dependency, and limited access to professional oral healthcare can also compromise the oral health of older people. To prevent rapid oral health deterioration, a comprehensive approach is required that involves effective communication between oral healthcare providers, other healthcare providers, and informal caregivers. Oral healthcare providers have a responsibility to advocate for the importance of maintaining adequate oral health and to raise awareness of the serious consequences of weakened oral health. By doing so, we can prevent weakened oral health from becoming a geriatric syndrome.

Keywords: oral health care; older people; multimorbidity; polypharmacy; frailty; sarcopenia; disability; care dependency

Citation: van der Putten, G.-J.; de Baat, C. An Overview of Systemic Health Factors Related to Rapid Oral Health Deterioration among Older People. *J. Clin. Med.* **2023**, *12*, 4306. https://doi.org/10.3390/jcm12134306

Academic Editor: Pia Lopez-Jornet

Received: 24 April 2023
Revised: 12 June 2023
Accepted: 19 June 2023
Published: 27 June 2023

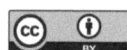

Copyright: © 2023 by the authors. Licensee MDPI, Basel, Switzerland. This article is an open access article distributed under the terms and conditions of the Creative Commons Attribution (CC BY) license (https://creativecommons.org/licenses/by/4.0/).

1. Introduction

The physical and psychological functions of many older adults are being negatively impacted by poor oral health. Difficulties with chewing, biting, swallowing, tasting, speaking, communicating, smiling, appearance, aesthetics, and self-esteem are common [1]. Among the frailest and most care-dependent older adults, dental caries, periodontal disease, tooth loss, and xerostomia are particularly prevalent [1–4]. Despite the fact that most chronic oral diseases are preventable and treatable, a variety of factors make it difficult to maintain good oral health as people age. This paper aims to present an overview of the published evidence on the systemic health factors that contribute to rapid oral health deterioration in older individuals, and to explore the implications of these factors for both general healthcare and oral healthcare provision.

2. Ageing

Ageing is typically viewed as a gradual decline in the functioning of various bodily systems, stemming from the accumulation of damaged tissue and substances caused by intrinsic or extrinsic mechanisms [5]. The process of biological ageing is a multifaceted and intricate phenomenon, and although the exact molecular mechanisms behind its onset and progression remain unclear, ample evidence suggests that oxidative stress may play a significant role [6]. Kinases, phosphatases, and transcription factors are particularly sensitive to changes in cellular redox status, and chronic or severe disruptions in this homeostasis can result in cell death or proliferation. Immune senescence, or the quantitative and qualitative changes in the immune system that accompany ageing, is another hallmark of this process. While immune senescence does not necessarily entail a progressive decline in immune function, it often leads to cytokine dysregulation, which can cause a chronic, low-grade inflammatory state. This inflammation may serve as a biological foundation for ageing and contribute to the onset of age-related diseases, increasing the risk of multimorbidity and mortality [6–9].

3. Ageing and Telomere Length

Telomere length is considered a useful biomarker of cellular ageing, as it reflects the repeated sequences of nucleotides that protect the ends of chromosomes [10]. With each replication of cells, telomeres shorten due to incomplete lagging strand replication, leading to cellular senescence once they reach a critically short length [11]. Studies have suggested that telomere length is sensitive to inflammation, as higher rates of telomere loss have been observed in a pro-inflammatory environment with increased blood cell replication [12]. This has prompted some researchers to explore the relationship between periodontal disease and telomere length [13–16]. In a NHANES study involving 21,000 participants aged 35–75 years, a significant correlation was found between periodontal disease and telomere length, particularly among women, overweight or obese individuals, and those with cardiometabolic comorbidities [17].

4. Diseases and Oral Health

Several studies have suggested a strong link between noncommunicable diseases and oral health, with demonstrated associations with oral diseases for various conditions including cancer, diabetes, cardiovascular diseases, depression, neurodegenerative conditions, rheumatic diseases, inflammatory bowel disease, gastric helicobacter pylori, obesity, and asthma [18]. The connection between oral health and these diseases is largely attributed to inflammation, although there are two other pathways that may explain the association [19–21]. Firstly, some systemic diseases have direct links to negative impacts on oral health and oral health-related quality of life (OHRQoL), such as Crohn's disease [22,23], Beçhet's disease [24–26], scleroderma [27,28], oral cancer [29–32], head and neck cancer [33], and Sjögren's syndrome [34–37]. Secondly, some chronic diseases may indirectly affect oral health, as they can lead to reduced motivation regarding oral hygiene and care. For example, psychiatric [38–47] and neurological diseases [48–53], as well as Alzheimer's disease [54,55], rheumatic [56], oncological [57], and cardiovascular diseases [58–63], can all have an impact.

Early diagnosis and treatment of oral conditions among older people with chronic diseases could prevent weak oral health and a decline in OHRQoL. However, individuals with cognitive disorders and those receiving palliative care may lose their ability to communicate their oral health needs, leading to under-reporting and underestimation of oral conditions [64]. This could result in healthcare providers failing to fully appreciate the extent of the problem, leading to untreated oral conditions and prolonged discomfort among these patients.

5. Multimorbidity and Polypharmacy

In 2013, a group of European researchers established a definition for multimorbidity, which refers to any combination of chronic disease with at least one other disease (acute or chronic), bio-psychosocial factor (associated or not), or somatic risk factor. This definition recognizes that any bio-psychosocial factor, somatic risk factor, social network, burden of diseases, healthcare consumption, and patient coping strategies may modify the effects of the multimorbidity. Multimorbidity can lead to increased disability, decreased quality of life, or frailty. While the concept of multimorbidity has been recognized and enhanced by European general practitioners [65], studies on its prevalence have not yet been conducted.

In populations of older adults with multimorbidities, the use of multiple medications is common, a phenomenon referred to as polypharmacy. Polypharmacy is associated with adverse outcomes, including medication–medication interactions, medication–disease interactions, decreased renal and hepatic function, and reduced lean body mass, hearing, vision, cognition, and mobility [66]. A meta-analysis showed that 38% of community-dwelling adults aged 60 years and older use five or more medications daily [67]. Additionally, almost half of care home residents are exposed to potentially inappropriate medications [66]. A systematic review identified 138 definitions of polypharmacy, but a numerical definition alone is insufficient to assess the safety and appropriateness of medication use. Therefore, a shift towards the term "appropriate polypharmacy", using a holistic approach that considers comorbidities present, is needed [68].

6. Frailty and Oral Health

The concept of frailty has become increasingly important in recent decades, but a consensus on its definition has not yet been reached. There are two main approaches to defining frailty: one that focuses solely on physical functioning, and another that takes into account other domains, such as memory and mood. For example, the Fried frailty phenotype considers unintentional weight loss, self-reported exhaustion, physical activity, hand grip strength, and walking speed, while the multidimensional frailty index by Rockwood et al. also considers cognitive and psychological factors (Figure 1) [69,70]. The prevalence of frailty varies depending on the approach used, with higher rates found for multidimensional assessments [71].

Clinical Frailty Scale*

1 **Very Fit** – People who are robust, active, energetic and motivated. These people commonly exercise regularly. They are among the fittest for their age.

2 **Well** – People who have **no active disease symptoms** but are less fit than category 1. Often, they exercise or are very **active occasionally**, e.g. seasonally.

3 **Managing Well** – People whose **medical problems are well controlled**, but are **not regularly active** beyond routine walking.

4 **Vulnerable** – While **not dependent** on others for daily help, often **symptoms limit activities**. A common complaint is being "slowed up", and/or being tired during the day.

5 **Mildly Frail** – These people often have **more evident slowing**, and need help in **high order IADLs** (finances, transportation, heavy housework, medications). Typically, mild frailty progressively impairs shopping and walking outside alone, meal preparation and housework.

6 **Moderately Frail** – People need help with **all outside activities** and with **keeping house**. Inside, they often have problems with stairs and need **help with bathing** and might need minimal assistance (cuing, standby) with dressing.

7 **Severely Frail** – **Completely dependent for personal care**, from whatever cause (physical or cognitive). Even so, they seem stable and not at high risk of dying (within ~ 6 months).

8 **Very Severely Frail** – Completely dependent, approaching the end of life. Typically, they could not recover even from a minor illness.

9. **Terminally Ill** – Approaching the end of life. This category applies to people with **a life expectancy <6 months**, who are **not otherwise evidently frail**.

Scoring frailty in people with dementia

The degree of frailty corresponds to the degree of dementia. Common **symptoms in mild dementia** include forgetting the details of a recent event, though still remembering the event itself, repeating the same question/story and social withdrawal.

In **moderate dementia**, recent memory is very impaired, even though they seemingly can remember their past life events well. They can do personal care with prompting.

In **severe dementia**, they cannot do personal care without help.

* 1. Canadian Study on Health & Aging, Revised 2008.
2. K. Rockwood et al. A global clinical measure of fitness and frailty in elderly people. CMAJ 2005;173:489-495.

© 2007-2009 Version 1.2. All rights reserved. Geriatric Medicine Research, Dalhousie University, Halifax, Canada. Permission granted to copy for research and educational purposes only.

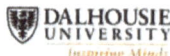

Figure 1. Clinical Frailty Scale (Dalhousie University, Halifax, NS, Canada), used with permission [69,70].

A systematic review investigated the link between oral health and frailty, focusing on five longitudinal studies that used Fried's frailty phenotype. These studies found that the number of teeth, oral functions, accumulation of oral health problems, and dry mouth symptoms were significantly associated with the incidence of frailty [72]. In community-dwelling older adults, oral pain was associated with weight loss and weak handgrip, while chewing problems were associated with low physical activity and low gait speed. Those who required dental prostheses were more likely to be prefrail or frail than others [73]. Further research is needed to determine whether oral health indicators can be used to assess frailty.

7. Sarcopenia and Oral Health

Sarcopenia is a condition that affects older individuals and causes a decline in muscle mass and strength. The prevalence of sarcopenia varies widely, between 3.2% to 40%, with the highest incidence in people above the age of 80 and those living in institutions [69–74]. Several risk factors have been identified, including age, chronic diseases, and physical activity levels. Chronic obstructive pulmonary disease, diabetes mellitus, and hypertension are among the chronic diseases that have been linked to sarcopenia [75]. Although it is a common issue in older adults, sarcopenia can be managed and even prevented with appropriate exercise and nutrition [74,76,77]. Interestingly, sarcopenia can also affect oral health in ways that are not well-known. As muscle mass declines, individuals may experience weaker temporomandibular and orofacial muscles, resulting in difficulty chewing and swallowing [78]. Figure 2 presents an overview of the associations between weak oral health, malnutrition, and sarcopenia [79].

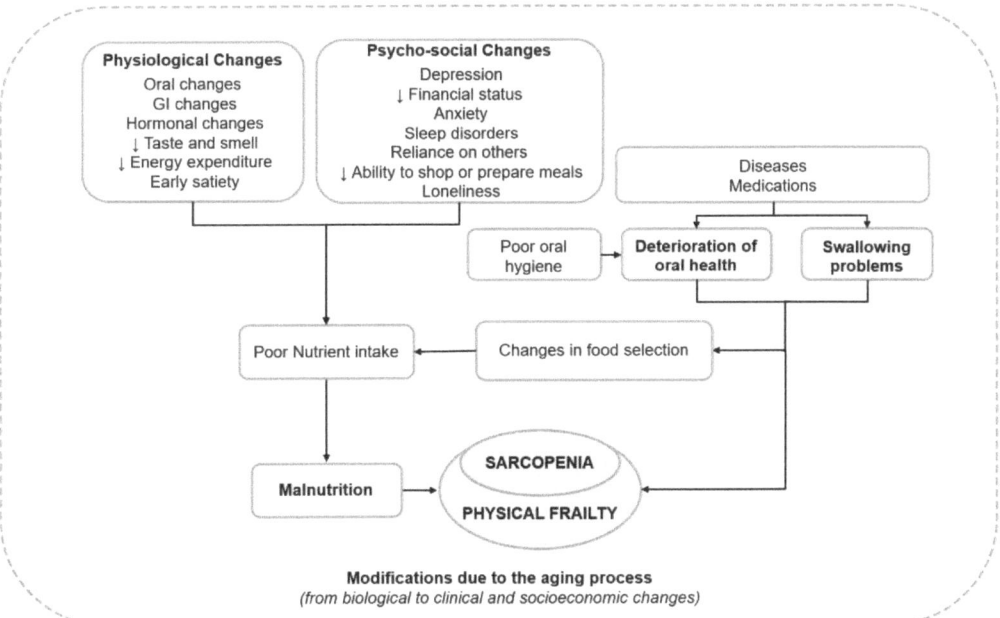

Figure 2. Overview of the associations between weak oral health, malnutrition, and sarcopenia, used with permission [79].

8. Disability and Oral Health

Among older adults, there are bidirectional associations between oral health and disability, where both health outcomes can impact each other. Tooth loss, for instance, may lead to disabilities such as limitations in activities of daily living, instrumental activities of daily living, and mobility [80–84]. Conversely, disability may be associated with chronic illnesses, weak oral health, and reduced quality of life among older people [85]. The World Health Organization defines disability as an impairment that may be physical, cognitive, mental, sensory, emotional, developmental, or a combination of these, and which may occur during a person's lifetime or from birth. Disabilities can cause physical and cognitive impairments, activity limitations, and participation restrictions [86]. To prevent disability among older adults, self-efficacy must be improved, and physical activity must be promoted [87]. Physical and cognitive functioning of older individuals can be assessed using several assessment instruments [88]. It is possible to analyze the order in which age-related declines occur by examining individuals and groups that are ageing physically and cognitively at different rates [89,90].

9. Impact of Ageing and Age-Related Diseases on General Healthcare Provision

There is a new trend in healthcare provision for older people which focuses on preventing premature admission to care homes. This trend offers various healthcare options, including the use of mobility aids, assistive technology devices, domiciliary healthcare, respite care, and telecare. By using assistive technology, the rate of functional decline in frail older people can be slowed down, while domiciliary healthcare aims to maximize independence, self-esteem, self-image, and quality of life [91,92]. Evidence suggests that domiciliary healthcare has positive outcomes, including improved quality of life, functional status, and reduced costs [93]. Informal care provision through visiting nurses, hospice carers, and physical therapists can also help older people live at home for a longer period. Respite care, which offers temporary relief to informal carers, has shown some positive effects, but more research is needed to support this claim [94–96].

Telecare, which involves the use of personal and environmental sensors in older people's homes, has been available for several decades. New options include sensors for falls, epilepsy, enuresis, and security monitoring for temperature, carbon monoxide, and smoke detection. Although the benefits of telecare are not yet fully understood due to limited research data, it presents an opportunity to identify what works best for each individual and in which circumstances [97]. Despite the new healthcare options, informal carers, such as spouses, children, relatives, and friends, still have to provide much of the domiciliary care to frail older people.

10. Impact of Multimorbidity and Polypharmacy on Oral Healthcare Provision

Multimorbidity can lead to a range of physical and psychosocial issues in older adults. The complexity of this condition means that symptoms may be difficult to diagnose, and diseases may be masked or exacerbated by other health problems. In addition, treatment of one disease may be affected by the presence of other diseases. This can result in a gradual decline in overall health. Oral healthcare providers who work with older adults should have a thorough understanding of geriatrics and pharmacology, and collaborate closely with physicians and pharmacists to provide individualized care [98]. Older adults are particularly susceptible to adverse reactions to medication due to age-related changes in pharmacokinetics and pharmacodynamics, as well as the prevalence of polypharmacy [99–101]. Many medications can cause a decrease in saliva secretion rate, leading to dry mouth and a range of oral health problems [100]. Oral healthcare providers should consider the impact of medication on oral health and be cautious in prescribing medication to patients with polypharmacy. The modified Summated Xerostomia Inventory (Table 1) can be used to assess xerostomia. Practical treatments are available to alleviate the symptoms of dry mouth and improve overall physical and psychosocial well-being [102,103].

Table 1. Modified summated xerostomia inventory.

		Never	Occasionally	Often
1	My mouth feels dry when eating a meal	1	2	3
2	My mouth feels dry	1	2	3
3	I have difficulty in eating dry foods	1	2	3
4	I have difficulties swallowing certain foods	1	2	3
5	My lips feel dry	1	2	3

Summated score < 8 no xerostomia; summated score ≥ 8 xerostomia.

11. Impact of Frailty, Disability, and Care Dependency on Oral Healthcare Provision

It is crucial for both formal and informal caregivers of older adults to understand that those who are frail or disabled are at significant risk of developing oral health problems. Caregivers should therefore take the responsibility of organizing a consultation with an oral healthcare provider. On the other hand, sudden deterioration of oral health in older individuals can be an early indicator of frailty and should prompt oral healthcare providers to arrange a consultation with a physician or geriatrician. Multiple epidemiological studies suggest that professional oral healthcare is urgently needed to address the unmet needs of older adults. To improve oral healthcare provision, there should be integration of oral healthcare into general healthcare, community programs that promote healthy behaviors, and access to preventive oral healthcare [104]. A crucial strategy is the development and implementation of an oral healthcare guideline to cater to older adults living in the community. As older adults prefer to age in place, new options for oral healthcare provision such as domiciliary oral healthcare, customised oral hygiene care aids, visiting dental hygienists and nurses, and oral hygiene telecare should be developed. Unfortunately, not all oral healthcare offices are easily accessible for older adults who are frail, disabled, or care dependent. Therefore, it is the responsibility of oral healthcare providers to make their premises easily and safely accessible for this group of individuals. Only when oral healthcare providers accept and face this responsibility can dentistry be transformed into medical oral healthcare and dentists be upgraded to oral physicians.

12. Epilogue

The risk of rapid deterioration in oral health is heightened by ageing, age-related diseases, multimorbidity, polypharmacy, frailty, disability, sarcopenia, and inappropriate oral hygiene care. Providing oral care to frail older people can be complex due to additional factors such as lifestyle (nutrition and smoking habits) and the motivation of the patient or caregivers to achieve adequate oral hygiene. Depending on the degree of frailty, the living environment, older people's preferences regarding oral health (shared decision making), and life expectancy, an individualized oral care plan must be made, in which the goals with regard to oral health are outlined. These goals should be formulated as concretely and measurably as possible and be realistic and acceptable to all parties, whereas the principles of palliative care should often be used for frail older people.

Furthermore, physicians should also be aware of the potential impact of risk factors of rapid deterioration on the oral health of their patients. Physicians should pay attention to their patients' oral health when developing diagnosis and treatment plans. Furthermore, physicians should be alert to the side effects of the medications they prescribe, as some medications can negatively impact oral health. They may consider prescribing alternative medications with less harmful effects on oral health. For example, medication with a negative effect on saliva secretion rates as a side-effect, can be replaced by other medication with a less xerogenic effect.

In general, it is important for physicians and dentists to view oral health as an integral part of a patient's overall health. By working together and providing proactive care, they can reduce the negative impact of these factors on oral health and improve patients' quality of life. Finally, it is crucial for all care providers to raise awareness about the importance of maintaining good oral health and the consequences of neglecting it, in order to prevent weakened oral health from becoming a geriatric syndrome [4].

Author Contributions: Writing—original draft, G.-J.v.d.P.; Writing—review & editing, C.d.B. All authors have read and agreed to the published version of the manuscript.

Funding: This research received no external funding.

Institutional Review Board Statement: Not applicable.

Informed Consent Statement: Not applicable.

Data Availability Statement: Not applicable.

Conflicts of Interest: The authors declare no conflict of interest.

References

1. van der Putten, G.J.; De Visschere, L.; van der Maarel-Wierink, C.; Vanobbergen, J.; Schols, J. The importance of oral health in (frail) elderly people—A review. *Eur. Geriatr. Med.* **2013**, *4*, 339–344. [CrossRef]
2. Kossioni, A.E.; Maggi, S.; Muller, F.; Petrovic, M. Oral health in older people: Time for action. *Eur. Geriatr. Med.* **2018**, *9*, 3–4. [CrossRef]
3. Marengoni, A.; von Strauss, E.; Rizzuto, D.; Winblad, B.; Fratiglioni, L. The impact of chronic multimorbidity and disability on functional decline and survival in elderly persons. A community-based, longitudinal study. *J. Intern. Med.* **2009**, *265*, 288–295. [CrossRef] [PubMed]
4. van der Putten, G.J.; de Baat, C.; De Visschere, L.; Schols, J. Poor oral health, a potential new geriatric syndrome. *Gerodontology* **2014**, *31* (Suppl. 1), 17–24. [CrossRef] [PubMed]
5. Strehler, B.L. Understanding aging. *Methods Mol. Med.* **2000**, *38*, 1–19. [CrossRef] [PubMed]
6. Michaud, M.; Balardy, L.; Moulis, G.; Gaudin, C.; Peyrot, C.; Vellas, B.; Cesari, M.; Nourhashemi, F. Proinflammatory cytokines, aging, and age-related diseases. *J. Am. Med. Dir. Assoc.* **2013**, *14*, 877–882. [CrossRef] [PubMed]
7. Miller, R.A. The aging immune system: Primer and prospectus. *Science* **1996**, *273*, 70–74. [CrossRef]
8. Sansoni, P.; Vescovini, R.; Fagnoni, F.; Biasini, C.; Zanni, F.; Zanlari, L.; Telera, A.; Lucchini, G.; Passeri, G.; Monti, D.; et al. The immune system in extreme longevity. *Exp. Gerontol.* **2008**, *43*, 61–65. [CrossRef]
9. Sadighi Akha, A.A. Aging and the immune system: An overview. *J. Immunol. Methods* **2018**, *463*, 21–26. [CrossRef]
10. Sanders, J.L.; Newman, A.B. Telomere length in epidemiology: A biomarker of aging, age-related disease, both, or neither? *Epidemiol. Rev.* **2013**, *35*, 112–131. [CrossRef]
11. Lu, W.; Zhang, Y.; Liu, D.; Songyang, Z.; Wan, M. Telomeres-structure, function, and regulation. *Exp. Cell Res.* **2013**, *319*, 133–141. [CrossRef] [PubMed]
12. Zhang, J.; Rane, G.; Dai, X.; Shanmugam, M.K.; Arfuso, F.; Samy, R.P.; Lai, M.K.; Kappei, D.; Kumar, A.P.; Sethi, G. Ageing and the telomere connection: An intimate relationship with inflammation. *Ageing Res. Rev.* **2016**, *25*, 55–69. [CrossRef]
13. Masi, S.; Gkranias, N.; Li, K.; Salpea, K.D.; Parkar, M.; Orlandi, M.; Suvan, J.E.; Eng, H.L.; Taddei, S.; Patel, K.; et al. Association between short leukocyte telomere length, endotoxemia, and severe periodontitis in people with diabetes: A cross-sectional survey. *Diabetes Care* **2014**, *37*, 1140–1147. [CrossRef] [PubMed]
14. Masi, S.; Salpea, K.D.; Li, K.; Parkar, M.; Nibali, L.; Donos, N.; Patel, K.; Taddei, S.; Deanfield, J.E.; D'Aiuto, F.; et al. Oxidative stress, chronic inflammation, and telomere length in patients with periodontitis. *Free Radic. Biol. Med.* **2011**, *50*, 730–735. [CrossRef] [PubMed]
15. Sanders, A.E.; Divaris, K.; Naorungroj, S.; Heiss, G.; Risques, R.A. Telomere length attrition and chronic periodontitis: An ARIC Study nested case-control study. *J. Clin. Periodontol.* **2015**, *42*, 12–20. [CrossRef] [PubMed]
16. Takahashi, K.; Nishida, H.; Takeda, H.; Shin, K. Telomere length in leukocytes and cultured gingival fibroblasts from patients with aggressive periodontitis. *J. Periodontol.* **2004**, *75*, 84–90. [CrossRef]
17. Song, W.; Yang, J.; Niu, Z. Association of periodontitis with leukocyte telomere length in US adults: A cross-sectional analysis of NHANES 1999 to 2002. *J. Periodontol.* **2021**, *92*, 833–843. [CrossRef]
18. Botelho, J.; Mascarenhas, P.; Viana, J.; Proenca, L.; Orlandi, M.; Leira, Y.; Chambrone, L.; Mendes, J.J.; Machado, V. An umbrella review of the evidence linking oral health and systemic noncommunicable diseases. *Nat. Commun.* **2022**, *13*, 7614. [CrossRef]
19. Gurenlian, J.R. Inflammation: The relationship between oral health and systemic disease. *Dent. Assist.* **2009**, *78*, 8–10, 12–14, 38–40; quiz 41–43. [PubMed]
20. Peric, M.; Marhl, U.; Gennai, S.; Marruganti, C.; Graziani, F. Treatment of gingivitis is associated with reduction of systemic inflammation and improvement of oral health-related quality of life: A randomized clinical trial. *J. Clin. Periodontol.* **2022**, *49*, 899–910. [CrossRef]
21. Bui, F.Q.; Almeida-da-Silva, C.L.C.; Huynh, B.; Trinh, A.; Liu, J.; Woodward, J.; Asadi, H.; Ojcius, D.M. Association between periodontal pathogens and systemic disease. *Biomed. J.* **2019**, *42*, 27–35. [CrossRef] [PubMed]

22. de Vries, S.A.G.; Tan, C.X.W.; Bouma, G.; Forouzanfar, T.; Brand, H.S.; de Boer, N.K. Salivary Function and Oral Health Problems in Crohn's Disease Patients. *Inflamm. Bowel Dis.* **2018**, *24*, 1361–1367. [CrossRef] [PubMed]
23. Rikardsson, S.; Jonsson, J.; Hultin, M.; Gustafsson, A.; Johannsen, A. Perceived oral health in patients with Crohn's disease. *Oral Health Prev. Dent.* **2009**, *7*, 277–282. [PubMed]
24. Ali, S.; Nagieb, C.S.; Fayed, H.L. Effect of Behcet's disease-associated oral ulcers on oral health related quality of life. *Spec. Care Dent.* **2022**, 1–8. [CrossRef]
25. Mumcu, G.; Ergun, T.; Inanc, N.; Fresko, I.; Atalay, T.; Hayran, O.; Direskeneli, H. Oral health is impaired in Behcet's disease and is associated with disease severity. *Rheumatology* **2004**, *43*, 1028–1033. [CrossRef] [PubMed]
26. Senusi, A.; Higgins, S.; Fortune, F. The influence of oral health and psycho-social well-being on clinical outcomes in Behcet's disease. *Rheumatol. Int.* **2018**, *38*, 1873–1883. [CrossRef]
27. Albilia, J.B.; Lam, D.K.; Blanas, N.; Clokie, C.M.; Sandor, G.K. Small mouths . . . Big problems? A review of scleroderma and its oral health implications. *J. Can. Dent. Assoc.* **2007**, *73*, 831–836.
28. Beaty, K.L.; Gurenlian, J.R.; Rogo, E.J. Oral Health Experiences of the Limited Scleroderma Patient. *J. Dent. Hyg.* **2021**, *95*, 59–69.
29. Chung, M.; York, B.R.; Michaud, D.S. Oral Health and Cancer. *Curr. Oral Health Rep.* **2019**, *6*, 130–137. [CrossRef]
30. Jobbins, J.; Bagg, J.; Finlay, I.G.; Addy, M.; Newcombe, R.G. Oral and dental disease in terminally ill cancer patients. *BMJ* **1992**, *304*, 1612. [CrossRef]
31. Vermaire, J.A.; Partoredjo, A.S.K.; de Groot, R.J.; Brand, H.S.; Speksnijder, C.M. Mastication in health-related quality of life in patients treated for oral cancer: A systematic review. *Eur. J. Cancer Care (Engl.)* **2022**, *31*, e13744. [CrossRef] [PubMed]
32. Zhang, J.; Bellocco, R.; Sandborgh-Englund, G.; Yu, J.; Sallberg Chen, M.; Ye, W. Poor Oral Health and Esophageal Cancer Risk: A Nationwide Cohort Study. *Cancer Epidemiol. Biomark. Prev.* **2022**, *31*, 1418–1425. [CrossRef] [PubMed]
33. Morimata, J.; Otomaru, T.; Murase, M.; Haraguchi, M.; Sumita, Y.; Taniguchi, H. Investigation of factor affecting health-related quality of life in head and neck cancer patients. *Gerodontology* **2013**, *30*, 194–200. [CrossRef] [PubMed]
34. Azuma, N.; Katada, Y.; Yoshikawa, T.; Yokoyama, Y.; Nishioka, A.; Sekiguchi, M.; Kitano, M.; Kitano, S.; Sano, H.; Matsui, K. Evaluation of changes in oral health-related quality of life over time in patients with Sjogren's syndrome. *Mod. Rheumatol.* **2021**, *31*, 669–677. [CrossRef]
35. Cartee, D.L.; Maker, S.; Dalonges, D.; Manski, M.C. Sjogren's Syndrome: Oral Manifestations and Treatment, a Dental Perspective. *J. Dent. Hyg.* **2015**, *89*, 365–371.
36. Enger, T.B.; Palm, O.; Garen, T.; Sandvik, L.; Jensen, J.L. Oral distress in primary Sjogren's syndrome: Implications for health-related quality of life. *Eur. J. Oral Sci.* **2011**, *119*, 474–480. [CrossRef]
37. Vujovic, S.; Desnica, J.; Stevanovic, M.; Mijailovic, S.; Vojinovic, R.; Selakovic, D.; Jovicic, N.; Rosic, G.; Milovanovic, D. Oral Health and Oral Health-Related Quality of Life in Patients with Primary Sjogren's Syndrome. *Medicina* **2023**, *59*, 473. [CrossRef] [PubMed]
38. Al-Mobeeriek, A. Oral health status among psychiatric patients in Riyadh, Saudi Arabia. *West Indian Med. J.* **2012**, *61*, 549–554. [CrossRef]
39. Bertaud-Gounot, V.; Kovess-Masfety, V.; Perrus, C.; Trohel, G.; Richard, F. Oral health status and treatment needs among psychiatric inpatients in Rennes, France: A cross-sectional study. *BMC Psychiatry* **2013**, *13*, 227. [CrossRef]
40. Buunk-Werkhoven, Y.A.; Dijkstra, A.; Schaub, R.M.; van der Schans, C.P.; Spreen, M. Oral health related quality of life among imprisoned Dutch forensic psychiatric patients. *J. Forensic Nurs.* **2010**, *6*, 137–143. [CrossRef]
41. Goud, V.; Kannaiyan, K.; Rao, B.V.; Abidullah, M.; Dharani, V.; Nayak, M. Oral Health Status and Treatment Needs of Psychiatric Outpatients Aged 18–64 Years in District Civil Hospital, Raichur, Karnataka: A Cross-Sectional Study. *J. Pharm. Bioallied Sci.* **2021**, *13*, S598–S601. [CrossRef] [PubMed]
42. Kisely, S.; Najman, J.M. A study of the association between psychiatric symptoms and oral health outcomes in a population-based birth cohort at 30-year-old follow-up. *J. Psychosom. Res.* **2022**, *157*, 110784. [CrossRef] [PubMed]
43. Kossioni, A.E.; Kossionis, G.E.; Polychronopoulou, A. Oral health status of elderly hospitalised psychiatric patients. *Gerodontology* **2012**, *29*, 272–283. [CrossRef]
44. Lewis, D. Summary of: Prevalence of oral diseases and oral-health-related quality of life in people with severe mental illness undertaking community-based psychiatric care. *Br. Dent. J.* **2012**, *213*, 462–463. [CrossRef]
45. Ngo, D.Y.J.; Thomson, W.M.; Subramaniam, M.; Abdin, E.; Ang, K.Y. The oral health of long-term psychiatric inpatients in Singapore. *Psychiatry Res.* **2018**, *266*, 206–211. [CrossRef]
46. Shah, V.R.; Jain, P.; Patel, N. Oral health of psychiatric patients: A cross-sectional comparision study. *Dent. Res. J.* **2012**, *9*, 209–214. [CrossRef] [PubMed]
47. Sjogren, R.; Nordstrom, G. Oral health status of psychiatric patients. *J. Clin. Nurs.* **2000**, *9*, 632–638. [CrossRef]
48. Auffret, M.; Meuric, V.; Boyer, E.; Bonnaure-Mallet, M.; Verin, M. Oral Health Disorders in Parkinson's Disease: More than Meets the Eye. *J. Parkinson's Dis.* **2021**, *11*, 1507–1535. [CrossRef]
49. Nakayama, Y.; Washio, M.; Mori, M. Oral health conditions in patients with Parkinson's disease. *J. Epidemiol.* **2004**, *14*, 143–150. [CrossRef]
50. Persson, M.; Osterberg, T.; Granerus, A.K.; Karlsson, S. Influence of Parkinson's disease on oral health. *Acta Odontol. Scand.* **1992**, *50*, 37–42. [CrossRef]

51. Ribeiro, G.R.; Campos, C.H.; Garcia, R.C. Oral Health in Elders with Parkinson's Disease. *Braz. Dent. J.* **2016**, *27*, 340–344. [CrossRef]
52. Saft, C.; Andrich, J.E.; Muller, T.; Becker, J.; Jackowski, J. Oral and dental health in Huntington's disease—An observational study. *BMC Neurol.* **2013**, *13*, 114. [CrossRef] [PubMed]
53. Manchery, N.; Henry, J.D.; Nangle, M.R. A systematic review of oral health in people with multiple sclerosis. *Community Dent. Oral Epidemiol.* **2020**, *48*, 89–100. [CrossRef] [PubMed]
54. Hamza, S.A.; Asif, S.; Bokhari, S.A.H. Oral health of individuals with dementia and Alzheimer's disease: A review. *J. Indian Soc. Periodontol.* **2021**, *25*, 96–101. [CrossRef] [PubMed]
55. Tiisanoja, A.; Syrjala, A.M.; Tertsonen, M.; Komulainen, K.; Pesonen, P.; Knuuttila, M.; Hartikainen, S.; Ylostalo, P. Oral diseases and inflammatory burden and Alzheimer's disease among subjects aged 75 years or older. *Spec. Care Dent.* **2019**, *39*, 158–165. [CrossRef] [PubMed]
56. Ahola, K.; Saarinen, A.; Kuuliala, A.; Leirisalo-Repo, M.; Murtomaa, H.; Meurman, J.H. Impact of rheumatic diseases on oral health and quality of life. *Oral Dis.* **2015**, *21*, 342–348. [CrossRef]
57. Carvalho, C.G.; Medeiros-Filho, J.B.; Ferreira, M.C. Guide for health professionals addressing oral care for individuals in oncological treatment based on scientific evidence. *Support. Care Cancer* **2018**, *26*, 2651–2661. [CrossRef]
58. Gianos, E.; Jackson, E.A.; Tejpal, A.; Aspry, K.; O'Keefe, J.; Aggarwal, M.; Jain, A.; Itchhaporia, D.; Williams, K.; Batts, T.; et al. Oral health and atherosclerotic cardiovascular disease: A review. *Am. J. Prev. Cardiol.* **2021**, *7*, 100179. [CrossRef]
59. Holmlund, A.; Lampa, E.; Lind, L. Oral health and cardiovascular disease risk in a cohort of periodontitis patients. *Atherosclerosis* **2017**, *262*, 101–106. [CrossRef]
60. Joshy, G.; Arora, M.; Korda, R.J.; Chalmers, J.; Banks, E. Is poor oral health a risk marker for incident cardiovascular disease hospitalisation and all-cause mortality? Findings from 172 630 participants from the prospective 45 and Up Study. *BMJ Open* **2016**, *6*, e012386. [CrossRef]
61. Kotronia, E.; Brown, H.; Papacosta, A.O.; Lennon, L.T.; Weyant, R.J.; Whincup, P.H.; Wannamethee, S.G.; Ramsay, S.E. Oral health and all-cause, cardiovascular disease, and respiratory mortality in older people in the UK and USA. *Sci. Rep.* **2021**, *11*, 16452. [CrossRef]
62. Meurman, J.H.; Bascones-Martinez, A. Oral Infections and Systemic Health—More than Just Links to Cardiovascular Diseases. *Oral Health Prev. Dent.* **2021**, *19*, 441–448. [CrossRef] [PubMed]
63. Najafipour, H.; Malek Mohammadi, T.; Rahim, F.; Haghdoost, A.A.; Shadkam, M.; Afshari, M. Association of oral health and cardiovascular disease risk factors "results from a community based study on 5900 adult subjects". *ISRN Cardiol.* **2013**, *2013*, 782126. [CrossRef] [PubMed]
64. Venkatasalu, M.R.; Murang, Z.R.; Ramasamy, D.T.R.; Dhaliwal, J.S. Oral health problems among palliative and terminally ill patients: An integrated systematic review. *BMC Oral Health* **2020**, *20*, 79. [CrossRef]
65. Le Reste, J.Y.; Nabbe, P.; Manceau, B.; Lygidakis, C.; Doerr, C.; Lingner, H.; Czachowski, S.; Munoz, M.; Argyriadou, S.; Claveria, A.; et al. The European General Practice Research Network presents a comprehensive definition of multimorbidity in family medicine and long term care, following a systematic review of relevant literature. *J. Am. Med. Dir. Assoc.* **2013**, *14*, 319–325. [CrossRef]
66. Le Reste, J.Y.; Nabbe, P.; Lazic, D.; Assenova, R.; Lingner, H.; Czachowski, S.; Argyriadou, S.; Sowinska, A.; Lygidakis, C.; Doerr, C.; et al. How do general practitioners recognize the definition of multimorbidity? A European qualitative study. *Eur. J. Gen. Pract.* **2016**, *22*, 159–168. [CrossRef]
67. Loya, A.M.; Gonzalez-Stuart, A.; Rivera, J.O. Prevalence of polypharmacy, polyherbacy, nutritional supplement use and potential product interactions among older adults living on the United States-Mexico border: A descriptive, questionnaire-based study. *Drugs Aging* **2009**, *26*, 423–436. [CrossRef]
68. Masnoon, N.; Shakib, S.; Kalisch-Ellett, L.; Caughey, G.E. What is polypharmacy? A systematic review of definitions. *BMC Geriatr.* **2017**, *17*, 230. [CrossRef]
69. Rockwood, K.; Mitnitski, A. Frailty in relation to the accumulation of deficits. *J. Gerontol. A Biol. Sci. Med. Sci.* **2007**, *62*, 722–727. [CrossRef] [PubMed]
70. Rockwood, K.; Song, X.; MacKnight, C.; Bergman, H.; Hogan, D.B.; McDowell, I.; Mitnitski, A. A global clinical measure of fitness and frailty in elderly people. *CMAJ* **2005**, *173*, 489–495. [CrossRef] [PubMed]
71. Collard, R.M.; Boter, H.; Schoevers, R.A.; Oude Voshaar, R.C. Prevalence of frailty in community-dwelling older persons: A systematic review. *J. Am. Geriatr. Soc.* **2012**, *60*, 1487–1492. [CrossRef]
72. Kamdem, B.; Seematter-Bagnoud, L.; Botrugno, F.; Santos-Eggimann, B. Relationship between oral health and Fried's frailty criteria in community-dwelling older persons. *BMC Geriatr.* **2017**, *17*, 174. [CrossRef] [PubMed]
73. de Andrade, F.B.; Lebrao, M.L.; Santos, J.L.; Duarte, Y.A. Relationship between oral health and frailty in community-dwelling elderly individuals in Brazil. *J. Am. Geriatr. Soc.* **2013**, *61*, 809–814. [CrossRef] [PubMed]
74. Ferreira, L.F.; Scariot, E.L.; da Rosa, L.H.T. The effect of different exercise programs on sarcopenia criteria in older people: A systematic review of systematic reviews with meta-analysis. *Arch. Gerontol. Geriatr.* **2023**, *105*, 104868. [CrossRef] [PubMed]
75. Cao, W.; Zhu, A.; Chu, S.; Zhou, Q.; Zhou, Y.; Qu, X.; Tang, Q.; Zhang, Y. Correlation between nutrition, oral health, and different sarcopenia groups among elderly outpatients of community hospitals: A cross-sectional study of 1505 participants in China. *BMC Geriatr.* **2022**, *22*, 332. [CrossRef]

76. Zhao, H.; Cheng, R.; Song, G.; Teng, J.; Shen, S.; Fu, X.; Yan, Y.; Liu, C. The Effect of Resistance Training on the Rehabilitation of Elderly Patients with Sarcopenia: A Meta-Analysis. *Int. J. Environ. Res. Public Health* **2022**, *19*, 15491. [CrossRef]
77. Yoo, J.I.; Ha, Y.C.; Cha, Y. Nutrition and Exercise Treatment of Sarcopenia in Hip Fracture Patients: Systematic Review. *J. Bone Metab.* **2022**, *29*, 63–73. [CrossRef]
78. Hatta, K.; Ikebe, K. Association between oral health and sarcopenia: A literature review. *J. Prosthodont. Res.* **2021**, *65*, 131–136. [CrossRef]
79. Azzolino, D.; Passarelli, P.C.; De Angelis, P.; Piccirillo, G.B.; D'Addona, A.; Cesari, M. Poor Oral Health as a Determinant of Malnutrition and Sarcopenia. *Nutrients* **2019**, *11*, 2898. [CrossRef]
80. Holm-Pedersen, P.; Schultz-Larsen, K.; Christiansen, N.; Avlund, K. Tooth loss and subsequent disability and mortality in old age. *J. Am. Geriatr. Soc.* **2008**, *56*, 429–435. [CrossRef]
81. Komiyama, T.; Ohi, T.; Miyoshi, Y.; Murakami, T.; Tsuboi, A.; Tomata, Y.; Tsuji, I.; Watanabe, M.; Hattori, Y. Association Between Tooth Loss, Receipt of Dental Care, and Functional Disability in an Elderly Japanese Population: The Tsurugaya Project. *J. Am. Geriatr. Soc.* **2016**, *64*, 2495–2502. [CrossRef] [PubMed]
82. Komiyama, T.; Ohi, T.; Tomata, Y.; Tanji, F.; Tsuji, I.; Watanabe, M.; Hattori, Y. Dental Status is Associated With Incident Functional Disability in Community-Dwelling Older Japanese: A Prospective Cohort Study Using Propensity Score Matching. *J. Epidemiol.* **2020**, *30*, 84–90. [CrossRef] [PubMed]
83. Matsuyama, Y.; Listl, S.; Jurges, H.; Watt, R.G.; Aida, J.; Tsakos, G. Causal Effect of Tooth Loss on Functional Capacity in Older Adults in England: A Natural Experiment. *J. Am. Geriatr. Soc.* **2021**, *69*, 1319–1327. [CrossRef] [PubMed]
84. Yin, Z.; Yang, J.; Huang, C.; Sun, H.; Wu, Y. Eating and communication difficulties as mediators of the relationship between tooth loss and functional disability in middle-aged and older adults. *J. Dent.* **2020**, *96*, 103331. [CrossRef]
85. Kotronia, E.; Brown, H.; Papacosta, O.; Lennon, L.T.; Weyant, R.J.; Whincup, P.H.; Wannamethee, S.G.; Ramsay, S.E. Oral health problems and risk of incident disability in two studies of older adults in the United Kingdom and the United States. *J. Am. Geriatr. Soc.* **2022**, *70*, 2080–2092. [CrossRef]
86. World Health Organization (WHO). *World Report on Disability*; WHO: Geneva, Switzerland, 2011.
87. Motl, R.W.; McAuley, E. Physical activity, disability, and quality of life in older adults. *Phys. Med. Rehabil. Clin. N. Am.* **2010**, *21*, 299–308. [CrossRef]
88. Clouston, S.A.; Brewster, P.; Kuh, D.; Richards, M.; Cooper, R.; Hardy, R.; Rubin, M.S.; Hofer, S.M. The dynamic relationship between physical function and cognition in longitudinal aging cohorts. *Epidemiol. Rev.* **2013**, *35*, 33–50. [CrossRef]
89. Bossers, W.J.; van der Woude, L.H.; Boersma, F.; Scherder, E.J.; van Heuvelen, M.J. Recommended measures for the assessment of cognitive and physical performance in older patients with dementia: A systematic review. *Dement. Geriatr. Cogn. Dis. Extra* **2012**, *2*, 589–609. [CrossRef]
90. Gill, T.M. Assessment of function and disability in longitudinal studies. *J. Am. Geriatr. Soc.* **2010**, *58* (Suppl. 2), S308–S312. [CrossRef]
91. Mann, W.C.; Ottenbacher, K.J.; Fraas, L.; Tomita, M.; Granger, C.V. Effectiveness of assistive technology and environmental interventions in maintaining independence and reducing home care costs for the frail elderly. A randomized controlled trial. *Arch. Fam. Med.* **1999**, *8*, 210–217. [CrossRef]
92. Parsons, J.; Rouse, P.; Robinson, E.M.; Sheridan, N.; Connolly, M.J. Goal setting as a feature of homecare services for older people: Does it make a difference? *Age Ageing* **2012**, *41*, 24–29. [CrossRef] [PubMed]
93. Ryburn, B.; Wells, Y.; Foreman, P. Enabling independence: Restorative approaches to home care provision for frail older adults. *Health Soc. Care Community* **2009**, *17*, 225–234. [CrossRef] [PubMed]
94. Evans, D. Exploring the concept of respite. *J. Adv. Nurs.* **2013**, *69*, 1905–1915. [CrossRef] [PubMed]
95. Shaw, C.; McNamara, R.; Abrams, K.; Cannings-John, R.; Hood, K.; Longo, M.; Myles, S.; O'Mahony, S.; Roe, B.; Williams, K. Systematic review of respite care in the frail elderly. *Health Technol. Assess.* **2009**, *13*, 1–246. [CrossRef]
96. Hogan, L.; Boron, J.B.; Masters, J.; MacArthur, K.; Manley, N. Characteristics of dementia family caregivers who use paid professional in-home respite care. *Home Health Care Serv. Q.* **2022**, *41*, 310–329. [CrossRef]
97. Parker, S.G.; Hawley, M.S. Telecare for an ageing population? *Age Ageing* **2013**, *42*, 424–425. [CrossRef]
98. Dolan, T.A. Professional education to meet the oral health needs of older adults and persons with disabilities. *Spec. Care Dentist.* **2013**, *33*, 190–197. [CrossRef]
99. Corsonello, A.; Pedone, C.; Incalzi, R.A. Age-related pharmacokinetic and pharmacodynamic changes and related risk of adverse drug reactions. *Curr. Med. Chem.* **2010**, *17*, 571–584. [CrossRef]
100. Liu, B.; Dion, M.R.; Jurasic, M.M.; Gibson, G.; Jones, J.A. Xerostomia and salivary hypofunction in vulnerable elders: Prevalence and etiology. *Oral Surg. Oral Med. Oral Pathol. Oral Radiol.* **2012**, *114*, 52–60. [CrossRef]
101. Ship, J.A.; Pillemer, S.R.; Baum, B.J. Xerostomia and the geriatric patient. *J. Am. Geriatr. Soc.* **2002**, *50*, 535–543. [CrossRef]
102. van der Putten, G.J.; Brand, H.S.; Schols, J.M.; de Baat, C. The diagnostic suitability of a xerostomia questionnaire and the association between xerostomia, hyposalivation and medication use in a group of nursing home residents. *Clin. Oral Investig.* **2011**, *15*, 185–192. [CrossRef] [PubMed]

103. Thomson, W.M.; van der Putten, G.J.; de Baat, C.; Ikebe, K.; Matsuda, K.; Enoki, K.; Hopcraft, M.S.; Ling, G.Y. Shortening the xerostomia inventory. *Oral Surg Oral Med. Oral Pathol. Oral Radiol. Endodontol.* **2011**, *112*, 322–327. [CrossRef] [PubMed]
104. Griffin, S.O.; Jones, J.A.; Brunson, D.; Griffin, P.M.; Bailey, W.D. Burden of oral disease among older adults and implications for public health priorities. *Am. J. Public Health* **2012**, *102*, 411–418. [CrossRef] [PubMed]

Disclaimer/Publisher's Note: The statements, opinions and data contained in all publications are solely those of the individual author(s) and contributor(s) and not of MDPI and/or the editor(s). MDPI and/or the editor(s) disclaim responsibility for any injury to people or property resulting from any ideas, methods, instructions or products referred to in the content.

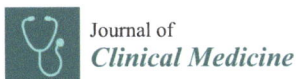
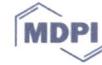

Review

The Impact of Xerostomia on Food Choices—A Review with Clinical Recommendations

Frauke Müller [1,2,*], Najla Chebib [1], Sabrina Maniewicz [1] and Laurence Genton [3]

[1] Division of Gerodontology and Removable Prosthodontics, University Clinics of Dental Medicine, 1205 Geneva, Switzerland
[2] Department of Rehabilitation and Geriatrics, Geneva University Hospitals, 1205 Geneva, Switzerland
[3] Clinical Nutrition, Geneva University Hospitals, University of Geneva, 1205 Geneva, Switzerland
* Correspondence: frauke.mueller@unige.ch

Abstract: Xerostomia and hyposalivation are highly prevalent conditions in old age, particularly among multimorbid elders, and are often attributed to the use of multiple medications. These conditions negatively affect oral functions, such as chewing, swallowing, speech, and taste. Additionally, the lack of lubrication of the oral mucosa frequently leads to super-infections with candida. Denture retention and comfort may also be compromised. The risk of dental caries and erosion of natural teeth increases since saliva, which is essential for repairing initial lesions in tooth structures, is insufficient. The dry sensation in the mouth also impacts the emotional and social well-being of elderly individuals. Patients experiencing xerostomia often avoid certain foods that are uncomfortable or difficult to consume. However, some foods may alleviate the symptoms or even stimulate salivation. This review discusses the limited available evidence on nutritional advice for patients with xerostomia and aims to provide insight into the patient's perspective while offering clinical recommendations. Future studies should focus on investigating the nutritional intake of individuals suffering from xerostomia or hyposalivation in order to ensure oral health comfort, prevent malnutrition, and minimize the impact on their quality of life.

Keywords: nutrition; nutritional counselling; food choice; xerostomia; hyposalivation; elders; geriatric; gerodontology

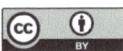

1. Introduction

Xerostomia and hyposalivation are conditions commonly observed in the elderly population, and their occurrence is increasing along with the growing number of elderly individuals in our societies [1]. Xerostomia refers to the subjective sensation of having a dry mouth, while hyposalivation is characterized by a measurable decrease in saliva production [2]. The reported prevalence of xerostomia varies widely, ranging from 5.5 to 78%. These significant differences may be attributable to variations in terminology, survey methods, and specific study populations [1]. In a systematic review with meta-analyses conducted by Pina et al., the prevalence of hyposalivation for unstimulated and stimulated methods was estimated to be 33% (95% CI 21.1–47.0, $p < 0.0001$, n = 2425 individuals) and 30% (95% CI 22.5–39.0, $p < 0.0001$, n = 1495 individuals), respectively [3].

The consequences of reduced saliva production are manifold. They range from difficulties in chewing and swallowing to digestive problems and impaired absorption of nutrients. Moreover, individuals with xerostomia experience a decrease in flavour perception, enjoyment of food, and appetite. Due to the lack of lubrication of the oral mucosa, people with xerostomia often face limitations in their food choices as certain foods become challenging to tolerate, chew, and swallow. The reduced flavour and texture perception can also affect their overall nutritional intake. These consequences may have a significant psychosocial impact and potentially lead to deficiencies in essential nutrients. Saliva plays a vital role in maintaining the health of hard and soft tissues in the oral cavity. It helps remove food debris, neutralize acids, and protect against bacterial infections, thereby preventing dental caries, periodontal disease, and mucositis [3,4]. Hyposalivation promotes the development of dental caries and eventual tooth loss, in particular when combined with poor oral hygiene and a diet rich in sugar and carbohydrates. Therefore, it not only directly affects oral health but also indirectly contributes to impaired masticatory efficiency via the avoidance of various foods with a reduced dentition, which may result in a poor diet and inadequate food intake [5–7].

From a patient's perspective, residents in Long-Term Care facilities who complain at times, or even constantly, of the sensation of a dry mouth state a severe limitation of their oral health-related quality of life [4,8]. Many readers may have personally experienced the unpleasant feeling of a "dry mouth" during stressful situations or while sleeping with an open mouth. The tongue seems to stick to the roof of the mouth, the lips are dry, and speaking is difficult. Eating and swallowing become more challenging, and the sensitive mucosa may limit food choices. Furthermore, even the taste sensation may be affected [9]. The emotional and social impact of xerostomia extends far beyond the oral cavity and undoubtedly has a profound effect on the patient's daily life and well-being [4].

The aetiology of a dry mouth can be quite diverse. The most severe cases of dry mouth, accompanied by significant hyposalivation, can arise from surgical removal of the salivary glands or radiation therapy as part of cancer treatment [10,11]. Pathologically reduced salivary secretion is also observed in conditions such as Sjogren's syndrome, diabetes, or Parkinson's patients [1,12,13]. Further risk factors for varying degrees of salivary deficiency or the sensation of a dry mouth are overall poor health and the use of certain medications. Numerous drugs can impact salivary production, such as antidepressants, anxiolytics, antihypertensives, diuretics, painkillers, medication for Parkinson's disease, and neuroleptics. Female gender, age, and obesity are other known risk factors in younger patients [14]. Smoking, excessive coffee consumption, heavy snoring, mouth breathing, or dehydration also foster hyposalivation [1,15,16]. Lastly, in elders, the reduced sensation of thirst should also be mentioned, which often leads to insufficient fluid intake and dehydration [17].

Despite ongoing advancements in medicine and dentistry, the available therapeutic options for treating dry mouth are unfortunately still very limited and often unsatisfactory for the patient. Various therapeutic approaches have been described, including saliva stimulation or substitution, medications, or even transcutaneous electrical stimulation, and acupuncture [18–20]. Drug intervention to increase salivation seems most adequate for multimorbid elders, but it should be administered by the attending physician rather than within a dental setting. Certain medications, such as pilocarpine or cevimeline, can stimulate the residual capacity of salivary gland tissue. However, improvement of salivary gland hypofunction may be limited [21]. Exciting prospects for future therapeutic options lie in the fields of developmental and stem cell biology [22]. Recently, guidelines for non-nutritional therapies for xerostomia have been published by The Multinational Association of Supportive Care in Cancer/International Society of Oral Oncology, and the American Society of Clinical Oncology [11].

The impact of xerostomia on food choices and dietary patterns is still not well understood. However, providing clinical recommendations can help individuals with xerostomia avoid pain, discomfort, and difficulties with swallowing. Avoiding certain foods may lead to an unbalanced and unhealthy diet, and it may even contribute to malnutrition. On the other hand, making appropriate dietary choices may not only help to alleviate symptoms but may even stimulate salivation. Therefore, the aim of this review is to summarize the impact of xerostomia and hyposalivation on patients' food preferences and propose clinical recommendations for an adapted diet that is comfortable and safe to chew and swallow, alleviates discomfort, and increases the natural flow of saliva.

2. Physiology of Salivation

Saliva primarily consists of water, but it also contains important components essential for maintaining the health of the oral cavity. Alongside electrolytes such as bicarbonate, calcium, fluoride, phosphate, potassium, and sodium, saliva contains various immunoglobulins. Saliva also contains immune factors and phagocytes. Additionally, amylase and growth proteins have been detected in the mucins. The saliva mixture may also contain microorganisms and epithelial cells [23,24]. The functions of saliva extend beyond simply moistening the oral mucosa. Saliva is involved in initiating food digestion, buffering the pH value, remineralising the tooth structure, diluting flavours, and increasing the lubrication of the food to facilitate swallowing. Saliva also has essential functions with regard to the digestive process in the upper parts of the gastrointestinal tract [7].

The major and minor salivary glands of the orofacial system collectively produce approximately 0.5–1.0 L of saliva every day. While the sublingual and submandibular salivary glands produce primarily viscous and highly mucinous saliva, the parotid gland secretes almost 90% of the total saliva of predominantly serous consistency [25]. At rest, without simultaneous chewing, the salivary flow rate is approximately 0.3–0.4 mL per minute. However, during chewing, the salivary flow increases to 1.5–2.0 mL per minute, especially when chewing on one side only [26]. This reflexive secretion of saliva is triggered by the periodontal receptors, which are mechanically stimulated by pressure exerted during chewing on the occlusal surfaces of the teeth [27]. Interestingly, this reflex salivary secretion also occurs in edentulous patients wearing full dentures, and increasing the occlusal force by restorative means can help to increase the salivary flow [28]. The saliva produced during mastication is rather serous and is mostly secreted by the parotid gland. Salivary secretion can also be triggered by gustatory or visual stimuli, such as appetizingly prepared and fragrant food. Thermal or painful stimuli can also stimulate the flow of saliva.

Interestingly, solid objects that are not food may also trigger increased saliva secretion in the oral cavity. This can be observed, for example, after the insertion of dentures [29]. Patients perceive this undesirable side effect of newly fitted dentures as often bothersome, as they may need to swallow more frequently and may have concerns about unnoticed drooling. However, if the stimulus—in this case, the prosthesis—is continuously present, i.e., if the prosthesis is worn consistently for extended periods of time, the reflex adapts, and the salivary flow typically normalizes within the first week after denture insertion. Moreover, replacement dentures can allow for higher chewing forces, which in turn can also increase salivary flow [28]. This effect may persist for a longer duration, although evidence to support this assumption is lacking.

3. Age-Related Changes

There is increasing debate regarding the notion that dry mouth is more prevalent in older individuals as a result of physiological age-related changes [30]. Throughout life, the number of glandular cells decreases by approximately 40%, i.e., the ratio of glandular cells to excretory ducts is shifted in favour of the latter [31,32]. Instead of glandular cells, connective tissue and individual fat cells are observed in older people [33]. The stimulation of salivation via the periodontal receptors is also diminished along with lower chewing forces and fewer natural teeth in older adults [34]. However, these changes seem to primarily affect the Stimulated Salivary Flow (SSFR), while resting saliva (RSFR) in healthy elders is equally diminished, but remains adequate to maintain proper oral mucosa moisture and the oral cavity healthy until old age [20]. With advancing age, the number of chronic diseases and the associated intake of medication increase [35], many of which have the undesired effect of causing hyposalivation [36]. Despite a higher prevalence of xerostomia and hyposalivation in old age, it has to be considered a pathological condition rather than a physiological one [37].

4. Definitions

Xerostomia refers to the subjective sensation of having a dry mouth, which can occur with or without an actual decrease in salivary flow. On the other hand, hyposalivation refers to an objectively reduced salivary flow. A resting saliva flow rate (RSFR) below 0.1 mL/min or a stimulated saliva flow rate (SSFR) lower than 0.7 mL is commonly regarded as pathological. Monitoring the salivary flow during routine dental check-up visits can be beneficial as a reference to assess impairment [20].

5. Clinical Symptoms

The clinical manifestations of hyposalivation comprise dry mucous membranes that may stick to the mirror during a dental examination. The mucosal membranes appear pale, thin, and lack lustre. The tongue often exhibits deep grooves, while the lips feel dry and sticky during speech, a phenomenon often accompanied by an inflammation of the corners of the mouth known as cheilitis angularis. Hyposalivation patients are more prone to candidiasis [38]. If natural teeth are present, they may exhibit a dull surface and fine hairline cracks on the enamel, resembling the appearance of an antique porcelain vase. Erosion, abrasion, and caries are common, with root caries being a particular concern in patients with receding gums, especially when combined with a diet rich in sugar and carbohydrates [39]. The saliva itself appears viscous and is difficult to extract by massaging the parotid gland. Clinically, one may observe whitish, sticky saliva with small bubbles at the corner of the mouth. Difficulties chewing and swallowing specific foods are also common signs of hyposalivation [40].

6. Quantifying Salivary Flow

Several methods have been described to test the salivary flow rate during chewing (SSFR) and at rest (RSFR). For the stimulation of saliva flow, Kohler and Winter described a simple test in 1985 by chewing a gauze sponge for 2 min and weighing it before-and-after mastication [41]. Another method proposed by the group of Wolf utilizes the weight loss of candy as a quick measure of hyposalivation [42]. Similarly, chewing gum or paraffin can also be used to stimulate the salivary flow, and the saliva can be collected by spitting into a measuring cup over a given period of time [43]. If specifically targeting the parotid gland, saliva can be collected using a Lashley cup [44]. Unstimulated saliva can be obtained through methods such as draining, spitting, or suction [2,20].

7. Patient's Perception

Patients with xerostomia commonly experience subjective difficulties in speaking due to dry lips and the sensation of the tongue sticking to the roof of the mouth. They also report a decreased sense of taste, leading to a preference for stronger seasonings in meals [45,46]. Chewing and swallowing can be affected, and the oral mucosa may become sensitive or even painful. Flavours are less diluted, making it challenging to tolerate hot spices and acids. Eating dry foods like bread, biscuits, or toast may be difficult. Swallowing becomes a challenge but can be facilitated by taking a sip of liquid along with the food. In denture wearers, the lack of sufficient salivary film can affect denture retention, and inflamed denture-bearing tissues can cause discomfort. In severe cases, denture intolerance may occur.

Validated instruments for assessing xerostomia from the patient's perspective are important in understanding the impact of dry mouth on their daily lives. As a gold standard, Thomson and co-workers described the "Xerostomia Inventory", in which 11 problems are rated on a scale from 1 (never) to 5 (very often) [47]. The questions on the Xerostomia Inventory are:

- My mouth feels dry.
- I have problems eating dry foods.
- I get up at night to drink.
- My mouth feels dry during a meal.
- I drink liquids to make swallowing easier.
- I suck on sweets to help with dry mouth.
- Some foods are hard for me to swallow.
- My facial skin feels dry.
- My eyes feel dry.

- My lips feel dry.
- The inside of my nose feels dry.

8. Dry Mouth and Nutrition

Reduced salivary flow and the subjective perception of a dry mouth can impair eating and swallowing and lead to oral discomfort, as shown by Dormenval and co-workers in 82 hospitalised geriatric patients [48]. Saliva deficiency can also significantly impact taste perception. The taste buds on the tongue detect taste stimuli and transmit signals to the central nervous system through the chorda tympani, a branch of the seventh facial nerve. When saliva is lacking, the transmission of taste signals may be compromised. Matsuo and co-workers conducted an animal experiment in which the salivary glands were surgically removed from some rats [49]. All four stimuli, salty, sour, bitter, and sweet, that were presented to the experimental animals showed lower activity potentials in the chorda tympani when the salivary glands had been removed.

Measuring the impact of xerostomia and hyposalivation on food choice in a medical setting requires one of the above-mentioned methods to quantify salivary flow. Other approaches comprise the use of questionnaires or monitoring the patient's nutritional intake over a given period of time. In most cases, no baseline information would be available as a reference; hence, a before-and-after questionnaire may be necessary, despite the shortcomings of retrospective reporting. In addition, psychological instruments and PROMs might evince the impact of the altered diet on the patient's well-being and quality of life.

Several studies relying on food questionnaires suggest that xerostomia affects the quantity and quality of food intake and ultimately the quality of life [50–52]. For instance, in 1405 adults living in Lithuania, xerostomia was associated with lower intakes of carbohydrates and proteins [51]. People aged > 65 years with xerostomia have reduced intakes of omega-3 fatty acids, micronutrients (vitamin E, folate, fluoride), and water [53]. Older studies reported that people with xerostomia tended to avoid crunchy, dry, and sticky foods [52] and had lower intakes of fibre, potassium, vitamin B6, iron, calcium, and zinc [50]. These changes in nutritional intake place people with xerostomia at risk of malnutrition. The European Society of Clinical Nutrition and Metabolism (ESPEN) guideline in geriatrics acknowledges this risk [54,55]. In cases of malnutrition or risk of malnutrition, this guideline provides guidance for nutritional support and recommends strategies such as reducing or replacing medications that contribute to xerostomia. Furthermore, it recognises xerostomia as a risk factor for dehydration. Dehydration can be treated by oral fluid intake in asymptomatic patients with a serum measured plasma osmolality > 300 mOsm/kg but may require subcutaneous or intravenous hydration in cases of more severe dehydration or failure of sufficient oral fluid intakes.

9. Nutritional Advise for Relief of Symptoms

While scientific evidence for nutritional recommendations specifically tailored to xerostomia may be limited, there are some general guidelines that can help alleviate symptoms and support overall oral health. In addition to ensuring adequate calorie, protein, and fluid intake, nutritional advice should aim to relieve symptoms. To date, these mostly rely on anecdotal evidence and testimonies of patients on the internet or recommendations on websites of learned societies, associations, or dental practices specialised in hyposalivation treatment, cancer associations, or simply derived from common sense. Hence, the derived recommendations listed in Tables 1 and 2 are non-exhaustive and not based on scientific evidence (Tables 1 and 2). Of note, smoking should be discouraged as it worsens xerostomia.

Table 1. Drinks and foods having an impact on xerostomia symptoms.

Drinks That May Alleviate Symptoms
Adequate hydration (sips of water, fruit juice or green tea during and outside of meals)
Cold fluids
Foods That May Alleviate Symptoms
Soft, moist foods, cool or at room temperature
High fat liquids (e.g., gravies, cream, milk, sauces, salad dressings)
Soups
Ice cream, yoghurt, nutritional supplements
Frozen pineapple lozenges, frozen grapes
Fruits with high water content (e.g., watermelon)
Baby food
Drinks That May Worsen Symptoms
Caffeine containing drinks (e.g., sodas, black tea and coffee)
Alcohol (including alcohol-containing mouthwashes), as they increase the risk of dehydration
Acidic beverages, as they may be painful for the mucosal membranes
Foods That May Worsen Symptoms
Dry foods (e.g., bread, biscuits, toasts, cake, crackers)
Hot, spicy and salty foods
Acidic foods (e.g., fresh fruits), as they may be painful for the mucosal membranes
Mechanically irritating foods
Mushy and sticky foods (e.g., banana, dried fruits, chocolate, honey, jams)

Table 2. Foods having stimulating saliva secretion.

Foods/Chewing Devices That May Foster Salivary Flow
Sugar-free herbal lozenges or liquorice
Moderately acidic and preferably sugar-free candies, beverages and sherbets
Non-acidic chewing-active visco-elastic foods (chewing gum or Chewy Tubes®)

Liquid intake is particularly important for dry mouth patients. Meals should be well-seasoned, although hot and spicy condiments that irritate the mucous membrane should be avoided. As a general rule, meals should be served with lots of gravy. Dry foods, such as biscuits, can be better enjoyed with fruit or green tea. Black tea and coffee, as well as alcohol, on the other hand, increase dehydration and should not be excessively consumed. Thick foods such as yoghurt or ice cream relieve dry mouth symptoms. Sucking lozenges should not be too acidic or contain sugar, as the latter increases the risk of caries and tooth loss. Although acidic fruits may be painful for inflamed mucous membranes, they can still be enjoyed when steamed or baked. High-water-content fruits like watermelon are also recommended. If the mucous membrane is already painfully inflamed, ice cream, an ice cube, or even lozenges from frozen pineapple can cool and soothe. For severe cases, like oncology patients, a viable option is baby food in jars, as it is easy to eat and provides essential nutrients.

Patients need to be advised that mushy and sticky foods should be avoided as they stick to the mucous membranes and the formation of a cohesive bolus may be difficult. When not cleared by the tongue and cheeks, the remaining food can also lead to tooth decay and inflammation of the periodontal tissues, especially if oral hygiene is not performed thoroughly because of the sensitivity and painfulness of the mucous membranes. It should also be avoided to treat the mucous membranes with petroleum-based ointments, such as Vaseline. These dry out the oral mucosa even further and prevent the natural washing away of pathogenic germs [56]. It is important to know that the combination of xerostomia and poor oral hygiene can lead to rapidly progressing root caries and tooth loss within a very short time. Patients with dry mouth should therefore always receive dental care and nutritional advice [57].

The last and probably least satisfactory relief for dry mouth is moistening the oral cavity with small sips or spray shots from a vaporizer of water. Tea, gels, or mouthwashes during the day may provide immediate, but not long-lasting, relief. Ultimately, replacement with artificial saliva is recommended. It is important to consult with a healthcare professional, such as a dentist or doctor, to determine the most suitable artificial saliva product and usage instructions based on individual needs and preferences. They can provide guidance on the appropriate application and frequency of artificial saliva use for optimal relief.

10. Nutritional Advise for Stimulating Saliva

Amidst all nutritional guidance, as aforementioned, the utmost important advice is to ensure an adequate intake of fluids, with small "reminders" encouraging the patient to drink a sufficient quantity throughout the day.

Furthermore, some other nutrients may help stimulate salivary flow, such as viscoelastic foods that increase salivation by stimulating the periodontal receptors via occlusal load during chewing (Table 2). Salivation can also be stimulated by unilateral chewing of sugar-free gum [27]. The salivation effect of chewing gum was mentioned already, but regrettably, the act of chewing gum is not particularly favoured by the elderly population. At the age of 85, 6 out of 10 Swiss people wear removable dentures [58]. In this regard, it is unfortunate that all chewing gums presently accessible on the market adhere to denture acrylic, thus rendering the act of chewing exceptionally arduous. This problem may be overcome by recommending silicone tubes of different hardness and surface textures with a large handle to hold. These tubes were conceived to train the chewing muscles during facial growth in children with Duchenne syndrome. However, they may also be used to stimulate salivary flow by unilateral mastication. In this regard, geriatric patients with poor chewing efficiency should not be promptly prescribed a mixed diet, as the benefits of chewing solid food are evident. Before doing so, a dental examination should verify if the patient's capacity to eat a normal diet can be regained by restorative means.

Salivation can also be stimulated by sucking on sweets, although sour drops may cause dental erosion and are therefore less suitable than aromatic lozenges or liquorice. Care should also be taken to ensure that they contain no sugar to prevent the development of tooth decay.

Recent trends in geriatric medicine confirm a strategy to prioritize medications to reduce the total number of prescribed drugs [59].

11. Summary of Recommendations

Saliva production is stimulated by a chewing-active diet. Chewing sugar-free chewing gum in addition to chewing-active main meals is therefore one of the most effective forms of therapy. Meals should be well-seasoned, avoiding excessive spiciness or acidity. Coffee and black tea should only be consumed in moderation. If the mucous membranes are already inflamed, soothing relief can be found in ice cream and frozen pineapple. It is essential to maintain excellent oral hygiene when consuming soft and sticky foods. Overall, it should be emphasised that sufficient fluid intake throughout the day is, in many ways, the most important food for the elderly.

12. Future Research

Given the little to no scientific evidence on the food choice of patients suffering from xerostomia or hyposalivation, clinical research, be it qualitative or clinical, is needed to provide evidence-based clinical recommendations, especially concerning a "chewing-active" diet that may help stimulate salivary function. Furthermore, future studies should explore the impact of xerostomia on nutritional status and, if substantiated, develop interventions based on scientific evidence. Last but not least, the patient's perspective should be addressed in a scientific manner, ensuring their experiences and viewpoints are considered and incorporated into the research findings.

Author Contributions: Conceptualization and manuscript F.M. and L.G.; critical review of manuscript N.C. and S.M. All authors have read and agreed to the published version of the manuscript.

Funding: This research received no external funding.

Institutional Review Board Statement: Not applicable.

Informed Consent Statement: Not applicable.

Data Availability Statement: Not applicable.

Conflicts of Interest: The authors have no conflict of interest.

References

1. Liu, B.; Dion, M.R.; Jurasic, M.M.; Gibson, G.; Jones, J.A. Xerostomia and salivary hypofunction in vulnerable elders: Prevalence and etiology. *Oral Surg. Oral Med. Oral Pathol. Oral Radiol.* **2012**, *114*, 52–60. [CrossRef] [PubMed]
2. Barbe, A.G. Medication-Induced Xerostomia and Hyposalivation in the Elderly: Culprits, Complications, and Management. *Drugs Aging* **2018**, *35*, 877–885. [CrossRef] [PubMed]
3. Pina, G.M.S.; Mota Carvalho, R.; Silva, B.S.F.; Almeida, F.T. Prevalence of hyposalivation in older people: A systematic review and meta-analysis. *Gerodontology* **2020**, *37*, 317–331. [CrossRef] [PubMed]
4. Gibson, B.; Periyakaruppiah, K.; Thornhill, M.H.; Baker, S.R.; Robinson, P.G. Measuring the symptomatic, physical, emotional and social impacts of dry mouth: A qualitative study. *Gerodontology* **2020**, *37*, 132–142. [CrossRef]
5. Millwood, J.; Heath, M.R. Food choice by older people: The use of semi-structured interviews with open and closed questions. *Gerodontology* **2000**, *17*, 25–32. [CrossRef] [PubMed]
6. N'Gom, P.I.; Woda, A. Influence of impaired mastication on nutrition. *J. Prosthet. Dent.* **2002**, *87*, 667–673. [CrossRef] [PubMed]
7. Pedersen, A.M.; Bardow, A.; Jensen, S.B.; Nauntofte, B. Saliva and gastrointestinal functions of taste, mastication, swallowing and digestion. *Oral Dis.* **2002**, *8*, 117–129. [CrossRef]
8. Locker, D. Dental status, xerostomia and the oral health-related quality of life of an elderly institutionalized population. *Spec. Care Dent.* **2003**, *23*, 86–93. [CrossRef]
9. Silva, I.M.V.; Donaduzzi, L.C.; Perini, C.C.; Couto, S.A.B.; Werneck, R.I.; de Araujo, M.R.; Kurahashi, M.; Johann, A.; Azevedo-Alanis, L.R.; Vieira, A.R.; et al. Association of xerostomia and taste alterations of patients receiving antineoplastic chemotherapy: A cause for nutritional concern. *Clin. Nutr. ESPEN* **2021**, *43*, 532–535. [CrossRef]
10. Jham, B.C.; Reis, P.M.; Miranda, E.L.; Lopes, R.C.; Carvalho, A.L.; Scheper, M.A.; Freire, A.R. Oral health status of 207 head and neck cancer patients before, during and after radiotherapy. *Clin. Oral Investig.* **2008**, *12*, 19–24. [CrossRef]
11. Mercadante, V.; Al Hamad, A.; Lodi, G.; Porter, S.; Fedele, S. Interventions for the management of radiotherapy-induced xerostomia and hyposalivation: A systematic review and meta-analysis. *Oral Oncol.* **2017**, *66*, 64–74. [CrossRef] [PubMed]
12. Lopez-Pintor, R.M.; Casanas, E.; Gonzalez-Serrano, J.; Serrano, J.; Ramirez, L.; de Arriba, L.; Hernandez, G. Xerostomia, Hyposalivation, and Salivary Flow in Diabetes Patients. *J. Diabetes Res.* **2016**, *2016*, 4372852. [CrossRef] [PubMed]
13. Turner, M.D. Hyposalivation and Xerostomia: Etiology, Complications, and Medical Management. *Dent. Clin. N. Am.* **2016**, *60*, 435–443. [CrossRef] [PubMed]
14. Flink, H.; Bergdahl, M.; Tegelberg, A.; Rosenblad, A.; Lagerlof, F. Prevalence of hyposalivation in relation to general health, body mass index and remaining teeth in different age groups of adults. *Community Dent. Oral Epidemiol.* **2008**, *36*, 523–531. [CrossRef]
15. Han, P.; Suarez-Durall, P.; Mulligan, R. Dry mouth: A critical topic for older adult patients. *J. Prosthodont. Res.* **2015**, *59*, 6–19. [CrossRef]
16. Rech, R.S.; Hugo, F.N.; Torres, L.; Hilgert, J.B. Factors associated with hyposalivation and xerostomia in older persons in South Brazil. *Gerodontology* **2019**, *36*, 338–344. [CrossRef]
17. Fischer, D.; Ship, J.A. The effect of dehydration on parotid salivary gland function. *Spec Care Dent.* **1997**, *17*, 58–64. [CrossRef]
18. Brito-Zeron, P.; Retamozo, S.; Kostov, B.; Baldini, C.; Bootsma, H.; De Vita, S.; Dorner, T.; Gottenberg, J.E.; Kruize, A.A.; Mandl, T.; et al. Efficacy and safety of topical and systemic medications: A systematic literature review informing the EULAR recommendations for the management of Sjogren's syndrome. *RMD Open* **2019**, *5*, e001064. [CrossRef]
19. Sivaramakrishnan, G.; Sridharan, K. Electrical nerve stimulation for xerostomia: A meta-analysis of randomised controlled trials. *J. Tradit. Complement. Med.* **2017**, *7*, 409–413. [CrossRef]
20. Villa, A.; Wolff, A.; Aframian, D.; Vissink, A.; Ekstrom, J.; Proctor, G.; McGowan, R.; Narayana, N.; Aliko, A.; Sia, Y.W.; et al. World Workshop on Oral Medicine VI: A systematic review of medication-induced salivary gland dysfunction: Prevalence, diagnosis, and treatment. *Clin. Oral Investig.* **2015**, *19*, 1563–1580. [CrossRef]
21. Cifuentes, M.; Del Barrio-Diaz, P.; Vera-Kellet, C. Pilocarpine and artificial saliva for the treatment of xerostomia and xerophthalmia in Sjogren syndrome: A double-blind randomized controlled trial. *Br. J. Derm.* **2018**, *179*, 1056–1061. [CrossRef]
22. Ikeda, E.; Ogawa, M.; Takeo, M.; Tsuji, T. Functional ectodermal organ regeneration as the next generation of organ replacement therapy. *Open Biol.* **2019**, *9*, 190010. [CrossRef]
23. Farnaud, S.J.; Kosti, O.; Getting, S.J.; Renshaw, D. Saliva: Physiology and diagnostic potential in health and disease. *Sci. World J.* **2010**, *10*, 434–456. [CrossRef] [PubMed]

24. Humphrey, S.P.; Williamson, R.T. A review of saliva: Normal composition, flow, and function. *J. Prosthet. Dent.* **2001**, *85*, 162–169. [CrossRef]
25. Kubala, E.; Strzelecka, P.; Grzegocka, M.; Lietz-Kijak, D.; Gronwald, H.; Skomro, P.; Kijak, E. A Review of Selected Studies That Determine the Physical and Chemical Properties of Saliva in the Field of Dental Treatment. *Biomed. Res. Int.* **2018**, *2018*, 6572381. [CrossRef] [PubMed]
26. Paszynska, E.; Linden, R.W.; Slopien, A.; Rajewski, A. Flow rates and inorganic composition of whole saliva in purging bulimic patients treated with fluoxetine. *World J Biol Psychiatry.* **2011**, *12*, 282–287. [CrossRef]
27. Hector, M.P.; Sullivan, A. Migration of erythrosin-labelled saliva during unilateral chewing in man. *Arch. Oral Biol.* **1992**, *37*, 757–758. [CrossRef] [PubMed]
28. Matsuda, K.; Ikebe, K.; Ogawa, T.; Kagawa, R.; Maeda, Y. Increase of salivary flow rate along with improved occlusal force after the replacement of complete dentures. *Oral Surg. Oral Med. Oral Pathol. Oral Radiol. Endod.* **2009**, *108*, 211–215. [CrossRef]
29. Tango, R.N.; Arata, A.; Borges, A.L.S.; Costa, A.K.F.; Pereira, L.J.; Kaminagakura, E. The Role of New Removable Complete Dentures in Stimulated Salivary Flow and Taste Perception. *J. Prosthodont.* **2018**, *27*, 335–339. [CrossRef]
30. Xu, F.; Laguna, L.; Sarkar, A. Aging-related changes in quantity and quality of saliva: Where do we stand in our understanding? *J. Texture Stud.* **2019**, *50*, 27–35. [CrossRef]
31. Sorensen, C.E.; Larsen, J.O.; Reibel, J.; Lauritzen, M.; Mortensen, E.L.; Osler, M.; Pedersen, A.M. Associations between xerostomia, histopathological alterations, and autonomic innervation of labial salivary glands in men in late midlife. *Exp. Gerontol.* **2014**, *57*, 211–217. [CrossRef]
32. Vissink, A.; Mitchell, J.B.; Baum, B.J.; Limesand, K.H.; Jensen, S.B.; Fox, P.C.; Elting, L.S.; Langendijk, J.A.; Coppes, R.P.; Reyland, M.E. Clinical management of salivary gland hypofunction and xerostomia in head-and-neck cancer patients: Successes and barriers. *Int. J. Radiat. Oncol. Biol. Phys.* **2010**, *78*, 983–991. [CrossRef]
33. Scott, J.; Flower, E.A.; Burns, J. A quantitative study of histological changes in the human parotid gland occurring with adult age. *J. Oral Pathol.* **1987**, *16*, 505–510. [CrossRef] [PubMed]
34. Wyatt, C.C.; So, F.H.; Williams, P.M.; Mithani, A.; Zed, C.M.; Yen, E.H. The development, implementation, utilization and outcomes of a comprehensive dental program for older adults residing in long-term care facilities. *J. Can. Dent. Assoc.* **2006**, *72*, 419.
35. Barnett, K.; Mercer, S.W.; Norbury, M.; Watt, G.; Wyke, S.; Guthrie, B. Epidemiology of multimorbidity and implications for health care, research, and medical education: A cross-sectional study. *Lancet* **2012**, *380*, 37–43. [CrossRef]
36. Marcott, S.; Dewan, K.; Kwan, M.; Baik, F.; Lee, Y.J.; Sirjani, D. Where Dysphagia Begins: Polypharmacy and Xerostomia. *Fed. Pr.* **2020**, *37*, 234–241.
37. Saleh, J.; Figueiredo, M.A.; Cherubini, K.; Salum, F.G. Salivary hypofunction: An update on aetiology, diagnosis and therapeutics. *Arch. Oral Biol.* **2015**, *60*, 242–255. [CrossRef]
38. Babu, N.A.; Anitha, N. Hyposalivation and oral candidiasis-A short review. *J. Oral Maxillofac. Pathol.* **2022**, *26*, 144–146. [CrossRef] [PubMed]
39. Arcella, D.; Ottolenghi, L.; Polimeni, A.; Leclercq, C. The relationship between frequency of carbohydrates intake and dental caries: A cross-sectional study in Italian teenagers. *Public Health Nutr.* **2002**, *5*, 553–560. [CrossRef] [PubMed]
40. Rogus-Pulia, N.M.; Gangnon, R.; Kind, A.; Connor, N.P.; Asthana, S. A Pilot Study of Perceived Mouth Dryness, Perceived Swallowing Effort, and Saliva Substitute Effects in Healthy Adults Across the Age Range. *Dysphagia* **2018**, *33*, 200–205. [CrossRef] [PubMed]
41. Kohler, P.F.; Winter, M.E. A quantitative test for xerostomia. The Saxon test, an oral equivalent of the Schirmer test. *Arthritis Rheum.* **1985**, *28*, 1128–1132. [CrossRef] [PubMed]
42. Wolff, A.; Herscovici, D.; Rosenberg, M. A simple technique for the determination of salivary gland hypofunction. *Oral Surg. Oral Med. Oral Pathol. Oral Radiol. Endod.* **2002**, *94*, 175–178. [CrossRef] [PubMed]
43. Navazesh, M.; Christensen, C.M. A comparison of whole mouth resting and stimulated salivary measurement procedures. *J. Dent. Res.* **1982**, *61*, 1158–1162. [CrossRef] [PubMed]
44. Schroder, S.A.; Bardow, A.; Eickhardt-Dalboge, S.; Johansen, H.K.; Homoe, P. Is parotid saliva sterile on entry to the oral cavity? *Acta Otolaryngol.* **2017**, *137*, 762–764. [CrossRef] [PubMed]
45. Rawal, S.; Hoffman, H.J.; Bainbridge, K.E.; Huedo-Medina, T.B.; Duffy, V.B. Prevalence and Risk Factors of Self-Reported Smell and Taste Alterations: Results from the 2011–2012 US National Health and Nutrition Examination Survey (NHANES). *Chem. Senses* **2016**, *41*, 69–76. [CrossRef]
46. Samnieng, P.; Ueno, M.; Shinada, K.; Zaitsu, T.; Wright, F.A.; Kawaguchi, Y. Association of hyposalivation with oral function, nutrition and oral health in community-dwelling elderly Thai. *Community Dent. Health* **2012**, *29*, 117–123. [PubMed]
47. Thomson, W.M.; Chalmers, J.M.; Spencer, A.J.; Williams, S.M. The Xerostomia Inventory: A multi-item approach to measuring dry mouth. *Community Dent. Health* **1999**, *16*, 12–17.
48. Dormenval, V.; Budtz-Jorgensen, E.; Mojon, P.; Bruyere, A.; Rapin, C.H. Associations between malnutrition, poor general health and oral dryness in hospitalized elderly patients. *Age Ageing* **1998**, *27*, 123–128. [CrossRef]
49. Matsuo, R.; Yamauchi, Y.; Morimoto, T. Role of submandibular and sublingual saliva in maintenance of taste sensitivity recorded in the chorda tympani of rats. *J. Physiol.* **1997**, *498 Pt 3*, 797–807. [CrossRef]

50. Rhodus, N.L.; Brown, J. The association of xerostomia and inadequate intake in older adults. *J. Am. Diet. Assoc.* **1990**, *90*, 1688–1692. [CrossRef]
51. Stankeviciene, I.; Aleksejuniene, J.; Puriene, A.; Stangvaltaite-Mouhat, L. Association between Diet and Xerostomia: Is Xerostomia a Barrier to a Healthy Eating Pattern? *Nutrients* **2021**, *13*, 4235. [CrossRef] [PubMed]
52. Loesche, W.J.; Bromberg, J.; Terpenning, M.S.; Bretz, W.A.; Dominguez, B.L.; Grossman, N.S.; Langmore, S.E. Xerostomia, xerogenic medications and food avoidances in selected geriatric groups. *J. Am. Geriatr. Soc.* **1995**, *43*, 401–407. [CrossRef] [PubMed]
53. Lee, K.A.; Park, J.C.; Park, Y.K. Nutrient intakes and medication use in elderly individuals with and without dry mouths. *Nutr. Res. Pract.* **2020**, *14*, 143–151. [CrossRef] [PubMed]
54. Volkert, D.; Beck, A.M.; Cederholm, T.; Cruz-Jentoft, A.; Goisser, S.; Hooper, L.; Kiesswetter, E.; Maggio, M.; Raynaud-Simon, A.; Sieber, C.C.; et al. ESPEN guideline on clinical nutrition and hydration in geriatrics. *Clin. Nutr.* **2019**, *38*, 10–47. [CrossRef]
55. Volkert, D.; Beck, A.M.; Cederholm, T.; Cruz-Jentoft, A.; Hooper, L.; Kiesswetter, E.; Maggio, M.; Raynaud-Simon, A.; Sieber, C.; Sobotka, L.; et al. ESPEN practical guideline: Clinical nutrition and hydration in geriatrics. *Clin. Nutr.* **2022**, *41*, 958–989. [CrossRef] [PubMed]
56. Schimmel, M.; Wiseman, M.A.; Sonis, S.T.; Müller, F. Palliative Care and Complications of cancer therapy. In *Oral Healthcare and the Frail Elder: A Clinical Perspective*; MacEntee, M., Müller, F., Wyatt, C.C., Eds.; Wiley-Blackwell: Ames, IA, USA, 2011.
57. Singh, M.; Tonk, R.S. Dietary considerations for patients with dry mouth. *Gen. Dent.* **2012**, *60*, 188–189.
58. Schneider, C.; Zemp, E.; Zitzmann, N.U. Oral health improvements in Switzerland over 20 years. *Eur. J. Oral Sci.* **2017**, *125*, 55–62. [CrossRef]
59. Hill-Taylor, B.; Sketris, I.; Hayden, J.; Byrne, S.; O'Sullivan, D.; Christie, R. Application of the STOPP/START criteria: A systematic review of the prevalence of potentially inappropriate prescribing in older adults, and evidence of clinical, humanistic and economic impact. *J. Clin. Pharm. Ther.* **2013**, *38*, 360–372. [CrossRef]

Disclaimer/Publisher's Note: The statements, opinions and data contained in all publications are solely those of the individual author(s) and contributor(s) and not of MDPI and/or the editor(s). MDPI and/or the editor(s) disclaim responsibility for any injury to people or property resulting from any ideas, methods, instructions or products referred to in the content.

MDPI AG
Grosspeteranlage 5
4052 Basel
Switzerland
Tel.: +41 61 683 77 34

Journal of Clinical Medicine Editorial Office
E-mail: jcm@mdpi.com
www.mdpi.com/journal/jcm

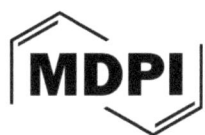

Disclaimer/Publisher's Note: The statements, opinions and data contained in all publications are solely those of the individual author(s) and contributor(s) and not of MDPI and/or the editor(s). MDPI and/or the editor(s) disclaim responsibility for any injury to people or property resulting from any ideas, methods, instructions or products referred to in the content.

www.ingramcontent.com/pod-product-compliance
Lightning Source LLC
LaVergne TN
LVHW072355090526
838202LV00019B/2551